# AIDS Vaccine Development
## Challenges and Opportunities

Edited by Wayne C. Koff, Patricia Kahn, and Ian D. Gust

*Caister Academic Press*

Copyright © 2007
Caister Academic Press
32 Hewitts Lane
Wymondham
Norfolk NR18 0JA
UK

www.caister.com

British Library Cataloguing-in-Publication Data
A catalogue record for this book is available from the British Library
ISBN: 978-1-904455-11-0

Printed and bound in Great Britain

# Contents

# Contributors

**Jim Ackland**
Managing Director and CEO
Global BioSolutions
Craigieburn
Victoria
Australia

jackland@globalbiosolutions.com

**Roy Anderson**
Department of Infectious Disease Epidemiology
Imperial College
London University
St Mary's Campus
London
UK

**Jon Kim Andrus**
Pan American Health Organization
Washington, DC
USA

**Rattan Banerjee**
PS&S Engineering
Warren, NJ
USA

**Seth Berkley**
International AIDS Vaccine Initiative
New York, NY
USA

**Chris Beyrer**
Department of Epidemiology
Johns Hopkins Bloomberg School of Public Health
Baltimore, MD
USA

cbeyrer@jhsph.edu

**J. Ties Boerma**
Department of Measurement and Health Information
Systems
World Health Organization
Geneva
Switzerland

**Johannes Antonie Bogaards**
Crucell
Leiden
The Netherlands

**Susan P. Buchbinder**
HIV Research Section
San Francisco Department of Public Health
San Francisco, CA
USA

spb@itsa.ucsf.edu

**Dennis R. Burton**
Department of Immunology
The Scripps Research Institute
La Jolla, CA
USA

burton@scripps.edu

**José Esparza**
HIV, TB and Reproductive Health
Global Health Program
Bill & Melinda Gates Foundation
Seattle, WA
USA

Jose.Esparza@gatesfoundation.org

**Jean-Louis Excler**
International AIDS Vaccine Initiative
New York, NY
USA

**Patricia E. Fast**
International AIDS Vaccine Initiative
New York, NY
USA

pfast@iavi.org

**Jonathan D. Fuchs**
HIV Research Section
San Francisco Department of Public Health
San Francisco, CA
USA

**Donald F. Gerson**
Dongchun-dong
Yeonsu-gu
Incheon
South Korea

dg@celltrion.com

**Marc Girard**
Université Paris 7 - Denis Diderot
Paris
France

**Jaap Goudsmit**
Crucell
Leiden
The Netherlands

j.goudsmit@crucell.com

**Ian D. Gust**
Department of Microbiology and Immunology
The University of Melbourne
Melbourne
Victoria
Australia

**Patricia Kahn**
International AIDS Vaccine Initiative
New York, NY
USA

**Nzeera Ketter**
International AIDS Vaccine Initiative
New York, NY
USA

**Wayne C. Koff**
Vaccine Research
International AIDS Vaccine Initiative
New York, NY
USA

wkoff@iavi.org

**Bette T. Korber**
Laboratory Fellow
Theoretical Biology and Biophysics
Los Alamos National Laboratory
Los Alamos, NM
USA

btk@lanl.gov

**Thomas K. Leitner**
Theoretical Division
Los Alamos National Laboratory
Los Alamos, NM
USA

**Margaret A. Liu**
Transgene
S.A. Strasbourg
France

**John R. Mascola**
Vaccine Research Center
NIAID
NIH
Bethesda, MD
USA

jmascola@nih.gov

**Catherine C. Miller**
Theoretical Division
Los Alamos National Laboratory
Los Alamos, NM
USA

**Bhawani Mukherjee**
PS&S Engineering
Warren, NJ
USA

**Gary J. Nabel**
Vaccine Research Center
NIAID
NIH
Bethesda, MD
USA

**Marjorie Opuni**
Population and Family Health Sciences
Johns Hopkins Bloomberg School of Public Health
Baltimore, MD
USA

mopuniak@jhsph.edu

**Stanley A. Plotkin**
Sanofi Pasteur
Doylestown, PA
USA

Stanley.Plotkin@sanofipasteur.com

**Ciro A. de Quadros**
Albert B. Sabin Vaccine Institute (SVI)
Washington, DC
USA

ciro.dequadros@sabin.org

**Kenneth L. Rosenthal**
Department of Pathology & Molecular Medicine
Institute for Molecular Medicine & Health
McMaster University
West Hamilton, ON
Canada

rosenthl@mcmaster.ca

**Sarah L. Rowland-Jones**
MRC Human Immunology Unit
Weatherall Institute of Molecular Medicine
John Radcliffe Hospital
Oxford
UK

sarah.rowland-jones@ndm.ox.ac.uk

**Nina D. Russell**
HIV, TB and Reproductive Health
Global Health Program
Bill & Melinda Gates Foundation
Seattle, WA
USA

**Bernhard Schwartländer**
The Global Fund to Fight AIDS, Tuberculosis and Malaria
Vernier-Genève
Switzerland

**Steven G. Self**
Statistical Center for HIV/AIDS Research & Prevention (SCHARP)
Fred Hutchinson Cancer Research Center
Seattle, WA
USA

sgs@scharp.org

**Suganya Selvarajah**
The Scripps Research Institute
Department of Immunology
La Jolla, CA
USA

**Robert F. Siliciano**
Johns Hopkins University School of Medicine
Broadway Research Building
Baltimore, MD
USA

rsiliciano@jhmi.edu

**Karen Stanecki**
Demographic and Related Data
UNAIDS
Geneva
Switzerland

**Paul Thottingal**
Department of Medical Microbiology
University of Nairobi
Nairobi
Kenya

**Britta Wahren**
Karolinska Institute
Stockholm
Sweden

Britta.Wahren@smi.ki.se

**Mitchell Warren**
International AIDS Vaccine Initiative
New York, NY
USA

**S.B. Justin Wong**
Department of Microbiology
Yong Loo Lin School of Medicine
National University of Singapore
Singapore
The Republic of Singapore

# Foreword

Over the past two decades, the human immunodeficiency virus has spread across the world. Today 40 million people are living with HIV/AIDS, and over 25 million have already died. Each day, another 14,000 become infected. Despite vigorous education and behavior change campaigns in many (although not all) parts of the world, the epidemic continues to spread, resulting in the worst infectious disease epidemic since the fourteenth century and creating a development catastrophe of unprecedented proportions.

Although we must do all we can using current tools to prevent further spread of the virus, treat those who are infected and mitigate the disastrous consequences wrought by HIV/AIDS, these tools are not enough to end the epidemic. So at the same time the world must, as a critical priority, do much more to develop new prevention technologies that can protect people at risk and ultimately end HIV transmission. While this is a difficult and ambitious goal, the world has a good track record in using technology to solve some of our worst global problems.

However, the world does *not* have a good track record in the search for an AIDS vaccine. Once HIV was identified in 1984 as the cause of AIDS, it was logical that a vaccine—the only way the world has ever effectively halted the spread of a virus—would be seen as the clear solution for ending the epidemic. At the time, there were bold pronouncements that a vaccine would be ready in short order. Of course we now know that this was incorrect, for reasons that range from the immense scientific challenges and very high development costs to the almost complete lack of constituencies advocating for vaccines—obstacles that soon turned AIDS vaccine development into an orphan effort. In the mid-1990s, the world was spending less than $125 million a year trying to solve this problem.

More recently, we are fortunate that AIDS, particularly in developing countries, is receiving renewed political and financial attention. Yet, although an AIDS vaccine is an international public good of the highest order, it still fails to receive the attention it deserves. Today, the world spends around $750 million per year on the vaccine effort, a mere 2% of the global health research dollars.

This book is timely. With the world now beginning to pay more attention to AIDS, including development of a vaccine, this volume comprehensively reviews the state of the effort and the many challenges still to be solved. Starting with the global context, it then lays out the scientific underpinnings, vaccine design challenges and controversies, followed by discussion of the complexities surrounding clinical trials and infrastructure for testing vaccines. Alongside these more traditional scientific concerns, it also probes issues of vaccine manufacture, scale-up and deployment, and finally what the public health impact of an effective (or partially effective) vaccine might be. To cover these topics, the editors have drawn from a wide range of experienced authors.

Taken together, these chapters make a case that the world needs a two-tiered scientific approach: testing the best available products as quickly as possible, and at the same time conducting highly focused applied research to resolve many of the remaining scientific hurdles and design new types of candidates. Encouraging data from humans and non-human primates give us confidence that immunologic protection from HIV is possible, but the world is a long way away from mobilizing the type of concerted scientific effort necessary to solve these challenges in a timely fashion. And beyond the science, we must do much more to tackle some of the non-scientific barriers to AIDS vaccine development, including financing, manufacture and, ultimately, ensuring rapid access to a successful vaccine in all parts of the world.

So the knowledge in this book may be power, but at the end of the day, success in the fastest time frame will require creating a worldwide movement for AIDS vaccines that combines not only top scientific expertise but also the highest level of political commitment. Given the magnitude of this global tragedy, future generations will judge how well we dealt with AIDS—and, until we have a vaccine, we will never fully control this epidemic. We have witnessed several major public health successes in our lifetime, including the eradication of smallpox, almost complete control of polio and massive reduction in deaths from measles. Let's do what it takes to replicate these successes so that we can also live to see a day without AIDS.

Seth Berkley, MD
International AIDS Vaccine Initiative

# Acknowledgments

The editors wish to acknowledge the dedicated and tireless efforts of Sandi Glass and Lisa Gieber at the International AIDS Vaccine Initiative for exemplary administrative support in the development of this book, and a special acknowledgment to Annette Griffin of Horizon Press for her patience and excellent advice in shepherding the book from conception to completion. Finally, we applaud the many global stakeholders in AIDS vaccine development: international leaders in the developing world willing to promote AIDS vaccine efforts; community activists mobilizing support for AIDS vaccine clinical trials; scientists and public health experts working to develop and test AIDS vaccines; public sector, private sector, and nongovernmental organizations supporting and promoting AIDS vaccine research; and the thousands of altruistic volunteers willing to participate in AIDS vaccine clinical trials, who collectively help to speed the search for a safe and effective AIDS vaccine.

# Part I

# Global Overview

# Introduction

Wayne C. Koff and Ian D. Gust

## Background

The need for a safe and effective vaccine to prevent AIDS is obvious. Twenty three years since HIV was identified as the etiologic cause of AIDS, the WHO-UNAIDS joint program estimates that nearly 40 million people were living with HIV/AIDS and over 3 million died in 2005 alone, and ten new infections occur every minute—the vast majority in the developing world. AIDS is having a dramatic effect on economic activity and life expectancy in many countries, while the pandemic continues its insidious spread: it is estimated that over 100 million more people will become infected in the next two decades if a safe and effective vaccine does not become available.

Although the current means of prevention and education plus the use of anti-viral drugs have contained the rate of infection in developed countries, these measures are difficult to implement in regions with poorly developed health systems and inadequate infrastructure—although a few developing countries, such as Thailand and Uganda, have made some gains in slowing the epidemic.

Since many other viral epidemics (e.g., measles, hepatitis, poliomyelitis) have been successfully controlled by immunization, great faith has been placed on the ability of the biomedical research and public health enterprise to develop and deliver an effective HIV vaccine. Despite more than $1.5 billion invested in HIV vaccine work over the last decade and over 30 candidate vaccines in the product development pipeline, the prospect that an HIV vaccine will be licensed in the next five years appears remote.

The process of developing, testing and registering a new vaccine is lengthy and expensive, even when undertaken by an experienced vaccine manufacturer using established processes. For example, although the hepatitis A virus was first identified in 1973, it took another 18 years to develop a licensed vaccine even though the virus is monotypic and grew readily in cell culture, animal models could be used for preliminary evaluation of the vaccine's safety and efficacy prior to large-scale clinical trials, and the manufacturing process was similar to that used by Jonas Salk for producing inactivated polio vaccine in the 1950s.

In contrast, HIV presents some formidable challenges for vaccine development, and it will take unprecedented mobilization of a broad range of resources to achieve success. This book addresses these challenges, and is divided into five principal areas: an epidemiological overview; expectations of what an HIV vaccine needs to do; challenges in vaccine design; clinical trials; and the challenges of vaccine manufacturing, regulatory oversight and global delivery.

## Epidemiologic overview

From the first observation of five patients with a puzzling immunodeficiency in June 1981 to the three million deaths from AIDS in 2005 alone, the HIV pandemic continues to expand. Sub-Saharan Africa has borne the major impact, with HIV prevalence rates greater than 30% in some populations and life expectancy decreased by nearly 50% in several countries. More recently, Asia and Eastern Europe have become new epicenters of the pandemic, with over 5 million people living with HIV/AIDS in India at the end of 2005, projections of millions of new infections in China in the next decade, and the former Soviet Union experiencing the world's fastest-growing infection rate. The pandemic thus encompasses a series of emerging and changing epidemics described by Opuni *et al.* (Chapter 2), involving transmission via various routes (sexual, intravenous, and breast milk) and fuelled by globally diverse and rapidly changing strains of HIV.

## Expectations for an HIV vaccine

The ideal HIV vaccine would have a host of desirable characteristics. It would be:

+ safe;
+ effective in preventing the establishment of HIV infection in a high percentage of immunized people;
+ provide long-lived protection;
+ effective against globally diverse HIV strains;
+ feasible for manufacture on a large scale;
+ stable;

+ relatively inexpensive per dose; and
+ easy to administer.

However, even a less than ideal vaccine—for example, one that does not necessarily prevent infection but suppresses viral load, slows the progression of disease and impedes HIV transmission—could have dramatic public health benefits, according to mathematical modeling studies.

Compared with polio, measles or hepatitis B, AIDS vaccine development faces a number of daunting scientific hurdles; first, although natural infection with HIV induces vigorous humoral and cellular immune responses, these responses are not effective in the long term: sooner or later the virus overwhelms the immune system, leading to opportunistic infections and eventually to death. Nor are there any definitive cases of recovery from HIV infection. Therefore, correlates of protective immunity to HIV remain unknown, and vaccine developers must design their candidates from a theoretical perspective and test each hypothesis in the clinic before they can move forward.

Second, like other lentiviruses, HIV integrates into the genome of the host, allowing the provirus to persist silently in cellular reservoirs where it is hidden from immune attack. Wong and Silicano (Chapter 3) review the early events following HIV transmission, from initial exposure and uptake of the virus by antigen-presenting cells through amplification in gastrointestinal and other mucosal sites, seeding of the immune system's cellular reservoirs and finally virus proliferation in the blood. For vaccines, this implies that the window of opportunity for mounting a localized immune response which prevents establishment of an HIV infection (before virus has seeded the cellular reservoirs) is quite short.

Among the most important insights behind the current generation of candidate vaccines are the consistent findings of a relationship between viral load and disease progression. A large body of data in both the monkey model system and HIV-infected people shows a strong correlation between blood levels of SIV or HIV, as measured by RNA copy number, and the rate of progression to AIDS. Many groups have also documented an inverse relationship between SIV- or HIV-specific cellular immune responses and virus levels, suggesting that vaccines which induce these responses may blunt viral load and slow disease progression or impede transmission. In Chapter 4, Goudsmit et al. review some of the evidence for this notion, drawing on information from both animal studies and natural history cohorts. While these data provides a strong rationale for accelerating the testing of vaccines based on this concept, they also reveal the potential limitations of CMI-based approaches.

They also raise two more obstacles to the development of an AIDS vaccine: the lack of definitive correlates for protective immunity against HIV and the limitations of current animal models for AIDS. Thottingal and Rowland-Jones (Chapter 5) review the current state of the art surrounding immune correlates of protection, including data from highly exposed yet HIV-seronegative sex workers, superinfection studies and natural history studies. Without known correlates of protection, which can be defined only after a vaccine candidate demonstrates at least some protection in well-designed human efficacy trials, there is a general but unproven notion that both humoral and cellular immune responses will ultimately be required for a successful AIDS vaccine. This will most likely require novel (and therefore unproven and unlicensed) adjuvant and vaccine delivery technologies.

## Challenges in vaccine design

In addition to not knowing which immune responses are required for protective immunity against HIV, vaccine developers debate which HIV antigens are needed for an effective vaccine. While data from animal models suggest that live-attenuated vaccines confer the greatest level of protection, attempts to mimic their efficacy in the SIV model using viral vectors, subunit proteins, whole inactivated vaccines or combination prime-boost modalities have not achieved the same levels of protection. Understanding the mechanism for the superior protection conferred by live vaccines would be likely to help answer the question of which antigens to include in AIDS vaccine candidates. Mascola and Nabel (Chapter 6) discuss the rationale for including specific HIV genes in today's candidates. While in general the inclusion of additional genes makes a vaccine more complex to develop and to manufacture consistently, there is also a general feeling (based on vaccines such as acellular pertussis) that more is better—the thinking behind the design of candidates containing combinations of structural (env, gag, pol) and regulatory/accessory (nef, tat, rev, vif) genes.

Another obstacle to AIDS vaccine development is the inability so far to develop candidates that elicit antibodies which neutralize the broad spectrum of globally diverse isolates in circulation. Selvarajah and Burton (Chapter 7) review the ways in which HIV has evolved mechanisms to evade neutralization and then discuss strategies for solving this major vaccine design problem, in particular those based on studies of effective neutralizing monoclonal antibodies isolated from infected people.

These difficulties, together with evidence for a role of cellular immunity in protection against HIV (as discussed in Chapters 4 and 5), have led AIDS vaccine developers to focus attention on candidates that elicit cellular immune responses—the approach behind nearly all products in the current clinical pipeline. Wahren and Liu (Chapter 8) describe the vaccine design challenges associated with inducing cellular immunity, from the strength and breadth of responses to their durability and to long-term memory, and they review the different strategies in development.

Recent observations demonstrating that SIV (and, by analogy, HIV) replicates in cells of the mucosal immune system early after infection, irrespective of the route of transmission, have raised interest in mucosally delivered vaccines as a way of eliciting strong mucosal responses. Oral or intranasal delivery also has obvious benefits for ease of vaccine administration in the developing world. Rosenthal (Chapter 9) reviews the evidence that mucosal immunity contributes to protection against HIV and describes some new approaches for designing mucosally based HIV vaccines, in particular through the use of novel adjuvants. Studies of these adjuvants are also pointing to a potentially important role of innate immunity in protection against HIV.

Returning to the list of challenges posed by AIDS vaccines compared with those against childhood diseases, yet another is the enormous genetic variability of HIV. This could mean that AIDS vaccines will need to contain multiple strains (like pneumococcal or influenza vaccines, which are "cocktails" of several strains), be regionally specific and/or regularly updated. However, it must be noted that regional specificity in an era of jet travel is a poor option for AIDS vaccine development, and recent epidemiologic trends in countries such as Thailand, China, and Cameroon suggest that predicting which viruses will be circulating a decade in advance is plagued with uncertainties. Korber *et al.* (Chapter 10) address the issue of extensive HIV diversity, from variability at the level of nucleotide sequence to its potential impact on immune recognition and vaccine design. Vaccine developers are addressing this diversity in different ways: for example, Merck has developed a monovalent CMI-based candidate which elicited cross-reactive responses in phase I/II trials and is now being tested for efficacy. Other developers have opted for epitope-based or cocktail approaches. Until the initial demonstration of protective immunity with a vaccine, the relative importance of genetic variability cannot be definitively determined.

## Clinical trials

Over the past 5 years, the pipeline of products entering and progressing through AIDS vaccine trials has dramatically increased. However, there appears to be significant duplication of effort among the major stakeholders in AIDS vaccine development, with numerous DNA and pox vector vaccines in development. Esparza amd Russell (Chapter 11), reviews the current pipeline and the criteria and debates associated with advancing candidates from safety and immunogenicity to efficacy testing, and the increasing role of developing countries (where the epidemic is most severe) in conducting clinical trials. Building on the latter theme, Fast *et al.* (Chapter 12) describe the extensive work required to prepare the ground for large-scale vaccine trials, particularly in the developing world. Among many steps, this requires feasibility studies to determine HIV incidence (information needed so that efficacy trials can be designed with enough statistical power), finding suitable trial populations in different parts of the world, building the necessary health care and laboratory infrastructure, addressing political issues at the national and community levels, and forming innovative partnerships to address these issues.

Efficacy trials of AIDS vaccines fall into two general categories: Proof of concept studies to test a scientific hypothesis, and large-scale efficacy trials that can lead to licensure.

Self (Chapter 13) discusses both types of trial designs and the challenges they raise, including the choice of endpoints and the impact of anti-retroviral therapy on these endpoints. He also describes study designs for various secondary trial objectives, such as measuring correlates of protection, assessing the effects of viral variation and analyzing subgroups. Two chapters (by Fuchs and Buchbinder, and by Beyrer) provide real case perspectives from the first two efficacy trials conducted of AIDS vaccines—VaxGen's B/B gp120 in gay men (and a small number of high-risk women) in the US, Canada, Netherlands (Chapter 14), and VaxGen B/E gp120 in injecting drug users in Thailand (Chapter 15). Although neither vaccine showed efficacy, the experience of conducting these trials provided valuable lessons for future phase III studies.

## From testing to deployment

The issues described above represent scientific questions, in the case of vaccine design, and logistic/social/ethical ones, in the case of clinical trials. However, a series of often under-appreciated challenges involve manufacturing and regulatory issues associated with the design, testing and licensure of vaccine candidates for use around the world.

Ackland (Chapter 16) reviews the regulatory challenges associated with developing AIDS vaccines, and maps out the steps for a regulatory strategy that should accompany the scientific and clinical development process. He also discusses the key issue of different risk–benefit considerations in different areas of the world—for example, in a population in Botswana where prevalence exceeds 30%, compared with one in rural Norway where prevalence is quite low–and which might lead to a different risk–benefit analysis regarding the potential use or testing of candidate vaccines. The endpoints for licensure are addressed in the context of risk–benefit, along with the practical challenge of enhancing the global regulatory landscape so it can best support accelerated vaccine development and, eventually, licensure of vaccines in the world's most affected regions.

Next, Gerson *et al.* (Chapter 17) reviews the many challenges associated with process development and manufacturing of candidate AIDS vaccines: the current lack of resources (both human and financial) dedicated to process development and the limited global capacity for manufacturing vaccine pilot lots (which has slowed the entry of candidates into the clinic) and for large-scale production of vaccines. Another is that hundreds of millions of vaccine doses will eventually be needed once a product is licensed, and the time required to build and validate manufacturing plants with large-scale capacity is about the same (5–7 years) as that needed for clinical testing of an AIDS vaccine candidate. Gerson describes strategies and risks associated with investing in large-scale manufacturing in an environment in which no vaccine has shown efficacy in human trials.

In a broader sense, the global effort to develop an AIDS vaccine also involves a tension between finding an approach which is successful—regardless of the complexity of the manufacturing process, the number of doses needed and to some extent the cost—and the need for a vaccine which is not only effective but inexpensive, stable and easy to deliver globally, especially in resource-poor settings. Many academic investigators are pursuing approaches which if successful, would provide vaccines suitable for use in the developing world. However, the history of vaccine development suggests that the ultimate product will depend upon what is possible, not what would be optimal, and that if an effective vaccine is developed, mechanisms can be established to increase the production scale and reduce the cost relatively quickly.

Certain strategies for making AIDS vaccines introduce additional obstacles though their dependence on as-yet unproven and unlicensed technologies, new classes of adjuvant or novel cell substrates. Since an effective AIDS vaccine would be administered to hundreds of millions of people, the need to demonstrate a high level of safety for each component is paramount. It is noteworthy that the HIV vaccine programs of the major vaccine producing companies are largely based on existing, proven technology.

## Delivering an AIDS vaccine

The history of vaccine development is filled with successes in designing and producing effective vaccines followed by decades-long delays in introducing them into developing countries for wide-scale use; most successful vaccines, such as hepatitis B and *Haemophilus* vaccines, eventually reach the south only after "trickling down" from the north. Kim-Andras and DeQuarras (Chapter 18) describe the challenges of achieving more rapid global access for AIDS vaccines, and review the infrastructure requirements and financing needs necessary to move from dream to reality. Finally, Anderson and Plotkin (Chapter 19) review the data on the public health impact of AIDS vaccines, and discuss "how good is good enough" for introduction of an AIDS vaccine. This turns out to be a much more complex issue than it initially appears, with very different public health outcomes depending on the specific properties of the vaccine and how it is used.

## Summary

The challenges associated with AIDS vaccine development are daunting, yet the global price of the pandemic in the absence of safe and effective AIDS vaccines are staggering. Solving the scientific challenges requires strategies for engaging the most talented scientists on specific applied research problems. But solutions to these challenges are, by themselves, unlikely to lead to a safe and effective AIDS vaccine since clinical testing and establishment of the requisite infrastructure for delivery of licensed AIDS vaccines are equally critical elements of success. Thus, novel synergies between academia, government and industry, particularly industry's skills in project and portfolio management, can facilitate the worldwide search for an effective AIDS vaccine. Engaging the vaccine development industry is also likely to require new strategies for leveraging risk and novel approaches to intellectual property, to ensure that effective vaccines will reach the populations in greatest need in

the developing world while concomitantly assuring companies a return on their investment, which will drive the necessary product improvements for next generation vaccines.

These needs have led to new models of partnership in public health, spearheaded by the International AIDS Vaccine Initiative (IAVI) and the Bill & Melinda Gates Foundation. New models for addressing the scientific challenges, such as IAVI's Neutralizing Antibody Consortium, ensuring that clinical site and process development and manufacturing capacity are ready for the leading candidates, and creating a positive global regulatory environment must all be pursued in parallel, to shorten the timeline until there is an AIDS vaccine. With ten new infections of HIV every minute and 3 million AIDS deaths per year, it is critical for the global biomedical and public health communities to address AIDS vaccine development as an urgent global priority. This book attempts to lay out the challenges, and to offer strategies for solutions.

## Editors' note

During the preparation of this book, new data likely to impact global efforts in AIDS vaccine R&D continued to emerge, and new initiatives were launched to accelerate the search for a safe and effective HIV vaccine. For example, preliminary observations suggest that host genotype plays an important role in susceptibility to HIV, that some transmitted strains of HIV may be more sensitive to virus neutralization than the viral populations circulating in chronically infected individuals, and that early virus–host interactions may be key for an individual's subsequent disease course. Findings like these helped spur the US National Institutes of Health to establish the Center for HIV/AIDS Vaccine Immunology (CHAVI), which will focus on acute HIV infection with the goal of elucidating correlates of protective immunity. The CHAVI is the first of a series of new initiatives, launched in 2005, aimed at addressing key scientific challenges applicable to HIV vaccine design, as part of an alliance of stakeholders termed the Global HIV/AIDS Vaccine Enterprise, committed to accelerating AIDS vaccine development.

Recent data also suggests that anti-vector immunity—i.e., pre-existing immunity to the virus that forms the backbone of a vector-based vaccine platform such as Adeno-type 5—may mitigate the immunogenicity of the vaccine candidate. With correlates of protection against HIV still undefined, these observations led Merck and the HIV Vaccine Trials Network to launch a phase IIB proof-of-concept trial to estimate the efficacy of its Adeno-5 gag-pol-nef vaccine in subjects with and without pre-existing immunity to the vaccine vector. It also led several programs, such as those at IAVI, Glaxo-SmithKline and Crucell to launch vaccine development projects focused on low-seroprevalent adeno-vector-based vaccines.

Moreover, preliminary clinical trials data recently presented by investigators from the NIH Vaccine Research Center suggest that DNA priming followed by Adeno-5 vector boosting elicits stronger cellular and antibody responses than either DNA or Adeno alone. These data have led to acceleration of this candidate to phase IIa trials in the developing world, to assess the immunogenicity of the vaccine in populations likely to have high levels of pre-existing anti-Ad5 antibodies (based on sero-epidemiological surveys). If its promise appears to hold, this candidate would likely be next in line for entry into efficacy trials.

Finally, recent findings that a human papillomavirus vaccine (HPV) candidate prevents cervical cancer provide further evidence that vaccines can protect against sexually transmitted diseases. Licensure and deployment of the HPV vaccine in the developing world should lay important groundwork for what we all hope will be followed by the development and deployment of a safe, effective HIV vaccine.

# The Global HIV/AIDS Epidemic

Marjorie Opuni, Bernhard Schwartländer, J. Ties Boerma, and Karen Stanecki

2

## Abstract

Since AIDS was first recognized 25 years ago, 65 million people have been infected with HIV and 25 million of them have died. The HIV/AIDS epidemic is thus one of the worst epidemics to strike humanity in recorded history. This chapter provides an overview of the HIV/AIDS epidemic by region, highlighting epidemiological trends, the genetic diversity of HIV and differences in the modes of HIV transmission. It then discusses the need for an AIDS vaccine as well as the components of expanded responses to HIV/AIDS and how these can curb the epidemic and its impact.

## Introduction

The HIV/AIDS epidemic is one of the worst epidemics to strike humanity in recorded history. An estimated 38.6 million (33.4–46.0 million) people worldwide are estimated to be living with HIV or AIDS including an estimated 4.1 million (3.4–6.2 million) adults and children newly infected in 2005 (UNAIDS, 2006). In addition, an estimated 25 million have already died, making a cumulative of 65 million HIV infections since the epidemic began (UNAIDS and WHO, 2005). And because these deaths have occurred predominantly among prime-aged adults who are often parents, an estimated 15.2 million (13.3–17.0 million) children today have lost one or both parents to AIDS (UNAIDS, 2006).

The impact of HIV/AIDS on individuals, households and communities so far is only a preview of what lies ahead, given the time lag between HIV infection and the onset of disease. The survival of the millions of people living with HIV will be prolonged only if they have access to antiretroviral therapy once they have advanced HIV infection or AIDS, and/or vaccine technology that mitigates the progression of HIV-related disease is developed.

And unless HIV prevention interventions are strengthened globally and an effective preventative vaccine is developed, HIV will continue its unrelenting spread. This was illustrated in a recent analysis projecting the future course of the epidemic in 125 low- and middle-income countries (Stover et al., 2006). According to this study, at current levels of HIV prevention interventions, a cumulative total of 62.3 million new infections will occur between 2005 and 2015.

This chapter provides an overview of the HIV and AIDS epidemic by region, highlighting epidemiological trends, the genetic diversity of HIV and differences in the modes of HIV transmission. It then discusses the need for an AIDS vaccine as well as the components of expanded responses to HIV/AIDS and how these can curb the epidemic and its impact.

## HIV and AIDS by region

### Sub-Saharan Africa

Sub-Saharan Africa is the region where the spread of HIV has been most unrelenting and where the impact of the epidemic has been most severe. An estimated 24.5 million (21.6–27.4 million) people in the region are living with HIV/AIDS—almost 64% of the global total (UNAIDS, 2006). This includes an estimated 2.7 million (2.3–3.1 million) adults and children who were newly infected with HIV in 2005 (UNAIDS, 2006). Sub-Saharan Africa also accounts for three-fourths of the 25 million people who have already died, although only about 10% of the world population resides in sub-Saharan Africa (UNAIDS and WHO, 2005).

HIV prevalence among adults 15–49 years old in sub-Saharan Africa is estimated to be 6.1% (5.4–6.8%) but there are important differences across the region (UNAIDS, 2006). Southern Africa has the highest HIV infection rates in the world. The sub-region includes eight countries where adult HIV prevalence is above 15%: Botswana, Lesotho, Mozambique, Namibia, South Africa, Swaziland, Zambia, and Zimbabwe (UNAIDS, 2006). Swaziland has the highest adult prevalence in the world with 33.4% (21.2–45.3%), followed by Botswana, Lesotho, and Zimbabwe, where prevalence estimates are 24.1% (23.0–32.0%), 23.2% (21.9–24.7%) and 20.1% (13.3–27.6%) respectively (UNAIDS, 2006). Prevalence in the countries of East Africa is markedly lower with the highest adult prevalence estimates of 6.7% (5.7–7.6%), 6.5 (5.8–7.2%) and 6.1% (5.2–7.0%) found in Uganda, Tanzania and Kenya respectively (UNAIDS, 2006). In most countries of West Africa, prevalence is under 3% (UNAIDS, 2006). Adult HIV prevalence is highest in Côte d'Ivoire, where it is estimated to be 7.1% (4.3–9.7%). And while HIV prevalence in Nigeria is estimated to be 3.9% (2.3–5.6%), Nigeria is home to more people living with HIV than any other country in the world except India and South Africa (UNAIDS, 2006). Prevalence estimates in Central Africa are higher. Adult HIV prevalence estimates in Cameroon, the Central African Republic, Congo, and Gabon are 5.4% (4.9–5.9%), 10.7% (4.5–17.2%), 5.3% (3.3–7.5%) and 7.9% (5.1–11.5%) respectively (UNAIDS, 2006).

In terms of trends over time, recent data suggest that, excluding Zimbabwe, where national adult HIV prevalence has declined, HIV prevalence in Southern Africa is either increasing slightly or stabilizing at very high levels (UNAIDS and WHO, 2005; WHO AFRO, 2005). HIV infection levels are generally remaining stable in West and Central Africa, with declines in HIV prevalence observed in certain areas, including urban Burkina Faso, and certain increases observed in other areas, including in Dakar, Senegal, and Accra, Ghana (UNAIDS and WHO, 2005; WHO AFRO, 2005). Declining HIV prevalence levels have been documented in some countries in East Africa with important declines recorded in Uganda since the mid-1990s and in Kenya more recently (UNAIDS and WHO, 2005).

Heterosexual HIV transmission is the major mode of spread among adults in sub-Saharan Africa. Available population-based surveys show that women aged 15–49 years are 1.3–2 times more likely to be infected than men (WHO AFRO, 2005). This gender difference is particularly pronounced at younger ages. Young women aged 15–24 years are 2–5 times more likely to be infected than young men of the same age reflecting sexual contact between older men and younger women (WHO AFRO, 2005). Dominant heterosexual transmission also means that there is a significant level of mother-to-child transmission. An estimated 2.0 million (1.5–3.0 million) children under 15 are living with HIV/AIDS in sub-Saharan Africa with almost all of them acquiring the virus from their mother (UNAIDS, 2006).

Differences in HIV prevalence levels between urban and rural areas vary by country (WHO AFRO, 2005). While there are important differences in HIV prevalence levels between urban and rural areas in most countries in East Africa, with urban rates being higher than those in rural areas, the distinction is not as evident in many of the countries of West, Central and Southern Africa.

An estimated 2.0 million (1.7–2.3 million) adults and children died of AIDS in sub-Saharan Africa in 2005—over 70% of the world total (UNAIDS, 2006). The impact of HIV/AIDS on adult and child mortality is becoming increasingly clear, with the most dramatic evidence coming from Southern Africa (WHO AFRO, 2005). Until the early 1990s (before the AIDS epidemic hit the region) several countries in Southern Africa reported the lowest mortality rates on the continent; however these advances are being reversed by HIV/AIDS (Dorrington *et al.*, 2004; Feeney, 2001; Hosegood *et al.*, 2004).

HIV-1 strains account for more than 98% of all infections in sub-Saharan Africa (WHO AFRO, 2005). However there is high genetic variability in HIV-1 in the region (Kijak and McCutchan, 2005; McCutchan, 2006). Subtype C is the overwhelmingly predominant subtype in Southern Africa and in the horn of Africa (Kijak and McCutchan, 2005; McCutchan, 2006). Subtypes A, C and D and their recombinants predominate in the rest of East Africa (Kijak and McCutchan, 2005; McCutchan, 2006). While subtype A dominates in Kenya, subtype C is more common in Tanzania and subtype D is dominant in Uganda (Kijak and McCutchan, 2005), Though circulating recombinant forms (CRF) are rare in the sub-region, unique recombinant forms (URF) are common (Kijak and McCutchan, 2005). In Kenya, Tanzania and Uganda, URFs constitute 30–50% of the strains (McCutchan, 2006). The recombinant CRF02_AG dominates in West Africa and in the western parts of Central Africa, with CRF02_AG constituting 95% and 50% of HIV-1 strains in Cote d'Ivoire and Cameroon respectively (Kijak and McCutchan, 2005; McCutchan, 2006). The genetic diversity of HIV-1 is most extreme in Central Africa, No subtype predominates and a number of rare subtypes and recombinants have been found only in this sub-region (Kijak and McCutchan, 2005; McCutchan, 2006).

HIV-2 with its two subtypes—A and B—is similar to HIV-1 but less readily transmitted and it accounts for about 2% of HIV infections in sub-Saharan Africa (McCutchan, 2006; WHO AFRO, 2005). It is found primarily in West Africa with prevalence levels as high as 10% documented in some parts of Guinea-Bissau (Schim van der Loeff and Aaby, 1999).

## Asia and Oceania

An estimated 8.3 million (5.7–12.5 million), and 78,000 (48,000–170,000) people are living with HIV/AIDS in Asia and Oceania respectively (UNAIDS, 2006). This includes an estimated 930,000 (620,000–2.4 million) and 7,200 (3,500–55,000) people newly infected with HIV in 2005 (UNAIDS, 2006). Most of these persons are men—with 72% of people living with HIV in East Asia, 70% in South and Southeast Asia and 53% in Oceania being men (UNAIDS, 2006).

Adult HIV prevalence is estimated at 0.1% or less in East Asia while ranging from less than 0.1% to 1.6% in South and Southeast Asia (UNAIDS, 2006). With an estimated HIV prevalence of 1.6% (0.9–2.6%), Cambodia has the highest prevalence in South and Southeast Asia, followed by Thailand and Myanmar where estimated adult prevalence levels are 1.4% (0.7–2.1%) and 1.3% (0.7–2.0%) respectively (UNAIDS, 2006). In the Oceania region, HIV prevalence is estimated at 0.1% for all countries except Papua New Guinea, where it is estimated to be 1.8% (0.9–4.4%) (UNAIDS, 2006).

In most of the countries in Asia, national adult HIV prevalence has remained low compared with some other parts of the world including sub-Saharan Africa. However, this is misleading given the very large populations of some of the countries in the region.

India, for example, is a country with a population larger than that of all of Africa. Though national adult HIV prevalence in India is estimated to be 0.9% (0.5–1.5%), this nevertheless translates into an estimated 5.6 million (3.4–9.3 million) adults living with HIV (UNAIDS, 2006). In China, while adult HIV prevalence is estimated at less than 0.1%, this translates into 650,000 (390,000–1.1 million) adults living with HIV (UNAIDS, 2006). Clearly, with well over 2 billion people living in China and India alone, what happens in India and China will profoundly impact the future of HIV/AIDS.

Central to many of the epidemics in Asia are injecting drug use, unprotected sex and the interplay between the two (UNAIDS and WHO, 2005). In India while in the southern states, the epidemics are driven by heterosexual sex, in the northeast, there are significant epidemics among injecting drug users (UNAIDS and WHO, 2005). In China, HIV epidemics to date have been concentrated among injecting drug users, sex workers, former plasma donors, and their partners within certain geographic areas (UNAIDS and WHO, 2005). Transmission of HIV among injecting drug users and commercial sex workers and their clients has accounted for a high proportion of cases in Cambodia, Myanmar and Thailand (UNAIDS and WHO, 2005). The interplay between injecting drug use and sex work underlies the epidemics of Indonesia, Vietnam and China.

Two well-documented success stories in the response to HIV/AIDS in this region are the responses in Thailand and Cambodia. The epidemic in Thailand has been extensively documented, and Thailand has been hailed as one of the success stories in the response to HIV/AIDS. In Thailand, national HIV prevalence has dropped to its lowest (UNAIDS and WHO, 2005). In Cambodia, after peaking at 3% in 1997, national adult HIV prevalence in Cambodia has fallen by almost half (UNAIDS and WHO, 2005).

The genetic variability in HIV-1 in Asia is also significant (Kijak and McCutchan, 2005). The predominant subtype in India is subtype C (Kijak and McCutchan, 2005; McCutchan, 2006). In China, though the predominant subtype in circulation is subtype B, a number of different subtypes circulate (McCutchan, 2006). Subtypes B, C, CRF01_AE and the recombinants CRF07_BC and CRF08_BC have all been identified in China (Kijak and McCutchan, 2005). In South-East Asia, subtype CRF01_AE is the dominant strain (Kijak and McCutchan, 2005). A variety of URFs have also been identified in China, Myanmar and Thailand (Kijak and McCutchan, 2005; McCutchan, 2006).

## Latin America and the Caribbean

There are an estimated 1.6 million (1.2–2.4 million) and 330,000 (240,000–420,000) people living with HIV/AIDS in Latin America and the Caribbean respectively (UNAIDS, 2006). This includes an estimated 140,000 (100,000–420,000) and 37,000 (26,000–54,000) persons newly infected with HIV in 2005 (UNAIDS, 2006). Adult HIV prevalence is estimated at 0.5% (0.4–1.2%) in Latin America and 1.6% (1.1–2.2%) in the Caribbean, making the Caribbean the second-most affected region after sub-Saharan Africa (UNAIDS, 2006).

Six of the seven countries in the Caribbean have adult HIV prevalence levels above 1%, with prevalence in Haiti estimated at 3.8% (2.2–5.4%) (UNAIDS, 2006). In the seventh country—Cuba—HIV prevalence is estimated to be 0.1% (< 0.2%) (UNAIDS, 2006). Although it should be noted that national HIV prevalence in Haiti has been declining (UNAIDS, 2006). In Central America, with an HIV prevalence of 2.5% (1.4–4.0%), Belize has the highest prevalence level in the subregion followed by Guyana, Suriname and Honduras with estimated prevalence levels of 2.4% (1.0–4.9%), 1.9% (1.1–1.3%), 1.5% (0.8–2.4%) respectively (UNAIDS, 2006). Point estimates for adult HIV prevalence in the countries of South America range between 0.1% and 0.7% (UNAIDS, 2006). Though estimated HIV prevalence for Brazil is 0.5% (0.3–1.6%), with 620,000 (370,000–1.0 million) Brazil is the country in Latin America and the Caribbean, with the largest number of people living with HIV/AIDS (UNAIDS, 2006).

While an estimated 53% of people living with HIV/AIDS in the Caribbean are women, women comprise 30% of persons living with HIV/AIDS in Latin America (UNAIDS, 2006). This reflects the diversity in the modes of transmission in the two regions. Heterosexual transmission is predominant in the Caribbean and some parts of Central America (UNAIDS and WHO, 2005). This has led to increases in mother-to-child transmission; with pediatric AIDS cases rising in parallel with the increase in HIV infection in women. In the Andean Region, parts of Central America (including Mexico) and Brazil, male-to-male sexual contact is the most important mode of transmission (UNAIDS and WHO, 2005). The spread of HIV through the sharing of injecting drug equipment is a concern in Argentina, Brazil, Chile, Paraguay and Uruguay, the northern parts of Mexico, Bermuda and Puerto Rico (UNAIDS and WHO, 2005).

Adult and child deaths due to AIDS in 2005 were estimated to total 59,000 (47,000–76,000) and 27,000 (19,000–36,000) and in Latin America and the Caribbean respectively (UNAIDS, 2006). AIDS mortality has declined in Brazil following similar patterns to those observed in high-income countries. Survival time for people living with AIDS has increased substantially as a result of antiretroviral treatment given the Brazilian policy of providing universal access to antiretroviral treatment (Berkman *et al.*, 2005; Teixeira *et al.*, 2004).

With the exception of Cuba, subtype B predominates in the Caribbean (Kijak and McCutchan, 2005). With subtype B, a variety of A, D and H recombinants, CRF18_cpx, in Latin America and the Caribbean, the genetic diversity of HIV-1 is most extreme in Cuba (Kijak and McCutchan, 2005). In Argentina, Chile, Paraguay and Uruguay, B and B/F recombinants predominate while in Brazil, subtypes B, C, F and B/F recombinants are found (Kijak and McCutchan, 2005). In the rest of Latin America, subtype B is predominant (Kijak and McCutchan, 2005; McCutchan, 2006).

## Eastern Europe and Central Asia

The HIV/AIDS epidemic in Eastern Europe and Central Asia continues to worsen. An estimated 1.5 million (1.0–2.3 million) people are living with HIV/AIDS in Eastern Europe and Central Asia (UNAIDS, 2006). This includes an estimated 220,000 (150,000–650,000) adults and children newly infected with HIV in 2005 (UNAIDS, 2006). Adult HIV prevalence in the region is estimated at 0.8% (0.6–1.4%) compared with 0.6% (0.4–1.0%) in 2003 (UNAIDS, 2006). Approximately 72% of adults living with HIV in the region are men but the number of women getting infected is increasing (UNAIDS, 2006; UNAIDS and WHO, 2005). An estimated 53,000 (36,000–75,000) persons died of AIDS in 2005 (UNAIDS, 2006).

With an estimated adult prevalence of 1.4% (0.8–4.3%), Ukraine is the most heavily affected country in the region followed by Estonia, the Russian Federation and Moldova with estimated prevalence levels of 1.3% (0.6–4.3%), 1.1% (0.7–1.8%) and 1.1% (0.6–2.6%) respectively (UNAIDS, 2006). The overwhelming majority of people living with HIV/AIDS in the region live in the two countries: the Russian Federation [940,000 (560,000–1.6 million) people] and Ukraine [410,000 (250,000–680,000) people] (UNAIDS, 2006).

Injecting drug use among young people is the predominant mode of HIV transmission in Eastern Europe and Central Asia. However, heterosexual sex is becoming an increasingly important mode of transmission in a number of countries in the region. This trend has been documented in Kazakhstan, Ukraine, Belarus and the Republic of Moldova where between 30% and 45% of newly diagnosed HIV cases occurred to persons infected through heterosexual sex (UNAIDS and WHO, 2005).

In terms of the genetic diversity of HIV-1 in Eastern Europe and Central Asia, subtype A and to a lesser extent subtype B as well as a variety of recombinant strains including CRF03_AB predominate in the region (Kijak and McCutchan, 2005; McCutchan, 2006; Osmanov *et al.*, 2002).

## North Africa and the Middle East

Relatively few cases of HIV and AIDS have been reported in the countries of North Africa and the Middle East. An estimated 440,000 (250,000–720,000) people are living with HIV/AIDS in the region (UNAIDS, 2006). This includes an estimated 64,000 (38,000–210,000) persons newly infected with HIV in 2005 (UNAIDS, 2006). Adult HIV prevalence in North Africa and the Middle East is estimated to be 0.2% (0.1–0.4%) with almost 48% of adults living with HIV in the region being women (UNAIDS, 2006). And an estimated 37,000 (20,000–62,000) adults and children died of AIDS in 2005 (UNAIDS, 2006).

Systematic surveillance in much of the region remains inadequate and more and better information is needed to better understand the epidemiology of HIV/AIDS in the region (UNAIDS and WHO, 2005). Available information indicates that except for Sudan where national adult HIV prevalence is estimated at 1.6% (0.8–2.7%), HIV prevalence in the region is very low albeit increasing in some countries including Algeria, Iran, Libya, and Morocco (UNAIDS, 2006; UNAIDS and WHO, 2005). Available data suggest that the main modes of transmission are heterosexual intercourse and increasingly injecting drug use especially in Iran and Libya (UNAIDS, 2006; UNAIDS and WHO, 2005). Only limited information exists on the genetic diversity of HIV-1 in North Africa and the Middle East (McCutchan, 2006). Existing data indicate that subtypes A and B predominate in this region (Osmanov *et al.*, 2002).

## North America, Western and Central Europe

An estimated 1.3 million (770,000–2.1 million) people and 720,000 (550,000–950,000) people are living with HIV/AIDS in North America and Western and Central Europe respectively (UNAIDS, 2006). This includes an estimated 43,000 (34,000–65,000) and 22,000 (18,000–33,000) persons newly infected with HIV in 2005 (UNAIDS, 2006). AIDS deaths in 2005 were estimated to total 18,000 (11,000–26,000) in North America and 12,000 (<15,000) in Western and Central Europe (UNAIDS, 2006). The widespread availability of antiretroviral therapy in these two regions over the last decade initially led to a dramatic reduction in HIV/AIDS related mortality which has more recently leveled off at a comparatively low level (Collaborative Group on AIDS Incubation and HIV Survival including the CASCADE EU Concerted Action. Concerted Action on SeroConversion to AIDS and Death in Europe, 2000; Lee *et al.*, 2001).

Preventing new HIV infections continues to be a challenge even in the richest countries. The number of new HIV cases has remained stable at about 40,000 in the United States (Centers for Disease Control and Prevention, 2005). The number of newly infected has been growing in Canada and in several Western European countries while remaining stable and contained in most of Central Europe (UNAIDS and WHO, 2005).

The epidemic is disproportionately affecting poorer and marginalized sections of society in rich countries. In the United States, African-Americans account for 49% of new HIV infections though they make up only 12% of the country's population (Centers for Disease Control and Prevention, 2006). Similarly, in some Western European countries, a larger proportion of new HIV cases diagnosed are occurring through heterosexual intercourse among persons who, themselves or their partner, originate from countries where HIV prevalence is high (Hamers and Downs, 2004).

Approximately 74% and 72% of adults estimated to be living with HIV in North America and Western and Central Europe are men (UNAIDS, 2006). Underlying these distributions is the fact that sex between men and in some countries injecting drug use are the most prominent modes of transmission in these countries (UNAIDS and WHO, 2005).

However, increasing numbers of people in North America and Western and Central Europe are being infected through heterosexual intercourse (UNAIDS and WHO, 2005).

Subtype B is the predominant subtype in both North America and Western and Central Europe (McCutchan, 2006). However, both in North America and to a greater extent in Western and Central Europe, the genetic diversity of HIV-1 is increasing as a result of travel and immigration (Kijak and McCutchan, 2005). In France and Belgium, for example, 25% and 50% of HIV-1 infections are non-B subtypes (Kijak and McCutchan, 2005).

## Expanded responses

Against this background, it is important to remember that a continually expanding AIDS epidemic is not inevitable. But ultimately, it is recognized that the spread of HIV infection will probably only be contained with an effective preventative vaccine and there is hope for vaccine technology that will mitigate progression of HIV-related disease.

In the meantime, expanded responses to HIV/AIDS, including strong prevention programs and increased access to treatment, will enable us to reverse the course of the epidemic and reduce its impact (UN General Assembly, 2001). As mentioned above, several countries have been successful in turning around the epidemic. For example, the results of Thailand's efforts to achieve universal condom use in commercial sex establishments have been well documented (Kilmarx *et al.*, 2000), and similar successes are being achieved in Cambodia. Strong responses have also led to decreases in HIV rates in some African countries, in particular Uganda. There are now well-recognized elements essential to a strong response in HIV/AIDS prevention and care (Fig. 2.1).

Immediate implementation of a comprehensive set of HIV prevention interventions could avert a large number of future infections and reverse the course of the AIDS epidemic. Estimates suggest that significant expansion of these existing, well-known measures would mean preventing 50% of projected new infections between 2005 and 2015 (Stover *et al.*, 2006).

The "3 by 5" initiative committed to have 3 million people in need of antiretroviral therapy in low- and middle-income countries on the drugs by the end of 2005 (WHO, 2003). Though this goal was not met, it is estimated that between 2001 and 2005, the number of people on antiretroviral therapy in resource-poor countries increased from 240,000 to 1.3 million (UNAIDS, 2006). It has been calculated that between 250,000 and 350,000 deaths were averted in 2005 as a result of increased access to antiretroviral therapy (WHO and UNAIDS, 2005).

The resources required to provide an expanded response to HIV/AIDS in low-income and middle-income countries have been estimated at US$14.9 billion, US$18.1 billion and US$22.1 billion annually from 2006 to 2008 respectively (UNAIDS, 2005). These estimates include not only funding for prevention, care and treatment and support to orphans and vulnerable children (UNAIDS, 2005). Also included are

*Prevention interventions*
Mass media campaigns
Community mobilization
Voluntary counseling and testing
School-based AIDS education
Peer education for out-of-school youth
Outreach programs for commercial sex workers and their Clients
Outreach programs for men who have sex with men
Harm reduction programs for injecting drug users
Workplace prevention programs
Prevention programs for people living with HIV
Prevention programs for special populations
Condom social marketing
Public and commercial sector condom provision
Treatment for sexually transmitted infections
Prevention of mother-to-child transmission
Blood safety
Post-exposure prophylaxis (health care setting, rape)
Safe medical injections
Universal precautions

*Care and support activities*
Palliative care
Diagnostic HIV-1 testing
Treatment of opportunistic infections
Prophylaxis for opportunistic infections
Antiretroviral therapy
Laboratory testing
Orphanage care
Community support for orphans
School fee support for orphans
Health-care support of orphans
Family/home support for orphans

**Figure 2.1** Prevention interventions and care and support activities of the expanded response program. Source: UNAIDS 2005. Resource needs for an expanded response to AIDS in low- and middle- income countries (Geneva: UNAIDS).

program costs and human resource costs associated with the implementation of the prevention, care and support interventions.

## Conclusions

The spread of HIV continues despite progress seen in a number of countries around the world. The increasing availability of antiretroviral therapy may lead to reduced morbidity and mortality rates, and contribute to a more efficient response to HIV overall. However, experience in even the richest countries suggests that without a protective vaccine, it will be difficult to eliminate or eradicate HIV.

Therefore, the development of an HIV/AIDS vaccine is probably one of the most important scientific research priorities of our time. An HIV/AIDS vaccine that reduces the spread of HIV infection and/or limits the clinical progression to AIDS in people already infected with HIV would significantly strengthen a comprehensive response to HIV/AIDS.

Yet, the very nature of the epidemiology of HIV poses important obstacles for vaccine researchers as highlighted above and described elsewhere in this volume. One of the most important challenges in the development of HIV/AIDS vaccine is the genetic diversity of HIV-1, the predominant type of HIV in the world. Also, patterns of HIV transmission differ and to be effective, a vaccine must protect against these different modes of transmission. Progress in vaccine research in recent years gives reason for some optimism. However, even in the most optimistic scenarios, there is no doubt that an effective vaccine that can be used on a large scale in those areas where incidence is highest will not be available in the next few years.

As the world waits for a vaccine, the financial and logistical obstacles faced by those working to scale up existing prevention, care and support interventions must be overcome. Countries such as Brazil, Thailand, and Uganda have shown us the way. It is critical to learn from these successful examples to effectively scale up the responses to HIV/AIDS internationally. While the responses now must focus on available interventions in prevention and care, we must also prepare societies and countries for an effective vaccine. As shown by the spectacular failures with certain other vaccine programs, such as Hepatitis B, this is not a trivial matter (Chapter 18). With millions of people living with HIV/AIDS dying every year, a broad and visionary strategy is needed now so policy makers and implementers will be prepared as technology advances.

## References

Berkman, A., Garcia, J., Munoz-Laboy, M., Paiva, V., and Parker, R. (2005). A critical analysis of the Brazilian response to HIV/AIDS: lessons learned for controlling and mitigating the epidemic in developing countries. Am. J. Publ. Hlth 95, 1162–1172.

Centers for Disease Control and Prevention (2005). HIV/AIDS Surveillance Report (Atlanta, GA: Centers for Disease Control and Prevention).

Centers for Disease Control and Prevention (2006). HIV/AIDS among African Americans (Atlanta, GA: Centers for Disease Control and Prevention).

Collaborative Group on AIDS Incubation and HIV Survival including the CASCADE EU Concerted Action. Concerted Action on SeroConversion to AIDS and Death in Europe (2000). Time from HIV-1 seroconversion to AIDS and death before widespread use of highly-active antiretroviral therapy: a collaborative re-analysis. Lancet 355, 1131–1137.

Dorrington, R., Moultrie, T., and Timaeus, I. (2004). Estimation of mortality using the South African Census 2001 data. University of Cape Town Centre for Actuarial Research Monograph No.11.

Feeney, G. (2001). The impact of HIV/AIDS on adult mortality in Zimbabwe. Population Dev. Rev. 27, 771–780.

Hamers, F.F., and Downs, A.M. (2004). The changing face of the HIV epidemic in western Europe: what are the implications for public health policies? Lancet 364, 83–94.

Hosegood, V., Vanneste, A., and Timaeus, I. (2004). Levels and causes of adult mortality in rural South Africa: the impact of AIDS. AIDS 18, 663–671.

Kijak, G.H., and McCutchan, F.E. (2005). HIV diversity, molecular epidemiology, and the role of recombination. Curr. Infect. Dis. Rep. 7, 480–488.

Kilmarx, P.H., Supawitkul, S., Wankrairoj, M., Uthaivoravit, W., Limpakarnjanarat, K., Saisorn, S., and Mastro, T.D. (2000). Explosive spread and effective control of human immunodeficiency virus in northernmost Thailand: the epidemic in Chiang Rai province, 1988–99. AIDS 14, 2731–2740.

Lee, L.M., Karon, J.M., Selik, R., Neal, J.J., and Fleming, P.L. (2001). Survival after AIDS diagnosis in adolescents and adults during the treatment era, United States, 1984–1997. J. Am. Med. Ass. 285, 1308–1315.

McCutchan, F.E. (2006). Global epidemiology of HIV. J. Med. Virol. 78 Suppl. 1, S7–S12.

Osmanov, S., Pattou, C., Walker, N., Schwardlander, B., and Esparza, J. (2002). Estimated global distribution and regional spread of HIV-1 genetic subtypes in the year 2000. J. Acq. Immun. Defic. Syndr. 29, 184–190.

Schim van der Loeff, M. F., and Aaby, P. (1999). Towards a better understanding of the epidemiology of HIV-2. AIDS 13, Suppl. A, S69–S84.

Stover, J., Bertozzi, S., Gutierrez, J.P., Walker, N., Stanecki, K.A., Greener, R., Gouws, E., Hankins, C., Garnett, G.P., Salomon, J.A., et al. (2006). The global impact of scaling up HIV/AIDS prevention programs in low- and middle-income countries. Science 311, 1474–1476.

Teixeira, P.R., Vitoria, M.A., and Barcarolo, J. (2004). Antiretroviral treatment in resource-poor settings: the Brazilian experience. AIDS 18, Suppl. 3, S5–7.

UN General Assembly (2001). Declaration of commitment on HIV/AIDS. (New York: United Nations).

UNAIDS (2005). Resource needs for an expanded response to AIDS in low- and middle- income countries (Geneva: UNAIDS).

UNAIDS (2006). Report on the global HIV/AIDS epidemic (Geneva: UNAIDS).

UNAIDS and WHO (2005). AIDS epidemic update: December 2005 (Geneva: UNAIDS and WHO).

WHO (2003). The 3 by 5 initiative, WHO Fact Sheet (Geneva).

WHO and UNAIDS (2005). Progress on global access to HIV antiretroviral therapy: An update on "3 by 5." (Geneva: WHO and UNAIDS).

WHO AFRO (2005). HIV/AIDS Epidemiological Surveillance Report for the WHO African Region, 2005 Update (Geneva: WHO AFRO).

# Part II

# What Does a Vaccine Need to Do?

# Biology of Early Infection and Impact on Vaccine Design

3

S.B. Justin Wong and Robert F. Siliciano

## Abstract
Recent studies are providing insights into the early events following exposure to HIV-1, knowledge that is important for the design of preventive vaccines. This chapter summarizes current understanding of these events, with the goal of defining more precisely the "point of no return" after which immune responses cannot eradicate HIV. One key early step is a rapid exponential expansion of the virus population, which occurs as soon as HIV reaches tissue sites with high concentrations of susceptible CD4+ T-cells. Preventing this initial expansion is likely to be critical for achieving sterilizing immunity with vaccines, since once high-level viremia is present, a stable virus reservoir is established in resting memory CD4+ T-cells, which precludes eradication even with potent antiretroviral drugs. For these reasons, vaccine development should focus on preventing HIV from initially accessing crucial tissue sites.

## Introduction

Many critical features of HIV-1 infection result from events that occur very early in the course of infection. These include the dissemination of virus to the peripheral lymphoid tissues, which serve as the principal sites of viral replication, and seeding a stable reservoir of latent virus in resting memory CD4+ T-cells. Knowledge of the early events following transmission is essential for the design of vaccines that can halt this chain of events before a stable HIV reservoir is established in the host. Given the extraordinary stability of the latent reservoir, such early intervention affords vaccines their only real chance of success in eradicating HIV. Although recent studies suggest that some vaccines which fail to prevent infection may nevertheless have a beneficial effect in delaying disease progression (see Chapter 4), this review will focus on the biology of early HIV-1 infection as it pertains to vaccines designed to induce sterilizing immunity.

## Early events following transmission

Conceptually, the early events in sexual transmission of HIV-1 can be divided into distinct steps (Fig. 3.1):

1. penetration through epithelial barriers;
2. transit to sites where susceptible target T-cells are present at high concentration;
3. rapid expansion governed by the basic reproductive ratio ($R_0$);
4. increasing viremia and systemic dissemination of the virus;
5. establishment of a latent reservoir; and
6. decline in viremia to a steady state level (viral set point).

Although these early events are difficult to investigate, a significant amount of information has become available from studies in the SIV system and from *in vitro* experiments. Our current understanding of each of these six steps is reviewed below.

### Penetration through epithelial barriers

The initial step in most forms of HIV-1 transmission involves penetration through an epithelial barrier. (The exception is intravenous inoculation, for example via contaminated needles or blood products, after which virus can directly infect susceptible cells present in the blood or tissues.) However, the most common form of transmission involves sexual contact with an infected person and requires that virus and/or virally infected cells in the infecting inoculum cross a layer of epithelial cells lining the genital mucosa (see Moore and Shattock, 2003, for an excellent review; Chapter 9). Similarly, epithelial barriers in the gastrointestinal tract must be crossed for mother to infant transmission at parturition or breast feeding and for infection through oral or anal sex.

An intact epithelium presents a significant barrier because epithelial cells cannot be infected by HIV-1, and therefore virus must cross the epithelial layer to reach susceptible cells such as CD4+ T-lymphocytes and macrophages. In the vagina, a layer of stratified squamous epithelium several cells thick serves as a barrier to infection. The vaginal epithelium thins in response to changes during the menstrual cycle or to exogenous progesterone. In contrast, the cervix is lined by

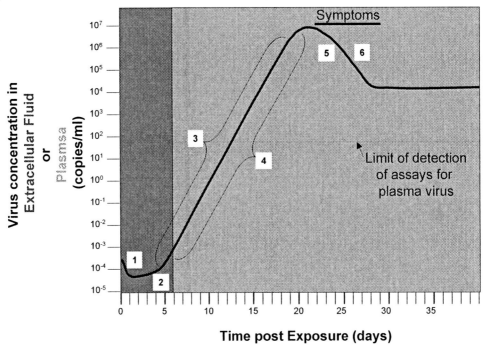

**Figure 3.1** Early events in HIV-1 transmission. A hypothetical plot of plasma virus levels over time is shown. Numbers refer to steps in the infection process, and correspond to sections in the text. Times and levels of viremia are representative values based on studies of acute HIV-1 infection in humans and SIV infection in rhesus macaques (see text for references). (1) Penetration through epithelial barriers. This process is likely to be inefficient. No replication can occur until virus reaches susceptible cells in the submucosal layer. (2) Transit to sites where susceptible targets T-cells are concentrated. The length of this phase has not been precisely measured and probably varies with transmission mode. If dense collections of lymphocytes are present in the submucosa, then rapid replication can begin immediately. If not, virus produced by initially infected cells or captured by local DC may be transported in the lymph to draining lymph nodes where rapid expansion can begin. (3) Rapid expansion governed by the basic reproductive ratio ($R_0$). Under conditions where target T-cells are not limiting, each productively infected cells can release enough virus to infect ~20 additional cells. (4) Viremia and systemic dissemination of the virus. Virus replicating at local sites or in draining lymph nodes enters the systemic circulation via the flow of lymph. Viremia becomes clinically detectable only after the level of 50 copies of HIV-1 RNA/ml is reached, by which time systemic distribution of virus is well under way. Symptoms of acute HIV-1 infection may occur as plasma virus levels peak. (5) Establishment of a latent reservoir. When large numbers of infected cells are present (e.g., at the peak of viremia), a fraction of the newly infected cells may survive the cytopathic effects of the infection and host effector mechanisms and revert back to a resting memory state while harboring integrated HIV-1 DNA. These cells form a stable latent reservoir for HIV-1. The formation of this reservoir is an inefficient process, as evidenced by the fact that latently infected cells are rare. It is likely to require substantial levels of viremia. (6) Decline in viremia to a steady state level. As target T-cells become limiting and immune responses to HIV-1 develop viremia levels off and then declines to a steady state level that varies from individual to individual and that determines the rate of disease progression. By this point, viral reservoirs in resting memory CD4+ T-cells and possibly other cells are well established.

simple columnar epithelium, which might be easier for HIV-1 to traverse. Both the vaginal and cervical epithelial layers can be compromised by concurrent inflammation (for example, due to a sexually transmitted disease), or by traumatic lesions such as microabrasions that occur during sexual intercourse. Interestingly, a major problem in the development of microbicides is that agents which lyse virus particles may also damage mucosal barriers, thereby actually facilitating transmission.

In the case of transmission across the gastrointestinal (GI) mucosa, it is possible that antigen-transporting M-cells overlying lymphoid follicles in the intestinal tract convey HIV-1 to underlying susceptible cells (Amerongen et al., 1991). In addition, transcytosis by epithelial cells may play a role. Transcytosis is an epithelial transcellular vesicular pathway that could transport virus across a tight epithelial barrier to susceptible cells underlying the mucosa (Bomsel, 1997). Primary cultures of intestinal cells express CCR5 but not CXCR4, and can selectively transfer R5 viruses to susceptible cells, possibly via transcytosis (Meng et al., 2002).

## Transit to sites where susceptible target T-cells are present at high concentration

Once mucosal barriers have been breached, virus replication begins as soon as HIV encounters susceptible cells. In the case of the GI tract, rapid initial expansion may be facilitated by the presence of dense collections of lymphocytes. This is not the case with the genital mucosa, which has only isolated lymphocytes plus numerous macrophages in the sub-mucosa. It was originally assumed that macrophages were the first cells to be infected in the genital tract. However, studies by Haase and colleagues suggest that even very early after mucosal (vaginal) inoculation of rhesus macaques with SIV, virus replicates mainly in CD4+ T-cells (Zhang et al., 1999). This may be partly due to the action of another important player: the networks of dendritic cells (DCs) that underlie all epithelial surfaces of the body and serve to capture antigens, transport them to lymph nodes, and present them to T-cells (Steinman et al., 2003; Barouch et al., 2000). Although DC are not readily infectable under most conditions, they may capture virus particles which then infect CD4$^+$ T-cells that come into contact with the virus-bearing DCs. In principle, this could take place either locally (if T-cells are present) or in the draining lymph node, if DC are induced to migrate there by inflammatory stimuli.

Recent studies are shedding light on the molecular mechanisms used by DCs to carry out this function, beginning with the viral attachment factors on certain DC populations that might contribute to virus uptake and transport. These factors include DC-specific ICAM-3-grabbing non-integrin (DC-SIGN) (Geijtenbeek et al., 2000), and related molecules. DC-SIGN is expressed on DC in the T-cell areas of lymphoid tissues and in mucosal lamina propria and skin. Since DCs are mobile cells that transport antigen to draining lymph nodes, it is conceivable that HIV-1 attached to DC via DC-SIGN or other surface proteins of similar function might be ferried from the initial site of encounter in the mucosa to susceptible cells in lymphoid tissue. Evidence for this notion comes from *in vitro* studies demonstrating that attachment of HIV-1 to DCs enhances the infection of co-cultured PBMCs in *trans*, even though these DC are not infectable or only poorly infected (Geijtenbeek et al., 2000). HIV-1 bound to DC can also remain infectious for up to 5 days (Geijtenbeek et al., 2000), a surprisingly lengthy period of time that might be related to viral internalization mediated by DC-SIGN. However, there is still no direct evidence that DC-SIGN plays an important role in HIV-1 transmission *in vivo*. It has also been suggested that Langerhans cells (a type of DC which do not express DC-SIGN in the genital mucosa) might be susceptible to infection by SIV and play a role in viral dissemination following vaginal inoculation (Miller and Hu, 1999).

Transmission across the mucosal barrier appears to initiate a local infection which disseminates systemically over the course of a few weeks. As discussed above, dense collections of lymphocytes underlie the mucosa in some sites, allowing immediate and rapid expansion of virus from the infecting inoculum. In contrast, the initial expansion may be slower at sites that are not rich in CD4$^+$ T-cells. This distinction may be critical for vaccines, because vaccine-induced immune responses have a much better chance of working before viral replication reaches its maximal rate. Local replication of virus in a small number of infected cells might permit enough time for a vaccine-primed memory response to develop effectively.

Systematic studies of the progression from local to systemic infection have been carried out mainly by infecting rhesus monkeys with pathogenic strains of SIV. These studies have shown that vaginal inoculation with SIVmac251 is followed within a few days by the appearance of detectable SIV RNA in endocervical intraepithelial lymphocytes and T-cells in the lamina propria of the endocervix (Zhang et al., 1999), and then by viral dissemination to lymphoid tissue. Between the first and second weeks of infection, the number of productively infected cells (nearly all CD4$^+$ T-cells) increases by 2–3 logs in the draining and distal lymph nodes, the gut-associated lymphoid tissue and the spleen (Zhang et al., 1999). Rapid depletion of CD4$^+$ T-cells occurs in the gut-associated lymphoid

tissue in the SIV model (Veazey et al., 1998). Several recent studies have shown that the gut mucosa is an important site of virus replication and CD4 depletion in acute HIV-1 infection (Guadalupe et al., 2003; Mehandru et al., 2004; Brenchley et al., 2004). A similar stepwise progression has been demonstrated during oral and intrarectal infection, with the local detection of SIV RNA-positive cells occurring at the initial site of infection within a few days, and the establishment of a systemic infection over the next few weeks (Stahl-Hennig et al., 1999). One study documented rapid systemic viral dissemination in rhesus macaques following vaginal infection with SIVmac251 (Hu et al., 2000). In humans, plasma HIV-1 can be detected 1–2 weeks after infection via the genital route (Daar et al., 1991). In other words, by the time HIV-1 infection is first symptomatic in humans, systemic infection is already well under way.

## Rapid expansion governed by the basic reproductive ratio ($R_0$)

Once HIV reaches a site where the number of susceptible target T-cells is not limiting, rapid expansion can occur. Virus released into the extracellular fluid during local infection at submucosal sites is delivered to regional nodes by the constant flow of lymph, while virus-bearing DC can potentially migrate to draining lymph nodes if stimulated by inflammatory mediators. Once in the node, rapid replication in activated CD4$^+$ T-cells can occur. These cells represent the main population of productively infected cells that maintain the infection chain until they are depleted (Zhang et al., 1999).

When target T-cells are not limiting, the expansion of the virus population is governed by the basic reproductive ratio ($R_0$), which is the number of newly infected cells generated from a single infected cell before target T-cell depletion. (For an excellent review of viral dynamics, see Wodarz and Nowak, 2002.) In acute HIV-1 infection, $R_0$ is estimated to be on the order of 20 (Little et al., 1999)—that is, each infected cell generates enough virus to infect 20 additional cells! This explosive expansion might occur in any T-cell-rich site, such as a lymph node draining the initial site of infection or (for transmission via the GI tract) in the gut-associated lymphoid tissue. To stop this expansion, $R_0$ must be reduced to <1. Put another way, by the time the rapid expansion stage is reached, vaccine-induced immune responses must block infection of susceptible cells with >95% efficacy to prevent the infection from becoming established (Little et al., 1999). Clearly, there is a much greater chance of success if the vaccine responses act before virus reaches sites rich in target T-cells, meaning that these responses must be fully operative very early in infection. Because of this time constraint, pre-formed antibodies and activated cytolytic effector mechanisms rather than memory B and T-cell responses may be required.

## Viremia and systemic distribution of HIV-1

High level viremia can be detected as early as 10–12 days after exposure to virus. By the time viremia rises above the detection limit of the most sensitive assays (50 copies of HIV-1

RNA/ml of plasma), virus is already in the rapid expansion phase, with plasma virus levels doubling every 10 hours (Little *et al.*, 1999). In theory, as target T-cells become limiting, the rate of viral replication slows, and viremia peaks and then declines (Wodarz and Nowak, 2002). Although total CD4 counts decrease somewhat during primary infection, the key factor in the declining viral load may be the availability of activated CD4$^+$ T-cells in which HIV-1 replicates most efficiently. However, this decline occurs at about the same time that immune responses to HIV-1 first become detectable, with CTL responses probably the most important component at this stage (Koup *et al.*, 1994; Schmitz *et al.*, 1999). Thus, it is likely that both decreased target T-cell availability and the developing immune response to HIV-1 cause viremia to level off and then decline.

Peak levels, usually reached about 3 weeks after exposure, are typically on the order of $10^7$ copies of HIV-1 RNA/ml but, can be up to 10-fold higher. During this phase, virus is disseminated throughout the body to all tissue sites the circulating virus can access. At about the same time, some patients experience a febrile illness that may lead them to seek medical attention. It is important to note that not all patients become symptomatic, and that by this stage the rapid expansion phase of infection is finished, or nearly so.

### Establishment of a latent reservoir

The establishment of a stable latent reservoir for HIV-1 represents a "point of no return" with respect to eradication via vaccination. A viral reservoir is a cell type or anatomical site in which a replication-competent form of the virus accumulates and persists with more stable kinetics than the main pool of actively replicating virus (Blankson *et al.*, 2002). Some viral reservoirs contain latent virus. Latency is a reversibly non-productive state of infection in which cells do not produce virus, but retain the capacity to do so under appropriate conditions. In HIV-1 infection, a latent reservoir is established in resting memory CD4$^+$ T-cells (Blankson *et al.*, 2002).

The establishment of this reservoir within resting CD4$^+$ memory cells appears to be an accident of nature, reflecting the tropism of HIV-1 for activated CD4$^+$ T-cells and the ability of these cells to revert to a profoundly quiescent state which is non-permissive for viral replication (reviewed in Blankson *et al.*, 2002). Our understanding of how this comes about begins with the fact that most CD4$^+$ T-cells in the body are in a resting state. About half are naïve in the sense that they have not yet encountered antigen, while the remainder are memory cells that have responded to antigen sometime in the past. Naïve CD4$^+$ T-cells are long-lived resting cells which express little CCR5 and are therefore poor targets for R5 HIV-1 infection. However, when they encounter cognate antigen in the context of appropriate co-stimulation, naïve cells proliferate and differentiate into effector CD4$^+$ T-cells. Over 90% of this expanded effector pool is destined to die, but the remaining cells revert back to a profoundly quiescent state and survive as long-lived resting memory CD4$^+$ T-cells that reside in the lymph nodes,

spleen and non-lymphoid organs. Upon secondary encounter with antigen, these memory cells differentiate rapidly into effector cells.

It is these activated CD4$^+$ effector cells that constitute the main targets for productive infection with HIV-1. The vast majority of productively infected cells die quickly from either the cytopathic effects of viral infection or the effects of host immune responses. However, a small proportion of infected cells containing a stably integrated copy of the HIV-1 genome revert back to a quiescent state and establish a latent reservoir of virus within resting memory CD4$^+$ T-cells (post-integration latency) (Chun *et al.*, 1997). In these cells, nuclear levels of activation-dependent T-cell transcription factors like NFκB decrease. Because these factors are also required to potentiate transcription from the HIV-1 promoter (Nabel and Baltimore, 1987), viral gene expression falls below the level needed to support productive viral replication. When these latently infected cells become reactivated, productive infection can ensue, leading to fresh rounds of viral replication and infection. Until then, these cells express little or no viral gene product, and they differ from other resting CD4$^+$ memory T-cells only by the small amount of extra DNA representing the HIV-1 genome.

Since memory T-cells are necessarily long-lived, this reservoir guarantees lifelong persistence of HIV-1 even in patients who have suppressed active viral replication via highly active antiretroviral therapy (HAART) (Finzi *et al.*, 1999; Siliciano *et al.*, 2003). These latently infected cells evade immune surveillance because they express little or no viral protein, which makes them a virtually insurmountable obstacle to viral eradication by the immune system, nor are they affected by antiretroviral drugs. Even in patients on HAART who have suppressed viremia below the limit of detection, latently infected memory CD4$^+$ T-cells demonstrate remarkably stable kinetics (half-life estimated at 44 months) (Siliciano *et al.*, 2003), and they probably persist for the lifespan of the infected individual. Timing thus becomes a critical issue for an effective prophylactic vaccine, which will need to act early in order to prevent a latent viral reservoir from becoming established. A stable reservoir can be found even in patients treated with HAART as early as 2 days following the onset of symptomatic primary HIV-1 infection (Finzi *et al.*, 1999). It is therefore imperative that vaccine-induced effector mechanisms prevent the high level viremia of acute HIV-1 infection, which in turn probably requires that they act before the rapid exponential expansion of the virus population begins. In other words, vaccines must exert antiviral effects in the first few days following exposure in order to be effective in generating sterilizing immunity.

### Decline in viremia to a steady state level

Within a few weeks of exposure, plasma virus levels decline coincident with the development of CTL responses to HIV-1. However, this decline does not continue until virus disappears; instead viremia stabilizes at a steady-state level, or "set point," typically between $10^4$ and $10^5$ copies of HIV-1 RNA/ml of plasma. This set point level strongly influences the subsequent rate of CD4 depletion and disease progression. Vaccines that modulate HIV-1 immunity without preventing infection may have a beneficial effect in delaying disease progression (Barouch et al., 2000), partly by lowering the set point. Nevertheless, by the time that a set point is reached, eradication is no longer possible.

## What a vaccine needs to do

Given the above considerations, we can speculate on what a vaccine must do to produce protective immunity against HIV-1 infection. Stimulating mucosal immunity might create an effective barrier to transmucosal spread of HIV-1, thereby abrogating infection before the exponential expansion phase. Notwithstanding the difficulties associated with designing vaccines that elicit high titers of broadly neutralizing antibodies reactive against primary HIV-1 isolates, an effective antibody response might prevent infection by interrupting the initial events during transmucosal viral spread. Support for this notion comes from the finding(s) that mucosal HIV-1-specific IgA can inhibit transcytosis of the virus across a tight epithelial barrier in vitro (Bomsel et al., 1998). Furthermore, studies with human monoclonal neutralizing antibodies directed against conserved regions in the HIV-1 envelope have demonstrated in principle what an efficacious anti-HIV-1 humoral response can achieve: Rhesus monkeys infused with high titers of these antibodies were protected against subsequent parenteral and mucosal challenge with chimeric SHIV viruses carrying HIV-1 envelope proteins (reviewed by Mascola, 2003). Protection from mucosal challenge with SHIV was linked to the detection of infused antibody at mucosal surfaces.

Whether HIV-1 specific CTL can contribute to protective immunity in the first few days of infection is less clear—although the role of primary CTL responses in controlling the viremia of acute HIV-1 infection is clear (Koup et al., 1994; Schmitz et al., 1999), as is the potential of vaccine-induced CTL to moderate the course of disease (Barouch et al., 2000; Chapter 4). In a rhesus macaque model of transient mucosal SIV infection, the induction of SIV envelope-specific CTL in the lamina propria was shown to be absolutely correlated with protection against subsequent colonic challenge with 10.000 TCID$_{50}$ of a heterologous primary SIV isolate (Murphey-Corb et al., 1999). However, a recent study suggests that CTL induced by systemic vaccination do not enhance protection afforded by suboptimal amounts of passive neutralizing antibodies (Mascola et al., 2003). Further work will therefore be needed to define the potential of CTL in the protective setting. The temporal considerations presented above suggest that CTL-based vaccines must give rise to the continuous presence of high levels of virus-specific CTL that remain in an activated state at mucosal sites.

## Conclusion

Without a clear picture of the early events following transmission of HIV-1, it may not be possible to rationally design a vaccine that can interrupt the chain of events leading from exposure to the establishment of a stable latent reservoir. Once such a reservoir has been established, particularly in resting memory CD4$^+$ T-cells, it may no longer be possible to eradicate HIV-1 infection.

## References

Amerongen, H.M., Weltzin, R., Farnet, C. M., Michetti, P., Haseltine, W.A., and Neutra, M.R. (1991). Transepithelial transport of HIV-1 by intestinal M cells: a mechanism for transmission of AIDS. J. Acquir. Immune. Defic. Syndr. 4, 760–765.

Barouch, D.H., Santra, S., Schmitz, J.E., Kuroda, M.J., Fu, T.M., Wagner, W., Bilska, M., Craiu, A., Zheng, X.X., Krivulka, G.R., et al. (2000). Control of viremia and prevention of clinical AIDS in rhesus monkeys by cytokine-augmented DNA vaccination. Science 290, 486–492.

Blankson, J.N., Persaud, D., and Siliciano, R.F. (2002). The challenge of viral reservoirs in HIV-1 infection. Annu. Rev. Med. 53, 557–93.

Bomsel, M. (1997). Transcytosis of infectious human immunodeficiency virus across a tight human epithelial cell line barrier. Nature Med. 3, 42–47.

Bomsel, M., Heyman, M., Hocini, H., Lagaye, S., Belec, L., Dupont, C., and Desgranges, C. (1998). Intracellular neutralization of HIV transcytosis across tight epithelial barriers by anti-HIV envelope protein dIgA or IgM. Immunity 9, 277–287.

Brenchley, J.M., Schacker, T.W., Ruff, L.E., Price, D.A., Taylor, J.H., Beilman, G.J., Nguyen, P.L., Khoruts, A., Larson, M., Haase, A.T., and Douek, D.C. (2004). CD4$^+$ T cell depletion during all stages of HIV disease occurs predominantly in the gastrointestinal tract. J. Exp. Med. 200, 749–759.

Chun, T.W., Carruth, L., Finzi, D., Shen, X., DiGiuseppe, J.A., Taylor, H., Hermankova, M., Chadwick, K., Margolick, J., Quinn, T.C., et al. (1997). Quantification of latent tissue reservoirs and total body viral load in HIV-1 infection. Nature 387, 183–188.

Daar, E.S., Moudgil, T., Meyer, R.D., and Ho, D.D. (1991). Transient high levels of viremia in patients with primary human immunodeficiency virus type 1 infection. N. Engl. J. Med. 324, 961–964.

Finzi, D., Blankson, J., Siliciano, J.D., Margolick, J.B., Chadwick, K., Pierson, T., Smith, K., Lisziewicz, J., Lori, F., Flexner, C., et al. (1999). Latent infection of CD4$^+$ T-cells provides a mechanism for lifelong persistence of HIV-1, even in patients on effective combination therapy. Nature Med. 5, 512–517.

Geijtenbeek, T.B., Kwon, D.S., Torensma, R., van Vliet, S. J., van Duijnhoven, G.C., Middel, J., Cornelissen, I.L., Nottet, H.S., KewalRamani, V.N., Littman, D. R., et al. (2000). DC-SIGN, a dendritic cell-specific HIV-1-binding protein that enhances trans-infection of T-cells. Cell 100, 587–597.

Guadalupe, M., Reay, E., Sankaran, S., Prindiville, T., Flamm, J., McNeil, A., and Dandekar, S. (2003). Severe CD4$^+$ T-cell depletion in gut lymphoid tissue during primary human immunodeficiency virus type 1 infection and substantial delay in restoration following highly active antiretroviral therapy. J. Virol. 77, 11708–11717.

Hu, J., Gardner, M. B., and Miller, C.J. (2000). Simian immunodeficiency virus rapidly penetrates the cervicovaginal mucosa after intravaginal inoculation and infects intraepithelial dendritic cells. J. Virol. 74, 6087–6095.

Koup, R.A., Safrit, J.A., Cao, Y., Andrews, C.A., McLeod, G., Borkowsky, W., Farthing, C., and Ho, D.D. (1994). Temporal association of cellular immune responses with the initial control of viremia in primary human immunodeficiency virus type 1 syndrome. J. Virol. 68, 4650–4655.

Little, S.J., McLean, A.R., Spina, C.A., Richman, D.D., and Havlir, D.V. (1999). Viral dynamics of acute HIV-1 infection. J. Exp. Med. 190, 841–850.

Mascola, J.R. (2003). Defining the protective antibody response for HIV-1. Curr. Mol. Med. 3, 209–216.

Mascola, J.R., Lewis, M.G., VanCott, T.C., Stiegler, G., Katinger, H., Seaman, M., Beaudry, K., Barouch, D.H., Korioth-Schmitz, B.,

Krivulka, G., *et al.* (2003). Cellular immunity elicited by human immunodeficiency virus type 1/simian immunodeficiency virus DNA vaccination does not augment the sterile protection afforded by passive infusion of neutralizing antibodies. J. Virol. *77*, 10348–10356.

Mehandru, S., Poles, M.A., Tenner-Racz, K., Horowitz, A., Hurley, A., Hogan, C., Boden, D., Racz, P., and Markowitz, M. (2004). Primary HIV-1 infection is associated with preferential depletion of CD4$^+$ T lymphocytes from effector sites in the gastrointestinal tract. J. Exp. Med. *200*, 761–770.

Meng, G., Wei, X., Wu, X., Sellers, M.T., Decker, J.M., Moldoveanu, Z., Orenstein, J.M., Graham, M.F., Kappes, J.C., Mestecky, J., Shaw, G.M., and Smith, P. D. (2002). Primary intestinal epithelial cells selectively transfer R5 HIV-1 to CCR5+ cells. Nature Med. *8*, 150–156.

Miller, C.J. and Hu, J. (1999). T-cell-tropic simian immunodeficiency virus (SIV) and simian-human immunodeficiency viruses are readily transmitted by vaginal inoculation of rhesus macaques, and Langerhans' cells of the female genital tract are infected with SIV. J. Infect. Dis. *179*, Suppl. 3, S413–S417.

Shattock, R.J., and Moore, J.P. (2003). Inhibiting sexual transmission of HIV-1 infection. Nature Rev. Microbiol. *1*, 25–34.

Murphey-Corb, M., Wilson, L.A., Trichel, A.M., Roberts, D.E., Xu, K., Ohkawa, S., Woodson, B., Bohm, R., and Blanchard, J. (1999). Selective induction of protective MHC class I-restricted CTL in the intestinal lamina propria of rhesus monkeys by transient SIV infection of the colonic mucosa. J. Immunol. *162*, 540–549.

Nabel, G. and Baltimore, D. (1987). An inducible transcription factor activates expression of human immunodeficiency virus in T-cells. Nature *326*, 711–713.

Schmitz, J.E., Kuroda, M.J., Santra, S., Sasseville, V.G., Simon, M. A., Lifton, M.A., Racz, P., Tenner-Racz, K., Dalesandro, M., Scallon, B.J., *et al.* (1999). Control of viremia in simian immunodeficiency virus infection by CD8$^+$ lymphocytes. Science *283*, 857–860.

Siliciano, J.D., Kajdas, J., Finzi, D., Quinn, T.C., Chadwick, K., Margolick, J.B., Kovacs, C., Gange, S.J., and Siliciano, R.F. (2003). Long-term follow-up studies confirm the stability of the latent reservoir for HIV-1 in resting CD4$^+$ T-cells. Nature Med. *9*, 727–728.

Stahl-Hennig, C., Steinman, R.M., Tenner-Racz, K., Pope, M., Stolte, N., Matz-Rensing, K., Grobschupff, G., Raschdorff, B., Hunsmann, G., and Racz, P. (1999). Rapid infection of oral mucosal-associated lymphoid tissue with simian immunodeficiency virus. Science *285*, 1261–1265.

Steinman, R.M., Granelli-Piperno, A., Pope, M., Trumpfheller, C., Ignatius, R., Arrode, G., Racz, P., and Tenner-Racz, K. (2003). The interaction of immunodeficiency viruses with dendritic cells. Curr. Top. Microbiol. Immunol. *276*, 1–30.

Veazey, R.S., DeMaria, M.A., Chalifoux, L.V., Shvetz, D.E., Pauley, D.R., Knight, H.L., Rosenzweig, M., Johnson, R.P., Desrosiers, R.C., and Lackner, A.A. (1998). Gastrointestinal tract as a major site of CD4þ T-cell depletion and viral replication in SIV infection. Science *280*, 427–431.

Wodarz, D. and Nowak, M.A. (2002). Mathematical models of HIV pathogenesis and treatment. Bioessays *24*, 1178–1187.

Zhang, Z.Q., Schuler, T., Zupancic, M., Wietgrefe, S., Staskus, K.A., Reimann, K. A., Reinhart, T.A., Rogan, M., Cavert, W., Miller, C.J., *et al.* (1999). Sexual transmission and propagation of SIV and HIV in resting and activated CD4$^+$ T-cells. Science *286*, 1353–1357.

# Cytotoxic T-Lymphocyte-Based Vaccines: Evidence for Efficacy in Animal Models and Humans

4

Jaap Goudsmit, Johannes Antonie Bogaards, and Marc Girard

## Abstract

Nearly all candidate AIDS vaccines now in clinical development are designed to stimulate the cellular arm of the immune
system, in particular the CD4$^+$ and CD8$^+$ T-cell compartments. Accumulated evidence suggests that these responses
will not prevent infection with HIV but may suppress viral
replication once infection has occurred, in turn delaying progression to clinical AIDS. In this article we review some of the
data from the rhesus macaque/SIV/SHIV model and from
natural history studies of HIV-infected people, and discuss
how useful cytotoxic T-lymphocyte (CTL)-based vaccines are
likely to be. Key uncertainties include the longevity of protection by, and the likelihood of viral escape from, HIV-specific
CTLs. From the data available we predict that effective suppression of viral load can provide significant clinical and public
health benefits, if an even modestly effective CTL-based vaccine is made available as early as possible.

## Introduction

The development of an effective AIDS vaccine is hampered
by the difficulty of designing candidates that stimulate broadly
neutralizing antibodies (reviewed in Chapter 7). On the other
hand, virus-specific CD4$^+$ and CD8$^+$ T-cell responses can be
readily induced by a wide variety of live vectors with and without DNA priming in both experimental animals and humans
(Letvin et al., 2002; Robinson et al., 2002; Priddy et al., 2004).
Whether or not these responses can confer protection against
AIDS is one of the most pressing questions facing the field.

Unfortunately only efficacy trials can unambiguously resolve this question, since there is no animal model for HIV;
the only reliable model system available to AIDS research is
the infection of rhesus macaques with either simian immunodeficiency virus (SIV) or laboratory hybrids of SIV and
HIV (called SHIV). Chimpanzees do not develop AIDS
disease and therefore are not a model of choice. Protection of
macaques against infection with SIV has so far been obtained
only with vaccines made from live attenuated virus (Daniel et
al., 1992). However, several different live vector-based vaccines
(with or without priming) are able to protect against disease

progression, with adenovirus-based approaches presently the
most promising (Priddy et al., 2004; Chapter 8). How well
either SIV or SHIV will predict the outcome in humans is
fiercely debated in the field. In general, it has proven easier to
protect against disease induced by SHIV strains than against
SIV. However, viral escape from vaccine-induced T-cell control of SHIV, leading to death from AIDS-related complica-
tion, has also been reported (Barouch et al., 2003).

The notion that T-cell-based vaccines may work by preventing disease progression rather than infection (unlike antibody-inducing vaccines, which under optimal conditions
can provide sterilizing anti-viral immunity), may have more
far-reaching consequences for HIV and AIDS than for "classical" viral infections in which virus does not typically establish
persistent infection. Most vaccines in widespread use today
provide high levels of protection from infectious diseases, even
though they usually do not prevent the initial infection of the
host and replication of the pathogen at the portal of entry. For
example, inactivated poliovirus vaccine (IPV) induces excellent
protection against poliomyelitis, yet poliovirus can multiply
actively in the intestinal tract of IPV vaccinees. But a vaccine-
induced immune barrier—in this case, antibodies that neutralize polio virus—prevents virus from spreading to the central
nervous system. Most vaccines are able to protect because at
least a few days elapse between the time of infection and the
development of overt disease, giving memory T- and B-cells
time to reactivate and the previously educated immune system
time to respond. This response is usually highly efficacious and
quickly leads to the elimination of the invading pathogen.

However, this type of vaccine-induced response may not
be sufficient for pathogens which can dodge the host immune
response and rapidly establish persistent infection, a group
that includes herpes simplex virus, cytomegalovirus and HIV.
The natural history of AIDS and the absence of even a single
documented case of recovery from HIV infection strongly argue that HIV infection is irreversible, due to the basic inability
of the immune system to eliminate the virus once it has integrated into the host genome—even though cellular immunity
can control the rate of virus multiplication and effectively slow

progression towards clinical AIDS. In the context of HIV vaccines, therefore, the key issue is to appraise the chances of success for the various T-cell-based vaccines now being developed.

## Evidence for efficacy of CTL-based vaccines in monkey models

Animal models can provide some insights into this issue. It has been repeatedly observed that macaques immunized with a variety of SIV and/or HIV antigens are not protected from infection when challenged with a high dose of pathogenic strains such as SHIV-89.6P. However, certain vaccine regimens lead to control of plasma viral loads, often to undetectable levels, and protection from SHIV-induced CD4$^+$ T-cell depletion and clinical disease. In contrast, unvaccinated control monkeys typically show high levels of viremia at the virological setpoint, a drastic loss of CD4$^+$ T-cells and progression to clinical disease, often leading to rapid death. The most immunogenic vaccination regimens stimulate strong HIV-specific CD8$^+$ T-cell responses, with up to 20% of the total CD8$^+$ cell population recognizing a single dominant epitope. Control of viral load in these animals can be readily abolished by depletion of their CD8$^+$ T-cells, and progressively resumes as the CD8$^+$ compartment is gradually restored.

Because these experiments often involved relatively limited numbers of monkeys kept in a pathogen-free environment and provided only short follow-up, they do not address either the long-term duration of vaccine-induced T-cell protection or the effects of immune system decline (for example, due to aging or to infection with an unrelated pathogen) on protection. Nor do most of them rigorously assess the often-documented phenomenon of viral escape—that is, the emergence of viral variants that evade HIV-specific CTLs, leading to virus breakthrough and the development of clinical symptoms.

The observation was first made in the early 1990s that a group of either vaccinated chimpanzees challenged with HIV or vaccinated macaques challenged with SIV show a subset of animals which initially appeared to have prevented infection by all criteria used at the time (including detection of infectious virus in PBMCs), but suddenly became viremic more than 6 months after challenge (Girard *et al.*, 1991). Since the primary endpoint in these early studies was protection against infection, these breakthrough animals were classified as vaccine failures and not analyzed further.

More than a decade later our views on the matter have evolved considerably, and the phenomenon of viral escape has received a great deal of attention. Directly relevant to T-cell-stimulating vaccines, viral escape from CTL responses has been found to occur during both acute and chronic SIV/HIV infection in macaques and in people (for review, see Goulder and Watkins, 2004). For example, an early, strong CTL response against the Tat protein was documented in acute SIV infection, but CTL-resistant variant viruses mutated in Tat emerged rapidly and went on to establish chronic, uncontrolled infection (Allen *et al.*, 2000; O'Connor *et al.*, 2002).

Turning to viral escape from CTL responses in vaccinated animals, different vaccines and challenges have yielded different outcomes (Barouch *et al.* 2003; McDermott, O'Connor *et al.* 2005). One study investigated a group of rhesus macaques vaccinated with DNA encoding SIVmac-gag and challenged with the heterologous SIVsm E660 strain (Barouch *et al.* 2003). Over a 3-year follow-up period, escape from Gag-specific CTLs occurred in seven of the nine vaccinated and control monkeys, including three that initially controlled viral replication below the study's level of detection (<500 copies of viral RNA/mL plasma). This high frequency of escape may reflect the narrow breadth of the CTL response to this relatively weak, single-antigen vaccine, perhaps combined with low-level viral replication, and hopefully would be lower with a more potent, multi-antigen or polyepitopic vaccine (Subbramanian *et al.*, 2003). Further studies are needed to understand these differences, and to resolve the factors—probably including completeness of viral suppression, breadth of the initial immune response, and/or degree of similarity between vaccine and challenge strains—that determine if, and how quickly, escape occurs. Still, the data suggest that viral escape from CTLs poses a potentially serious hurdle for T-cell-stimulating vaccines in HIV infection (Barouch and Letvin, 2004).

Extrapolating from these and other macaque protection data to HIV vaccine protection in humans is difficult, not least because the outcome of monkey studies depends heavily on the virus used for challenge. Highly pathogenic SHIVs such as SHIV-89.6P cause a profound depletion of circulating CD4$^+$ T-cells within 2–3 weeks of infection, and can lead to AIDS and death of the monkeys within a year. In contrast, SIV strains induce AIDS over a 1- to 2-year period without wiping out the CD4$^+$ T-cell compartment. Paradoxically, vaccine regimens that protect SHIV-89.6P-challenged rhesus macaques from rapid CD4$^+$ cell loss and clinical AIDS are unable to prevent the more gradual CD4$^+$ T-cell depletion and disease progression following challenge with SIVmac239, even though they induce broad SIV-specific T-cell responses and a reduction in peak virus load (reviewed in Horton, 2002). Thus, while they seem more aggressive initially, SHIV strains are easier than SIV to control by T-cell-stimulating vaccination.

The reasons for this are not well understood, but might reflect the different T-cell tropism of the two types of virus, which in turn reflects their different co-receptor usage (Nishimura *et al.*, 2005). Pathogenic SHIV strains usually enter target T-cells via the CXCR4 receptor (abbreviated as X4), whereas SIVs use the CCR5 receptor (also called R5; Igarashi *et al.*, 2003). The majority of X4+ CD4$^+$ T-cells are circulating naïve T-cells, whereas a large fraction of R5+ CD4$^+$ T-cells are memory T-cells localized in lymphoid tissues, including the gut-associated lymphoid tissue (GALT). Thus, infection by pathogenic X4-tropic SHIV leads to rapid elimination of CD4$^+$ T-cells in the blood and peripheral lymphoid organs, while infection by R5-tropic SIV depletes the pool of activated memory T-cells in the GALT and other lymphoid tissues (Brenchley, Schacker *et al.* 2004; Veazey *et al.*, 1998, 2000).

The propensity of SIV to destroy memory T-cells—exactly the cells needed for durable vaccine protection—might explain why these viruses are not contained by vaccination regimens that readily control pathogenic X4-tropic SHIVs (Igarashi et al., 2003). This raises the question of whether pathogenic SHIVs are a useful model for the development of HIV vaccines in humans (Feinberg and Moore, 2002; Nishimura et al., 2005).

The inability of most T-cell-stimulating vaccination regimens to control SIV infection in monkeys (Horton et al., 2002), along with emerging clinical data that generally find lower levels of T-cell responses to candidate HIV vaccines in humans, is fostering efforts to develop more potent vaccines and more innovative approaches. Indeed, some newer vaccines are beginning to demonstrate partial control of SIVmac infection in macaques (Murphy et al., 2000; Wang et al., 2000; Crotty et al., 2001; Pal et al., 2002; Zhao et al., 2003; Casimiro et al. 2005). However, it is likely that a wider range of immune responses will be needed for robust protection against R5 viruses, as proved to be the case for optimal protection in the retroviral Friend virus mouse model (Dittmer et al., 1999; Chapter 5). It would not be surprising to learn in the end that CD4+ T-helper cells, B lymphocytes and CD8+ CTL all contribute to protective immunity against HIV-1.

## Evidence for efficacy of CTLs in natural HIV infection

Natural history studies of HIV infection in humans have provided valuable data on the relationship between viral control and disease progression (Dorak et al. 2004; Quinn and Overbaugh, 2005). There is, however, a crucial caveat: immunity to HIV might differ in qualitative ways between infected people (whose responses are triggered by natural infection, and who may have suffered early immune system damage) and vacci-

nated individuals, where immunity would be well established prior to a first encounter with HIV.

Among the different studies that have addressed issues of viral control and disease progression in detail (including those in the MAC and Rakai Cohorts and the Harvard University Acute Infection Cohort), we focus here on the Amsterdam Cohort Study (ACS) of HIV infection and AIDS among homosexual men, which in 1984 began to recruit and prospectively follow high-risk gay men. The 138 cohort participants who seroconverted between 1984 and 1999 have provided valuable data on the prognosis of individuals with the lowest viral loads, and on the risk of viral escape from immune control in natural HIV infection.

Earlier studies (De Wolf et al., 1997) found that better control of viremia shortly after infection was associated with a longer lag until the onset of immune suppression and AIDS. Only 14% of individuals with high viral load at seroconversion and low load one year later developed AIDS within 7 years, compared with 29% of people with low virus load and 60% of those with high virus load at both time points (Fig. 4.1).

Looking in more detail at the 123 seroconverters who did not start antiretroviral therapy within the first year following seroconversion, only 17 (14%) had a virological setpoint below 1,000 HIV-1 RNA copies/mL plasma one year after the first positive antibody test (Goudsmit et al., 2002). To estimate the sustainability of this low viral load beyond 1 year, we calculated the time from setpoint until viral load rose either above 1,000 or above 10,000 copies/mL and found this interval to be 2.1 years and 7.0 years, respectively (Table 4.1). Antiretroviral therapy was initiated in nine patients after viral load had increased above 10,000 copies/mL, with a median time of 7.7 years.

We also monitored CD4+ T-cells in each of these 17 individuals. Only the one person with a sustained low viral load had

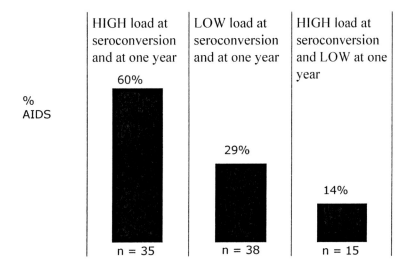

F. de Wolf et al, AIDS 1997;11:1799

**Figure 4.1** Percentage of individuals from the Amsterdam cohort study showing various levels of viral load at seroconversion and one year later, and who progressed to clinical AIDS within 7 years. Low viral load: <1,000 HIV-1 RNA copies per ml plasma; High: >10,000 copies.

**Table 4.1** Low viral load is maintained relatively short among individuals with best prognosis and low viral load at setpoint

| Probability* | Increase to above 1,000 cp/ml | Increase to above 10,000 cp/ml |
| --- | --- | --- |
| | Time (95% confidence interval) (years) | Time (95% confidence interval) (years) |
| 0.25 | 1.0 (0.6–2.1) | 4.8 (2.2–7.0) |
| 0.50 | 2.1 (1.0–3.0) | 7.0 (4.8–9.1) |
| 0.75 | 3.0 (2.1–6.2) | 9.1 (7.0–NA) |

* Probability of HIV-1 RNA increase over time.

stable CD4+ T-cell counts over 14 years of follow-up without antiretroviral therapy. The other 16, all of whom showed a rise in viral load at different times, experienced a gradual decline in CD4+ T-cell counts. These data indicate that long-term control of viremia is rare in naturally infected individuals and that a steady loss of CD4+ T-cells—a sure sign of progression towards immunodeficiency—occurs even in people with low initial viral loads.

Since several lines of evidence link control of viremia to CD8+ virus-specific CTLs, this loss of control over virus replication may be related to repeated escapes from the immune control exerted by CTLs that recognize particular T-cell epitopes. However, important details remain unclear: the minimum set of epitopes that CTLs must recognize to limit HIV infection is still undefined, nor is it known whether these

epitopes must be localized on a single viral protein or on multiple proteins. In a general sense HIV-1 escape is thought to reflect the interplay of selective pressure exerted by HIV-specific CTLs, their tolerance for specific mutations in the epitope they each recognize, and the cost of these mutations to the virus in terms of fitness (Friedrich *et al.*, 2004; Leslie *et al.*, 2004). In one in-depth analysis of a single seroconverter, we found a sequential accumulation of CTL-escape mutations during disease progression, suggesting that multiple combinations of T-cell epitopes are required to control viremia (Geels *et al.*, 2003).

To consider the potential public health effects of vaccines that do not prevent HIV-1 infection but control viremia (Chapter 19), we designed a mathematical model relating the level of viremia to disease progression and to HIV transmission (Van Ballegooijen *et al.*, 2003). Parameters for disease progression were estimated from ACS longitudinal data on untreated HIV-1 infection. The model distinguishes three types of disease progression following primary HIV-1 infection: slow, intermediate and fast, as defined by the virological setpoint (Fig. 4.2). The authors made the conservative assumption that vaccinated individuals have a virological setpoint comparable to that of natural slow progressors and subsequently follow a similar disease progression. In addition, it was assumed that vaccinated individuals would have reduced viremia in the primary phase of infection. Viral load was modeled as a discrete variable, and rise in viral load—incorporated

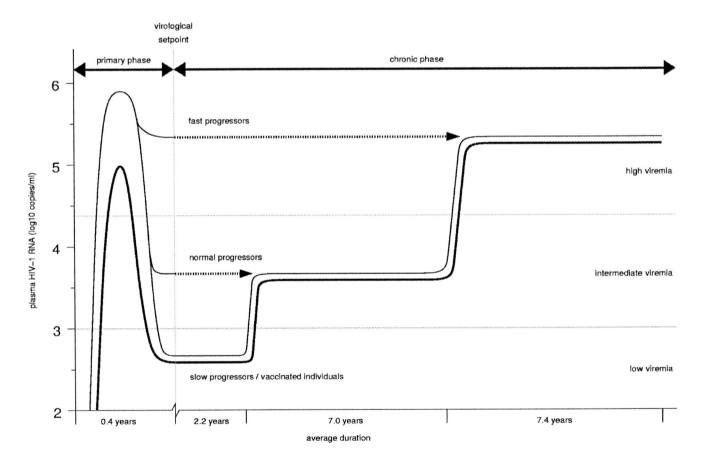

**Figure 4.2** Vaccine model based on natural history.

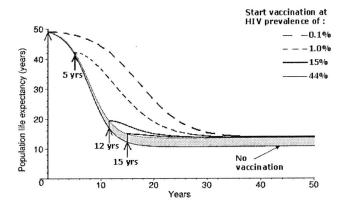

**Figure 4.3** Effects of CTL-based vaccination on life expectancy.

into the model as a step function—reflected viral escape from vaccine-induced CTLs.

The results of this analysis were revealing. First, they showed that a sexually active population can ultimately be reduced to 26% of its original size as a result of AIDS-induced mortality, in case $R_0 = 3$ (i.e. the average HIV-1 infected individual transmits the virus to three partners over his or her lifetime, assuming all contacts are with susceptible partners; in an endemic situation, the average infected individual infects one other person). Timely introduction of a CTL-based vaccine then postpones the peak incidence of HIV-1 and the dramatic decline in population size by as much as 22 years. This delay provides the opportunity to intensify prevention programs, increase access to antiretroviral therapy, and—last but not least—develop more immunogenic vaccines. In addition, early mass vaccination would delay the drop in life expectancy and help to maintain the socio-economic fabric of societies at high risk of AIDS. The effects of CTL-based vaccination on life expectancy would be most beneficial when the vaccine is widely applied early in an epidemic (Fig. 4.3).

## Conclusions

From the data available it appears that CTL-based vaccines will postpone and possibly prevent AIDS, but will not protect against HIV infection. This novel type of disease-modifying vaccine, when broadly applied, may change the course of an AIDS epidemic by increasing the number of long-term non-progressors in an HIV-infected population. In addition, such vaccines might slow the spread of HIV by lowering viral load in sexually active, asymptomatic individuals, and by doing so, increase the number of exposures needed to acquire HIV. These results emphasize that the earlier an even modestly effective CTL-based vaccine is used globally, the more impact it will have. With 14,000 new HIV-1 infections a day, we as a global community are moving far too slowly.

## References

Allen, T.M., O'Connor, D.H., Jing, P., Dzuris, J.L., Mothe, B.R., Vogel, T.U., Dunphy, E., Liebl, M.E., Emerson, C., Wilson, N., Kunstman, K.J., Wang, X., Allison, D.B., Hughes, A.L., Desrosiers, R.C., Altman, J.D., Wolinsky, S.M., Sette, A., and Watkins, D.I. (2000). Tat-specific cytotoxic T lymphocytes select for SIV escape variants during resolution of primary viraemia. Nature *407*, 386–390.

Barouch, D.H., Kuntsman, J., Glowczwskic, J., Kunstman, K.J., Egan, M.A., Peyerl, F.W., Santra, S., Kuroda, M.J., Schmitz, J.E., Beaudry, K., Krivulka, G.R., Lifton, M.A., Gorgone, D.A., Wolinsky, S.M., and Letvin, N.L. (2003). Viral escape from dominant simian immunodeficiency virus epitope-specific cytotoxic T-lymphocytes in DNA vaccinated rhesus monkeys. J. Virol. *77*, 7367–7373.

Barouch, D.H. and Letvin, N.L. (2004). HIV escape from cytotoxic T lymphocytes: a potential hurdle for vaccines? Lancet *364*, 10–11.

Barouch, D.H., Kunstman, J. *et al.* (2003). Viral escape from dominant simian immunodeficiency virus epitope-specific cytotoxic T lymphocytes in DNA-vaccinated rhesus monkeys. J. Virol. *77*, 7367–7375.

Brenchley, J.M., Schacker, T.W. *et al.* (2004). CD4+ T cell depletion during all stages of HIV disease occurs predominantly in the gastrointestinal tract. J. Exp. Med. *200*, 749–759.

Casimiro, D.R., Wang, F. *et al.* (2005). Attenuation of simian immunodeficiency virus SIVmac239 infection by prophylactic immunization with DNA and recombinant adenoviral vaccine vectors expressing Gag. J. Virol. *79*, 15547–15555.

Cornelissen, M., Mulder-Kampingo, G., Veenstra, J., Zorgdrager, F., Kuiken, C., Hartman, S., Dekker, J., van der Hoek, L., Sol, C., and Coutinho, R. (1995). Syncytium-inducing (SI) phenotype suppression at seroconversion after intramuscular inoculation of a non-syncytium-inducing/SI phenotypically mixed human immunodeficiency virus population. J. Virol. *69*, 1810–1818.

Crotty, S., Miller, C.J., Lohman, B.L., Neagu, M.R., Compton, L., Lu, D., Lü, F.X.-S., Fritts, L., Lifson, J.D., and Andino, R. (2001). Protection against simian immunodeficiency virus vaginal challenge by using Sabin poliovirus vectors. J. Virol. *75*, 7435–7452.

Daniel, M.D., Kirchhoff, F., Czajak, S.C., Seghal, P.K., and Desrosiers, R.C. (1992). Protective effects of a live attenuated SIV vaccine with a deletion in the nef gene. Science *258*, 1938–1941.

De Wolf, F., Spijkerman, I., Schellekens, P.T., Langendam, M., Kuiken, C., Bakker, M., Roos, M., Coutinho, R., Miedema, F., and Goudsmit, J. (1997). AIDS prognosis based on HIV-1 RNA, CD4+ T-cell count and function: markers with reciprocal predictive value over time after seroconversion. AIDS *11*, 1799–1806.

Dittmer, U., Brooks, D.M., and Hasenberg, K.J. (1999). Requirements for multiple lymphocyte subsets in protection by a live attenuated vaccine against retroviral infection. Nature Med. *5*, 189–193.

Dorak, M.T., Tang, J., *et al.* (2004). Transmission of HIV-1 and HLA-B allele-sharing within serodiscordant heterosexual Zambian couples. Lancet *363*, 2137–2139.

Goulder, P.J., and Watkins, D.I. (2004). HIV and SIV CTL escape: implications for vaccine design. Nature Rev. Immunol. *4*, 630–640.

Feinberg, M.B., and Moore, J.P. (2002). AIDS vaccine models: Challenging challenge viruses. Nat. Med. *8*, 207–210.

Friedrich, T.C., Dodds, E.J., Yant, L.J., Vojnov, L., Rudersdorf, R., Cullen, C., Evans, D.T., Desrosiers, R.C., Mothe, B.R., Sidney, J., Sette, A., Kunstman, K., Wolinsky, S., Piatak, M., Lifson, J., Hughes, A.L., Wilson, N., O'Connor, D.H., Watkins, D.I. (2004). Reversion of CTL escape-variant immunodeficiency viruses *in vivo*. Nature Med. *10*, 275–81.

Geels, M.J., Cornelissen, M., Schuitemaker, H., Anderson, K., Kwa, D., Maas, J., Dekker, J.T., Baan, E., Zorgdrager, F., van den Burg, R., van Beelen, M., Lukashov, V.V., Fu, T.-M., Paxton, W.A., van der Hoek, L., Dubey, S.A., Shiver, J.W., and Goudsmit, J. (2003). Identification of sequential viral escape mutants associated with altered T-cell responses in a human immunodeficiency virus type 1-infected individual. J. Virol. *77*, 12430–40.

Girard, M., Kieny, M-P., Pinter, A., Girard, M., Kieny, M., Pinter, A., Barre-Sinoussi, F., Nara, P., Kolbe, H., Kusumi, K., Chaput, A., Reinhart, T., Muchmore, E., Ronco, J., Kaczorek, M., Gomard, E., Gluckman, J., and Fultz, P.N. (1991). Immunization of chimpanzees confers protection against challenge with human immunodeficiency virus. Proc. Natl. Acad. Sci. USA *88*, 542–546.

Goudsmit, J., Bogaards, J.A., Jurriaans, S., Schuitemaker, H., Lange, J.M., Coutinho, R.A., and Weverling, G.J. (2002). Naturally HIV-1 seroconverters with lowest viral load have best prognosis, but in time lose control of viraemia. AIDS *16*, 791–793.

Horton, H., Vogel, T.U., Carter, D.K., Vielhuber, K., Fuller, D.H., Shipley, T., Fuller, J.T., Kunstman, K.J., Sutter, G., Montefiori, D.C., Erfle, V., Desrosiers, R.C., Wilson, N., Picker, L.J., Wolinsky, S.M., Wang, C., Allison, D.B., and Watkins, D.I. (2002). Immunization of rhesus macaques with a DNA prime/modified vaccinia virus Ankara boost regimen induces broad simian immunodeficiency virus (SIV)-specific T-cell responses and reduces initial viral replication but does not prevent disease progression following challenge with pathogenic SIVmac239. J. Virol. 76, 7187–7202.

Igarashi, T., Endo, Y., Nishimura, Y., Buckler, C., Sadjadpour, R., Donau, O.K., Dumaurier, M.-J., Plishka, R.J., Buckler-White, A., and Martin, M.A. (2003). Early control of highly pathogenic simian immunodeficiency virus/human immunodeficiency virus chimeric virus infections in rhesus monkeys usually results in long-lasting asymptomatic clinical outcomes. J. Virol. 77, 10829–10840.

Leslie, A.J., Pfafferott, K.J., Chetty, P., Draenert, R., Addo, M.M., Feeney, M., Tang, Y., Holmes, E.C., Allen, T., Prado, J.G., Altfeld, M., Brander, C., Dixon, C., Ramduth, D., Jeena, P., Thomas, S.A., St. John, A., Roach, T.A., Kupfer, B., Luzzi, G., Edwards, A., Taylor, G., Lyall, H., Tudor-Williams, G., Novelli, V., Martinez-Picado, J. Kiepiela, P., Walker, B.D., and Goulder, P.J. (2004). HIV evolution: CTL escape mutation and reversion after transmission. Nature Med. 10, 282–289.

Letvin, N.L., Barouch, D.H., and Montefiori, D.C. (2002). Prospects for vaccine protection against HIV-1 infection and AIDS. Annu. Rev. Immunol. 20, 73–99.

Letvin, N.L., and Walker, B.D. (2003). Immunopathogenesis and immunotherapy in AIDS virus infections. Nat. Med. 9, 861–866.

McDermott, A.B., O'Connor, D.H. et al. (2005). Cytotoxic T-lymphocyte escape does not always explain the transient control of simian immunodeficiency virus SIVmac239 viremia in adenovirus-boosted and DNA-primed Mamu-A*01-positive rhesus macaques. J. Virol. 79, 15556–15566.

Murphy, C.G., Lucas, W.T., Means, R.E., Czajak, S., Hale, C.L., Lifson, J.D., Kaur, A., Johnson, R.P., Knipe, D.M., and Desrosiers, R.C. (2000). Vaccine protection against simian immunodeficiency virus by recombinant strains of herpes simplex virus. J. Virol. 74, 7745–7754.

Nishimura, Y., Brown, C.R., et al. (2005). Resting naive CD4+ T cells are massively infected and eliminated by X4-tropic simian-human immunodeficiency viruses in macaques. Proc. Natl. Acad. Sci. USA 102, 8000–8005.

O'Connor, D.H., Allen, T.M., Vogel, T.U., Jing, P., DeSouza, I.P., Dodds, E., Dunphy, E.J., Melsaether, C., Mothe, B., Yamamoto, H., Horton, H., Wilson, N., Hughes, A.L., and Watkins, D.I. (2002). Acute phase cytotoxic T lymphocyte escape is a hallmark of simian immunodeficiency virus infection. Nature Med. 8, 493–499.

Pal, R., Venzon, D., Letvin, N.L., Santra, S., Montefiori, D.C., Miller, N.R., Tryniszewska, E., Lewis, M.G., VanCott, T.C., Hirsch, V., Woodward, R., Gibson, A., Grace, M., Dobratz, E., Markham, P.D., Z. Hel, Z., Nacsa, J., Klein, Tartaglia, M.J., and Franchini, G. (2002). ALVAC- SIV gag-pol-env- based vaccination and macaque major histocompatibility complex class I (A*01) delay SIVmac-induced immunodeficiency. J. Virol. 76, 292–302.

Priddy, F., Wright D., Lalezari J., Santiago, S., Novak, R, Brown, S., Lally, M., Marmor, M., Kublin, J., R Leavitt, R., Isaacs, R., Mehrotra, D., Shiver, J., Brown, D., and V520 Protocol 016 Study Group. (2004). Safety and immunogenicity of the MRK adenovirus type-5 gag/pol/nef HIV-1 (Trivalent) vaccine in healthy adults. 12th Conference on Retroviruses and Opportunistic Infections. Abstract #135. www.retroconference.org.

Quinn, T.C., and Overbaugh, J. (2005). HIV/AIDS in women: an expanding epidemic. Science 308, 1582–1583.

Robinson, H.L. (2002). New hopes for an AIDS vaccine. Nature Rev. Immunol. 2, 239–250.

Schmitz, J.E., Kuroda, M.J., Santra, S., Simon, M.A., Lifton, M.A., Lin, W., Khunkhun, R., Piatak, M., Lifson, J.D., Grosschupff, G., Gelman, R.S., Racz, P., Tenner-Racz, K., Mansfield, K.A., Letvin, N.L., Montefiori, D.C., and Reimann, K.A. (2003). Effect of humoral immune response on controlling viremia during primary infection of rhesus monkeys with simian immunodeficiency virus. J. Virol. 77, 2165–2173.

Subbramanian, R.A., Kuroda, M.J., Charini, W.A., Barouch, D.H., Costantino, C., Santra, S., Schmitz, J.E., Martin, K.L., Lifton, M.A., Gorgone, D.A., Shiver, J.W., and Letvin, N.L. (2003). Magnitude and diversity of cytotoxic-T-lymphocyte responses elicited by multiepitope DNA vaccination in rhesus monkeys. J. Virol. 77, 10113–10118.

Van Ballegooijen W.M., Bogaards J.A., Weverling G.J., Boerlijst M.C., and Goudsmit J. (2003). AIDS vaccines that allow HIV-1 to infect and escape immunologic control: a mathematic analysis of mass vaccination. J. Acquir. Immune Defic. Syndr. 34, 214–220.

Veazey, R.S., DeMaria, M., Chalifoux, L.V., Shvetz, D.E., Pauley, D.R., Knight, H.L., Rosenzweig, M., Johnson, R.P., Desrosiers, R.C., A. A. and Lackner, A.A. (1998). Gastrointestinal tract as a major site of CD4+ T-cell depletion and viral replication in SIV infection. Science 280, 427–431.

Veazey, R.S., Tham, I.C., Mansfield, K.G., DeMaria, M.A., Forand, A.E., Shvetz, D.E., Chalifoux, L.V., Sehgal, P.K., and Lackner, A.A. (2000). Identifying the target T-cell in primary simian immunodeficiency virus (SIV) infection: Highly activated memory CD4+ T-cells are rapidly eliminated in early infection in vivo. J. Virol. 74, 57–64.

Wang, S.W., Kozlowski, P.A., Schmeltz, G., Manson, K., Wyand, M.S., Glickman, R., Montefiori, D., Lifson, J.D., Johnson, R.P., Neutra, M.R., and Aldovini, A. (2000). Effective induction of simian immunodeficiency virus-specific systemic and mucosal immune responses in primates by vaccination with proviral DNA producing intact but non-infectious virions. J. Virol. 74, 10514–10522.

Zhao, J., Pincjewski, J., Gómez-Roman, V.R., David Venzon, D., Kalyanaraman, V.S., Markham, P.D., Aldrich, K., Moake, M., Montefiori, D.C., Lou, Y., Pavlakis, G.N., and Robert-Guroff, M. (2003). Improved protection of rhesus macaques against intrarectal simian immunodeficiency virus SIVmac251 challenge by a replication-competent Ad5hr-SIVenv/rev and Ad5hr-SIVgag recombinant priming/gp120 boosting regimen. J. Virol. 77, 8354–8365.

# What Does a Vaccine Need to do to Elicit Protective Immunity Against HIV Infection?

5

Paul Thottingal and Sarah L. Rowland-Jones

Abstract

The unique challenges of generating an effective vaccine to prevent HIV-1 infection have led immunologists to consider in detail the mechanisms of protective immunity that a successful candidate must elicit. This article reviews our current understanding of protective immunity to HIV-1 infection, based on studies of animal models and of exposed but apparently uninfected people.

## Introduction

The need to identify the key components of a protective immune response is a relatively new concept in vaccinology, which for much of its 200-year history has been a largely empirical science. The fundamental principle underlying most modern vaccines is that if a person survives an initial encounter with a pathogen, then they experience long-term protection from subsequent infection with that same pathogen, and often from closely related organisms. This observation can be traced back as long ago as 430 BC, when Thucydides wrote about the plague afflicting Athens, commenting that "during the times of epidemic, the sick and dying were cared for by those who had recovered as they were themselves free from apprehension." The concept of "immunity" (from the Latin "immunitas") developed over the next two millennia, culminating in the historic experiments of Edward Jenner using exudates from individuals infected with cowpox (who experienced only mild disease) to protect against the far more deadly smallpox infection.

Most of the vaccines used today in the global Extended Programme of Immunization, the cornerstone of the outstanding public health benefits of human vaccination, follow similar principles: Introduce small amounts of either killed whole organisms or live organisms that have been attenuated so they still elicit immunity but cannot cause disease. Such an empirical approach to HIV vaccine development, whilst predominantly successful in animal models, has largely been discounted because of the unacceptable risks that inadequately attenuated or inactivated HIV would pose when used in healthy, seronegative people (Daniel *et al.*, 1992). Thus for the first time, vaccinologists must consider what components of the HIV-specific immune response are essential to protect against HIV infection and disease (Koff *et al.*, 2006). At the same time, immunologists face the immense challenge of defining protective immunity for an infection that, in the overwhelming majority of infected people, will cause progressive disease and death. But, if no one "recovers" from or ultimately controls HIV infection, then the fundamental principle of vaccination is undermined. In this chapter, we review the data on the nature of immune responses that appear to be protective in animal models and in humans.

## Lessons learned from animal models

In the absence of unequivocal data for protective immunity in humans, animal models have been the mainstay of HIV vaccine studies. The principal weakness of these models is that they do not provide a faithful replication of HIV-1 disease in humans; however, mouse and nonhuman primate models of immunity to viral infections do offer the potential for immunologists to dissect out and manipulate those responses identified as essential in vaccine and natural history studies. Though small animal models are limited by the inability of HIV to replicate in rodent T-cells, Lymphocytic choriomeningitis virus (LCMV) infection in mice has become the landmark model for characterizing both cellular- and humoral-mediated immune responses in persistent viral infections. Although primate studies may be limited by the shortage of suitable animals and containment facilities worldwide, infection of non-human primates with HIV-1/SIV or the SHIV chimeric virus provide experimental models of viral infections more closely related to HIV-1 in humans, and information gleaned from these studies may help lead to a therapeutic or protective vaccine for HIV-1.

### Lymphocytic choriomeningitis virus (LCMV) infection in the mouse

Lymphocytic choriomeningitis virus (LCMV) is an arenavirus, an ambisense RNA virus thought to be a noncytopathic pathogen infecting its murine host. LCMV infection is primarily transmitted from mother to young via a placental route. Infection of adults results in an immunodeficiency syndrome that varies in its severity, largely in relation to the initial dose, route and kinetics of the viral challenge. In some cases persistent infection can occur, providing an important parallel with HIV-1 infection in humans (Buchmeier et al., 1980; Klenerman and Zinkernagel, 1997; Traub, 1935). The immune response to LCMV has been examined in unprecedented detail, leading to a thorough appreciation of the features of a successful immune response to this virus and of the properties that allow it to establish persistent infection (Buchmeier et al., 1980). These data provide some insights into what may be required for protective immunity in humans against persistent virus infections, with the important caveat that both the infecting virus and the immune system of humans may reveal essential differences from the murine model.

### Other murine models

Another valuable mouse model is the humanized severe combined immunodeficient (SCID)-hu mouse model, which has been employed to study protective immunity in the context of individuals who, despite regular exposure to HIV-1, remain seronegative over years and may be resistant to infection with HIV-1. Lymphocytes from these highly exposed persistently seronegative (HEPS) people can be used to reconstitute the mouse immune system, where they are then susceptible to HIV-1 infection. In such studies, a human monoclonal antibody (mAb) that neutralizes primary strains of HIV was shown to protect animals from HIV-1 challenge (Gauduin et al., 1997). However, in already-infected mice, even a potent cocktail of human mAbs made little impression on viral load, and viral isolates resistant to all three antibodies emerged within days of infection (Poignard et al., 1999). In another study, mice reconstituted with the peripheral blood mononuclear cells (PBMCs) of HEPS individuals were resistant to challenge with HIV-1, although the PBMCs themselves were readily infected in cell cultures. In contrast, mice reconstituted with the PBMCs of individuals not previously exposed to HIV-1 were readily infected with challenge virus. Depletion of $CD8^+$ cells from mice initially resistant to infection resulted in infection upon re-challenge, providing clear experimental evidence that in vivo protection against HIV-1 infection is $CD8^+$ T-cell dependent (Zhang et al., 1996).

### Nonhuman primate lentivirus models

More directly relevant to HIV-1 in humans is the study of nonhuman primate (NHP) models of the lentiviruses simian immunodeficiency virus (SIV), HIV-1, HIV-2 and the chimeric SHIV. Among NHP, HIV-1 infects only chimpanzees (a protected species) but causes no immunodeficiency or disease in this host, thereby limiting its value as a model. HIV-2 can infect macaques, but again, does not cause severe disease. In contrast, while different SIV strains in their natural African monkey hosts (such as sooty mangabeys, African green monkeys) are also only rarely associated with disease, inoculation

of SIV into Asian macaque species such as the Rhesus (*Macacca mulatta*), cynomolgus (*Macaca fascicularis*) or pigtailed macaques (*Macaca nemestrina*) leads to immunosuppression and immunodeficiency disease in a manner similar to—although much more rapid than—HIV-1 infection in humans (Gardner, 1996; Smith, 2002). This makes the SIV macaque system the most valuable and widely used model for HIV vaccines. Natural history studies of SIV in macaques have demonstrated several more valuable parallels to HIV-1 infection in humans, including viral tropism for macrophages, lifelong infection, virus evasion of host defenses via frequent mutations, and hidden reservoirs of latent proviral DNA. Another similarity is that infection is not eradicated despite vigorous cellular and humoral immune responses (Gardner, 1996; Smith, 2002). (Chapter 4).

Challenge systems, other than SIV, are sometimes used in NHP. The development of pathogenic SIV/HIV-1 hybrid strains called the simian-human immunodeficiency virus (SHIV) involves the design and manufacture of chimeric lentiviruses that incorporate the *gag, pol, vif, vpr* and *LTR* of the SIV virus, and the *tat, rev* and *env* of HIV-1. The advantage of the SHIV model is that these strains encode HIV-1 *env*, and therefore provide a potential system to test the importance of vaccine-induced antibodies against the HIV-1 envelope for protection. A further advantage is that the chimeric SHIVs can employ either coreceptor (CCR5 or CXCR4 or both depending on which HIV-1 envelope gene is inserted). However, pathogenic SHIV strains cause a much more rapid, profound immunosuppression than that seen during in natural HIV-1 infection.

In addition to the pathogenic SIV models, insights into viral control also come from studying non-pathogenic infections by lentiviruses in their natural hosts. In the case of SIV, its long co-evolution with African monkeys seems to have led to genetic and immunologic adaptations that allow both host and virus to co-exist. For example, recent studies in the sooty mangabey (*Cercocebus atys*) show that animals with SIV infection of their $CD4^+$ T-lymphocytes and very high viral loads nevertheless retain immuno-competence and show no apparent signs of disease (Silvestri et al., 2003). In contrast to human HIV-1 infection, SIV infection in the sooty mangabey has been shown to be associated with lower levels of immune activation, with both narrow focus of cellular immune response and attendant effector activity. This is an interesting finding, as though immune responses to natural SIV infection in the sooty mangabey are present, they are much less prominent than those seen in human HIV-1 infection. (Dunham et al., 2006). Similarly, the benign course of HIV-1 in experimentally infected chimpanzees (*Pan troglodytes*), which do not develop viremia or disease, can probably be explained by the likelihood that naturally infected central African chimpanzees were the reservoir from which HIV-1 entered the human population (Gao et al., 1999).

Perhaps even more intriguing, and only recently explored by the HIV research community, is the model of HIV-2 in humans. HIV-2 shows an extraordinarily high degree of homology to SIV in sooty mangabeys and is endemic in parts of West Africa, with a particular (and unexplained) predilection for countries with former social and economic ties to Portugal. HIV-2 cannot reasonably be thought of as an attenuated form of HIV-1 since it can, in a minority of people, cause the same devastating immunodeficiency as HIV-1 infection, leading to AIDS and death; moreover the proviral load is similar in the two infections (Ariyoshi *et al.*, 1996; Berry *et al.*, 2002). However, the majority of HIV-2-infected people die of causes other than AIDS, with a preserved CD4$^+$ T-cell count and a low plasma viral load (the latter in striking contrast to the sooty mangabey story). The reasons for the good outcome of most HIV-2-infected people are not well understood (Whittle *et al.*, 1998) although a recent study has demonstrated the preservation of CD4$^+$ T-cell help in HIV-2-infected people with no evidence of disease progression (Duvall *et al.*, 2006).

## Components of protective immunity in animal models—the need for a coordinated immune response

The murine LCMV model demonstrates that vertebrate hosts vary in their ability to successfully control or eradicate non-cytopathic viruses, with success dependent on a coordinated, complex immune response. Like many persistent viruses, LCMV is able to evade immune surveillance by generating both CTL escape mutants and escape variants from neutralizing antibodies, providing a reference point for studying similar phenomena in HIV-1 infection (Ciurea *et al.*, 2001a–c, 2000; Pircher *et al.*, 1990). In mice the dominant immune response to LCMV infection is through virus-specific cytotoxic T-lymphocytes (CTLs), while virus-specific antibodies do not appear to provide sterilizing immunity. However, at very high titer some LCMV-specific antibodies can protect against disease, suggesting that antibody-mediated mechanisms other than neutralization may be important for protection.

### Animal studies of virus-specific neutralizing antibody

At present, the correlate of protection for most successful human vaccines is the induction of protective neutralizing antibodies (nAb). Some vaccines may also elicit cell-mediated immunity, which is likely to be important in maintaining the overall protective response, but this is less well-studied. Neutralizing antibodies are generally directed at surface determinants such as envelope proteins, and therefore both free virions and infected host T-cells can become nAb targets. Passive transfer of antibody to uninfected hosts can protect against viral challenge, and protection generally correlates well with *in vitro* neutralizing capacity. However, in the absence of memory B- or T-lymphocytes, protection of this type is short-lived.

Animal models have been helpful in elucidating mechanisms by which antibodies can protect against infection other than through direct neutralizing capacity (Spear *et al.*, 1990).

Binding of antibody to the infected cell can trigger effector functions (such as Fc-mediated cell lysis, antibody-dependent cellular cytotoxicity (ADCC) or complement-dependent cytotoxicity) through two mechanisms: antibody-triggered signaling mechanisms which interfere with viral processes intracellularly, and interference with cell–cell transmission of free virions (Spear *et al.*, 1990, 1991, 2001). In mouse studies of yellow fever virus, specific subclasses of IgG (particularly IgG2a) can trigger effector functions that result in protection against disease (but not against infection)—in contrast to IgG1 molecules of the same specificity (Schlesinger and Chapman, 1995). Protection in this system is dependent on the Fc portion of IgG and mediated by complement-independent methods of viral control, most likely ADCC directed at infected cells. In the mouse model of dengue virus infection, it has been shown that virus-specific antibodies are not induced against proteins expressed on free virions, but rather against those on the host cell surface, such as dengue virus NS1 protein (Henchal *et al.*, 1988). The presence of non-neutralizing antibodies have also been observed in SHIV/SIV vaccine models but contributions of these antibodies to immune response have yet to be as well characterized (Hirsch *et al.*, 1996; Ourmanov *et al.*, 2000a,b; Patterson *et al.*, 2004). It is not known whether similar mechanisms may provide protection against HIV-1 infection.

Many authorities have seen antibodies with neutralizing capacity as the "holy grail" of a protective response. But inducing such antibodies may be difficult to achieve for HIV infection (Chapter 7), as suggested by the fact that only a handful of human monoclonal antibodies able to neutralize a broad range of primary HIV-1 strains have been isolated. The capacity of passively transferred neutralizing antibodies (the well-known panel of human IgG1-neutralising monoclonal antibodies F105, 2G12 and 2F5) to prevent intravenous infection of pregnant macaques and mucosal infection in their neonates has been clearly demonstrated (Baba *et al.*, 2000). However, what has emerged from animal models is that relatively high titers of antibodies must be present to neutralize challenge virus, often higher than seem likely to be achievable in current vaccine models. For example, studies in SHIV-challenged macaques found that nAb titers of 1 in 38 (99%) were required to maintain sterilizing immunity (Nishimura *et al.*, 2002; Parren *et al.*, 2001; Parren *et al.*, 1998).

The potential lack of coordinated effective support for maintenance of Nab may be what ultimately leads to failure of Nab to protect against HIV-1 infection. What is clear from studies of neutralizing antibodies is their relatively limited ability to prevent infection unless present very early in infection and at high titer, and that the potential for Nab to sustain their effect is marred by very rapid viral escape mechanisms. It is widely held that CTL is employed to control chronic disease progression where Nab have failed. What is less clear is what the potential role of antibody response is in control of chronic infection and the effect on disease progression, as there is some evidence that Nab may help influence steady state viremia in the SIV model (Miller et al., 1997).

## Animal studies of virus-specific cytotoxic T-lymphocytes (CTL)

Virus-specific CTLs play a major part in eradicating infections such as influenza, and in controlling viral replication in persistent infections like EBV and CMV. These CTLs have several effector functions, including lysis of infected cells (which in HIV-1 infection is likely to kill the cell before infectious progeny are produced) (Klenerman et al., 1996) and secretion of anti-viral cytokines and chemokines that control viral replication (Yang et al., 1997). Murine knock-out studies have shown that these effector functions differ in importance in different virus infections. For example perforin-mediated cytotoxicity is essential for the clearance of LCMV (Kagi et al., 1994) but less important for infections such as vaccinia and vesicular stomatitis virus. It is not known which aspects of CTL function are most important for controlling HIV infection, although the secretion of CC chemokines that compete with HIV-1 for the CCR5 receptor might be particularly valuable (Price et al., 1998). CTL lysis of target T-cells that are already infected (although they may not have actively replicating virus); (Buseyne et al., 2001), would therefore be expected at best to control viral replication and prevent further infection of target T-cells rather than to achieve sterilizing immunity. It has been demonstrated that SIV specific CTL are present at multiple sites other than the systemic circulation(gut, genital tract, and lymphoid tissues) during acute SIV infection, implying that these CTL may have distinct early roles in blunting rapid virus propagation on multiple fronts (Reynolds, 2006). Vaccines that induce only CTL have been shown to protect against high-dose challenge with pathogens such as influenza, LCMV and paramyxovirus in the absence of neutralizing antibody (Daniel et al., 1992; Fu et al., 1997; Hsu et al., 1998; Kagi and Hengartner, 1996; Oehen et al., 1992; Stott and Almond, 1995; Ulmer et al., 1993). Under these circumstances, the presence of CTL is likely to lead to transient infection that is contained and cleared rapidly. In other cases, CTLs alone do not lead to complete eradication of infection and serve principally to control the spread of virus and subsequent development of disease. (See also discussion in Chapter 4.)

Several lines of evidence suggest that SIV- or HIV-specific CTL can also mediate protection in macaques. In one set of studies, macaques exposed to low doses of HIV-2 were protected from subsequent challenge with virulent SIV (Putkonen et al., 1997), and this protection was associated with the presence of virus-specific CTL. Macaques exposed repeatedly to subinfectious doses of SIV generated strong proliferative responses to SIV which correlated with protection from challenge (Clerici et al., 1994). Similarly, macaques exposed to SIV mucosally can develop mucosal CTL responses and are then protected against viral challenge (Murphey-Corb et al., 1999), which brought about a transient but controlled

infection in these experiments. In macaques chronically infected with attenuated forms of SIV, CTL responses are associated with protection against superinfection by more aggressive strains of SIV (Daniel et al., 1992; Stott and Almond, 1995). Likewise, brief treatment of SIV-infected macaques with highly active antiretroviral drugs can facilitate control of infection by inducing strong immune responses that mediate resistance to subsequent infection with other SIV subtypes or with SHIV (Lifson et al., 2000). This protection can be completely abrogated by removing the CD8[+] subset, implying that CTLs are the essential component of overall viral control (Jin et al., 1999; Schmitz et al., 1999).

These data suggest that it may be possible for CTL responses to bring about containment and even eradication of an HIV/SIV challenge. However, the more frequent outcome of challenging vaccinated animals that show virus-specific CTL responses is a persistent infection with reduced viral loads and significantly delayed disease progression (Amara et al., 2001; Barouch et al., 2002; Barouch et al., 2000). If this holds true in humans, would protection against disease rather than sterilizing immunity be an acceptable outcome for an HIV vaccine? One parallel would be the example of tuberculosis in immunocompetent hosts, most of whom control initial infection and remain healthy. However, disease develops readily when the delicate balance between immune control and the host organism is disturbed. In macaque studies, prevention of disease in vaccinated animals with strong CTL responses has not been tested by subjecting vaccinated animals to therapeutic immuno-suppression (or by monitoring the effects of normal ageing on the immune system)—circumstances that model the immune system decline which might occur in some members of vaccinated human populations (and which can cause previously controlled tuberculosis to become active). A further caution for CTL-inducing vaccines is the great potential of HIV to generate variants that escape immune responses, including CTL (McMichael and Phillips, 1997). This has been clearly shown in naturally infected humans and macaques, and may also be seen in vaccinated animals with narrowly focused T-cell responses.

Recent animal data have emphasized the need for virus-specific T-lymphocyte-mediated help at the time of CTL induction if there is to be a re-expansion of memory CTL later, in response to challenge (Shedlock and Shen, 2003; Sun and Bevan, 2003; Zajac et al., 1998). Studies in the LCMV model have shown that the absence of T-cell help (in the MHC class II knock-out mouse) leads to the generation of CTL that lack normal effector functions and do not protect against challenge (Zajac et al., 1998). These studies have particular resonance for HIV-1 infection, in which virus-specific T-helper cells are preferentially infected (Douek et al., 2002). In light of such findings, a reasonable strategy is to develop vaccines that induce both virus-specific CD4 and CD8 responses. Macaques immunized with a vaccine construct that included target CD4 and CD8 epitopes and subsequently challenged with an aggressive SHIV89.6P chimera demonstrated viral loads which were 1,000-fold lower than their unvaccinated counterparts (Barouch *et al.*, 2000, 2001). This startling finding is tempered by the later appearance of escape from the immune control induced by the SHIV strain. In this case it took only a single amino acid change to generate escape variants, since the vaccine was based predominantly on a single immunodominant T-cell epitope, findings which amplified fears that viral escape mechanisms can still function at very low levels of viral persistence (Barouch *et al.*, 2002).

## Persistent antigen stimulation may be the key to a long-lasting immune response: so how can that be replicated by a vaccine?

Studies of macaques show that beneficial immune responses can be generated by vaccines, but they are not necessarily long-lasting. By analogy with the scenario of persistent virus infection, vaccines are only effective if they can induce long-term immunological memory that can be rapidly recruited upon re-exposure to virus (Oehen *et al.*, 1992). Repeated experiments with various prime-boost regiments (plasmid-encoded SIV gag/MVA-SIVgag boost, DNA prime/adenovirus boost or DNA/IL-2 prime) can stimulate very strong and early CTL responses, all of which decline quickly. (Allen *et al.*, 2000; Amara *et al.*, 2001; Hanke *et al.*, 1999). Macaque studies show that DNA alone is not a potent stimulator of CTL immune responses. However, prime-boost regimens that deliver "boost" DNA in recombinant viral vectors such as modified vaccinia Ankara (a replication-deficient vaccinia virus) and several similar viral vectors, have much better results than the prime vaccine itself (Amara *et al.*, 2001; Hanke *et al.*, 1999). The benefit of T-cell direction by the DNA component of the vaccine likely directs the immune response to the vaccine immunogen in subsequent rechallenge with the recombinant virus vector—which also redirects the immune response away from the immunodominant epitopes of the much larger vaccine vector. This approach greatly enhances DNA vaccination in macaques, inducing CTL responses which protect against challenge with SIV (Hanke *et al.*, 1999). Continued macaque studies with a variety of immunogens and adjuvants are under study to improve delivery and durability of immune responses to viral challenge.

What is important to keep in mind here is that success of any SIV or HIV-1 vaccine is measured by its ability to ensure that immunologically relevant proteins/epitopes are presented in a way that will induce effective cell-mediated and (hopefully) humoral responses, and that memory of these responses can be generated and recruited quickly enough to hold virus in check immediately in case of exposure to HIV, and for a long period thereafter. If a sterilizing effect is not achieved as a primary endpoint, then an acceptable secondary endpoint must be effective immune control with a goal of preventing or delaying disease.

## Mucosal immunity

One important drawback of the animal models described above is that the practical need to make most efficient use of the fewest possible subjects per study demands a highly effective challenge regimen that results in infection of 100% of the control animals; in most cases this means a single high-dose intravenous challenge. This may be a very poor surrogate for the most common scenarios of HIV-1 exposure in humans, which usually involve repeated low-dose exposure at mucosal surfaces. What potential mechanisms uncovered in animal studies offer clues to mucosal immunity against HIV-1 infection?

Animal models demonstrate clearly that transmission of SIV infection can be quite rapid. Studies in macaques have shown that infected dendritic cells can be found in the vaginal mucosa within 60 minutes of intravaginal exposure to SIV, and in the draining lymph node within 18 hours (Hu *et al.*, 2000). Further studies have shown that SIV replicates predominantly in CD4$^+$ T-cells at the portal of entry and in local lymph nodes. Of great interest, is that infection is propagated both from activated proliferating cells and resting cells. More recently, rapid and profound depletion of memory CD4$^+$ T-cells has been shown to occur, predominantly in mucosal lymphoid tissue after SIV infection in rhesus macaques. Immediate and widespread destruction of CD4$^+$ T-cell effector functions in mucosal lymphoid tissues may have an immediate consequence of blunting CTL and/or humoral immune responses, leaving viral dissemination largely unchecked (Mattapallil *et al.*, 2005). Populations of infected resting cells in lymphoid tissue have been shown to persist even after antiretroviral therapy, and are the likely source of chronic, latently persisting SIV-infected cells (Zhang *et al.*, 1999). Vaccine induced immune control, if not eradication of virus, in the early period of exposure/infection in lymphoid tissue may influence the outcome of SIV challenge, with important parallels in HIV exposure in humans (Koff *et al.*, 2006; Reynolds *et al.*, 2005; Veazey *et al.*, 1998). It is known in human infection that heterosexual transmission is an infrequent event once acute infection is past (Gray *et al.*, 2001), raising the important question of whether and how the local mucosal immune system could influence events taking place during transmission in a way that prevents infection.

Several pathogens gain access to the body through mucosal surfaces, and passive transfer studies have shown that compartmentalized mucosal antibodies present before viral exposure can protect against later challenge (Kato *et al.*, 2001; Ogra *et al.*, 2001). Mouse models of rotavirus challenge have shown that even non-neutralizing antibodies may have protective effects, perhaps through some intracellular mechanism (Burns *et al.*, 1996). Exposure of macaques to low doses of SIV through the colonic epithelium led to priming of both systemic and mucosal CTL responses (in the absence of persistent infection) that were associated with protection from subsequent high-dose virus challenge (Murphey-Corb *et al.*, 1999).

It is difficult to truly delineate the roles of neutralizing antibody and CTL in the immune response to viruses *in vivo*. Mouse models have shown that intra-rectal vaccination with an HIV peptide immunogen/HIV-1 gp160 expression recombinant vaccinia virus can protect against viral challenge, and that this response depends not on antibodies but on mucosal CTL at the site of exposure. Both resistance and CTL responses were amplified by local mucosal IL-12 delivery. CD8 depletion studies confirmed that immunity was dependent on the presence of mucosal CTL as opposed to splenic CTL, which were unable to protect against mucosal infection (Belyakov *et al.*, 1998). Other studies employing mucosal immunization (nasal, oral) have been conducted with a vaccine composed of live attenuated VSV (vesicular stomatitis virus) carrying the SIV *gag* and *env* genes. Subsequent SHIV 89.6 intravenous challenge led to infection and eventual disease progression of control animals, but low or absent viral titers in the vaccinees (Rose *et al.*, 2001). These examples illustrate that mucosal vaccination, or systemic vaccination that generates mucosal immunity, is an important consideration in HIV-1 vaccine design (Chapter 9).

## Lessons from highly exposed uninfected humans

Despite the extraordinarily rapid spread of HIV to tens of millions of people around the world in the past 20 years, virus transmission on an individual basis is relatively inefficient. This is illustrated by the high rate of serodiscordance in couples in stable long-term relationships in which, even with frequent unprotected intercourse, usually no more than 10–15% of partners of HIV-infected people become infected themselves. However, recent data suggest that the likelihood of HIV-1 transmission is substantially higher from partners with acute HIV-1 infection (Wawer *et al.*, 2005). Several investigators have studied potential mechanisms of resistance to HIV-1 infection in people who remain apparently uninfected despite a great deal of exposure to the virus. Many potential mechanisms that could account for resistance to HIV-1 infection do not necessarily reflect protective immunity—for example, homozygosity for the well-described deletion in CCR5 (the target receptor for primary strains of HIV-1), which renders CD4+ T-cells highly resistant to HIV-1 infection (Liu *et al.*, 1996). However, other genetic associations with resistance to HIV infection, such as HLA Class I and II types are in keeping with cell-mediated immune mechanisms. Resistance to HIV-1 infection is most striking in commercial sex workers (CSWs) with unusually high degrees of HIV exposure. Kenyan CSWs living in the Pumwani slum of Nairobi experience amongst the highest documented levels of HIV-1 exposure anywhere in the world, while studies on a long-standing cohort of these women found most of them become infected within three years of entering the cohort (Fowke *et al.*, 1996). In this Nairobi CSW cohort, HIV resistance is associated with HLA-A2, A*6802, B18 and DR1, while HLA-A23 is associated with increased rates of HIV infection (MacDonald *et al.*, 2000).

## Immunological mechanisms of HIV resistance

The associations of HLA type with HIV resistance imply that immunological mechanisms may be contributing to resistance in the HEPS women, and that the T-cells using these particular HLA molecules may be especially efficient at controlling HIV replication. Studies of people in a variety of HEPS cohorts have consistently detected the presence of a cellular immune response to HIV, in particular HIV-specific CTL and T-helper responses (Kaul and Rowland-Jones, 1999). HIV-specific CTL responses have also been detected in babies born to infected mothers, in occupationally exposed health care workers, the regular sexual partners of infected people and highly exposed CSWs.

The strongest links between these CTLs and protection come from the CSW cohorts, in whom immune responses without detectable infection probably indicate genuine HIV resistance. In the Nairobi CSW cohort, over 50% of women meeting the definition of HIV resistance have HIV-specific CD8+ T-cell responses detectable by interferon gamma-based ELISpot assays, and the likelihood of detecting these responses increases the longer the women remain highly exposed to HIV (Kaul *et al.*, 2001a). This observation is consistent with HIV resistance being acquired through increasing exposure to HIV, leading eventually to immunity to the virus. Similarly, with reduced exposure, CD8+ T-cell effector responses decline, and in these circumstances infection of women previously considered HIV resistant can occur (Kaul *et al.*, 2001b). These data are consistent with a model in which repeated genital exposure to HIV, perhaps as a result of initial exposure to only small amounts of virus or an attenuated strain, in a minority of individuals (possibly with particular host genetic advantages) can lead to cellular immune responses in the absence of infection and to circulating antibodies associated with resistance to infection. However, these data also suggest that this is not a particularly efficient way of generating protective immunity and that at best this immunity is only partial, requiring repeated stimulation to maintain effector T-cell responses. One way of interpreting these data is that it is relatively hard to achieve protection against repeated exposure to multiple strains of HIV, as would be the case in the Nairobi slums.

In contrast, intermittent exposure to the same strain of virus in a regular sexual partner may be more efficient at generating protective immunity. We have found much higher levels of CD4+ and CD8+ T-cell responses in the HIV-negative partners of infected people than we see in the CSW cohort (S. Pinheiro *et al.*, unpublished). Other investigators have reported similar findings in women exposed to a single HIV-infected partner (Promadej *et al.*, 2003). HIV-specific CD4+ T-cells have also been described in HEPS donors by many investigators. In one recent detailed study the presence of p24-specific CD4+ T-cells secreting MIP-1β, interferon gamma (IFNγ) and IL-2 was described in HEPS subjects but not in unexposed controls, and these CD4+ T-cells showed relative resistance to HIV-1 infection *in vitro* (Eyeson *et al.*, 2003). No differences were seen in either the presence or the magnitude of responses between HEPS subjects exposed parenterally or mucosally to HIV-1 (Makedonas *et al.*, 2005). However, although suggestive, this kind of data does not prove causation, and it remains entirely possible that these cellular responses are simply a marker of HIV exposure. Moreover, a prospective study in the Nairobi cohort found no association between the presence of env-specific CTL responses and protection from seroconversion (Kaul *et al.*, 2004).

It is also important to note that not all investigators have found T-cell responses in exposed uninfected donors (Hladik *et al.*, 2003). These inconsistencies may reflect methodological differences in the studies or—given the close relationship between exposure and the detection of responses in the Nairobi cohort—differences in the extent of exposure in the study cohorts.

In human HEPS studies the observed cellular immune responses have most likely been generated in response to transient infection, possibly with defective strains of HIV-1. However, a careful review of possible cases of transient HIV-1 infection in infants of infected mothers has not confirmed any documented cases to date (Frenkel *et al.*, 1998), so this remains speculative. Recent painstaking studies involving the leucopheresis of HEPS donors and sensitive PCR analysis to look for the presence of HIV-1 DNA showed that very low levels of conserved HIV-1 *gag* and *env* sequences were detectable in 2 of 10 HEPS subjects (Zhu *et al.*, 2003). The extraordinarily low levels of virus and the absence of sequence variation suggest that the virus is not replicating to any significant extent in these people, but the presence of HIV-1 DNA could be sufficient to prime HIV-specific immune responses. If this scenario was confirmed in a larger number of HEPS individuals, it would raise concerns about the potential of persistent and apparently contained infection to become reactivated under circumstances of immune dysfunction.

Other features of the immune response in HEPS individuals that may be relevant to vaccine design include the presence of HIV-specific CD8+ T-cells in genital secretions, where they appear to be enriched relative to HIV-infected donors (Kaul *et al.*, 2000). The finding of HIV-specific IgA responses at mucosal surfaces (Mazzoli *et al.*, 1997) has been controversial (Dorrell *et al.*, 2000), but may also highlight the importance of mucosal immunity in protection against HIV-1 infection. More recently, resistance to HIV-1 in the Nairobi CSW cohort has been shown to be linked to increases in the numbers of both CD4+ and CD8+ T-cells in the genital mucosa, together with increased RANTES expression (Iqbal *et al.*, 2005).

If the data from HEPS cohorts suggest that CTL provide an important protective mechanism in HIV infection, then other fundamental questions remain about the responses in exposed seronegative donors. How is a cellular response to HIV stimulated without simultaneously generating a systemic antibody response?—a very rare event in viral immunology, although not unheard of (under very particular circumstances).

Even harder to explain is why the low levels of CTL responses detected in HEPS subjects could lead to protection whilst the much higher CTL levels seen in infected people do not prevent eventual clinical progression. One possible explanation is that the responses generated in HEPS individuals have qualitative aspects of the responses linked with viral control and distinct from those in seropositive people (Rowland-Jones *et al.*, 2001).

## Conclusions

Taken together, the data from animal models show that whilst neutralizing antibodies clearly can offer protection against viral challenge with SIV and HIV strains, the high titers required for neutralization and the relatively rapid development of escape variants may present problems for vaccine strategies based on eliciting antibodies—not withstanding the considerable technical difficulties in generating neutralizing antibodies with candidate vaccines. However, non-neutralizing antibodies may play a role in controlling initial infection through effector mechanisms such as ADCC. If antibodies indeed help blunt initial infection, this may serve to allow other arms of the immune response to either eradicate infection or control persistent infection, thereby delaying disease. Cellular immune responses in the absence of antibodies are rarely associated with sterilizing immunity in animal models, but at best may lead to transient infection in some cases or to controlled viremia with delayed disease progression in other instances.

Immune responses in highly exposed persistently seronegative (HEPS) human subjects may be more like the desired vaccine response, but it remains unclear whether the responses detected in many such people are truly protective or simply a marker of HIV-1 resistance achieved by some other as-yet unidentified mechanism. These studies indicate that cellular immune responses in the absence of circulating antibody may be a correlate of protective immunity, which has provided support for current vaccine strategies that aim to elicit strong and persistent helper and cytotoxic T-cell responses against HIV-1 (Hanke and McMichael, 2000).

## References

Allen, T.M., Vogel, T.U., Fuller, D.H., Mothe, B.R., Steffen, S., Boyson, J.E., Shipley, T., Fuller, J., Hanke, T., Sette, A., *et al.* (2000). Induction of AIDS virus-specific CTL activity in fresh, unstimulated peripheral blood lymphocytes from rhesus macaques vaccinated with a DNA prime/modified vaccinia virus Ankara boost regimen. J. Immunol. *164*, 4968–4978.

Amara, R.R., Villinger, F., Altman, J.D., Lydy, S.L., O'Neil, S.P., Staprans, S.I., Montefiori, D.C., Xu, Y., Herndon, J.G., Wyatt, L.S., *et al.* (2001). Control of a mucosal challenge and prevention of AIDS by a multiprotein DNA/MVA vaccine. Science *292*, 69–74.

Ariyoshi, K., Berry, N., Wilkins, A., Ricard, D., Aaby, P., Naucler, A., Ngom, P.T., Jobe, O., Jaffar, S., Dias, F., *et al.* (1996). A community-based study of human immunodeficiency virus type 2 provirus load in rural village in West Africa. J. Infect. Dis. *173*, 245–248.

Baba, T.W., Liska, V., Hofmann-Lehmann, R., Vlasak, J., Xu, W., Ayehunie, S., Cavacini, L.A., Posner, M.R., Katinger, H., Stiegler, G., *et al.* (2000). Human neutralizing monoclonal antibodies of the IgG1 subtype protect against mucosal simian-human immunodeficiency virus infection. Nature Med. *6*, 200–206.

Barouch, D.H., Craiu, A., Santra, S., Egan, M.A., Schmitz, J.E., Kuroda, M.J., Fu, T.M., Nam, J.H., Wyatt, L.S., Lifton, M.A., et al. (2001). Elicitation of high-frequency cytotoxic T-lymphocyte responses against both dominant and subdominant simian-human immunodeficiency virus epitopes by DNA vaccination of rhesus monkeys. J. Virol. 75, 2462–2467.

Barouch, D.H., Kunstman, J., Kuroda, M.J., Schmitz, J.E., Santra, S., Peyerl, F.W., Krivulka, G.R., Beaudry, K., Lifton, M.A., Gorgone, D.A., et al. (2002). Eventual AIDS vaccine failure in a rhesus monkey by viral escape from cytotoxic T lymphocytes. Nature 415, 335–339.

Barouch, D.H., Santra, S., Schmitz, J.E., Kuroda, M.J., Fu, T.M., Wagner, W., Bilska, M., Craiu, A., Zheng, X.X., Krivulka, G.R., et al. (2000). Control of viremia and prevention of clinical AIDS in rhesus monkeys by cytokine-augmented DNA vaccination. Science 290, 486–492.

Belyakov, I.M., Ahlers, J.D., Brandwein, B.Y., Earl, P., Kelsall, B.L., Moss, B., Strober, W., and Berzofsky, J.A. (1998). The importance of local mucosal HIV-specific CD8(+) cytotoxic T lymphocytes for resistance to mucosal viral transmission in mice and enhancement of resistance by local administration of IL-12. J. Clin. Invest. 102, 2072–2081.

Berry, N., Jaffar, S., Schim van der Loeff, M., Ariyoshi, K., Harding, E., N'Gom, P.T., Dias, F., Wilkins, A., Ricard, D., Aaby, P., et al. (2002). Low level viremia and high CD4% predict normal survival in a cohort of HIV type-2-infected villagers. AIDS Res. Hum. Retroviruses 18, 1167–1173.

Buchmeier, M.J., Welsh, R.M., Dutko, F.J., and Oldstone, M.B. (1980). The virology and immunobiology of lymphocytic choriomeningitis virus infection. Adv Immunol 30, 275–331.

Burns, J.W., Siadat-Pajouh, M., Krishnaney, A.A., and Greenberg, H.B. (1996). Protective effect of rotavirus VP6-specific IgA monoclonal antibodies that lack neutralizing activity. Science 272, 104–107.

Buseyne, F., Le Gall, S., Boccaccio, C., Abastado, J.P., Lifson, J.D., Arthur, L.O., Riviere, Y., Heard, J.M., and Schwartz, O. (2001). MHC-I-restricted presentation of HIV-1 virion antigens without viral replication. Nature Med. 7, 344–349.

Ciurea, A., Hunziker, L., Klenerman, P., Hengartner, H., and Zinkernagel, R.M. (2001a). Impairment of CD4(+) T cell responses during chronic virus infection prevents neutralizing antibody responses against virus escape mutants. J. Exp. Med. 193, 297–305.

Ciurea, A., Hunziker, L., Martinic, M.M., Oxenius, A., Hengartner, H., and Zinkernagel, R.M. (2001b). CD4+ T-cell-epitope escape mutant virus selected in vivo. Nature Med. 7, 795–800.

Ciurea, A., Hunziker, L., Zinkernagel, R.M., and Hengartner, H. (2001c). Viral escape from the neutralizing antibody response: the lymphocytic choriomeningitis virus model. Immunogenetics 53, 185–189.

Ciurea, A., Klenerman, P., Hunziker, L., Horvath, E., Senn, B.M., Ochsenbein, A.F., Hengartner, H., and Zinkernagel, R.M. (2000). Viral persistence in vivo through selection of neutralizing antibody-escape variants. Proc. Natl. Acad. Sci. USA 97, 2749–2754.

Clerici, M., Clark, E.A., Polacino, P., Axberg, I., Kuller, L., Casey, N.I., Morton, W.R., Shearer, G.M., and Benveniste, R.E. (1994). T-cell proliferation to subinfectious SIV correlates with lack of infection after challenge of macaques. AIDS 8, 1391–1395.

Daniel, M.D., Kirchhoff, F., Czajak, S.C., Sehgal, P.K., and Desrosiers, R.C. (1992). Protective effects of a live attenuated SIV vaccine with a deletion in the nef gene. Science 258, 1938–1941.

Dorrell, L., Hessell, A.J., Wang, M., Whittle, H., Sabally, S., Rowland-Jones, S., Burton, D.R., and Parren, P.W. (2000). Absence of specific mucosal antibody responses in HIV-exposed uninfected sex workers from the Gambia. AIDS 14, 1117–1122.

Douek, D.C., Brenchley, J.M., Betts, M.R., Ambrozak, D.R., Hill, B.J., Okamoto, Y., Casazza, J.P., Kuruppu, J., Kunstman, K., Wolinsky, S., et al. (2002). HIV preferentially infects HIV-specific CD4+ T cells. Nature 417, 95–98.

Dunham, R., Pagliardini, P., Gordon, S., Sumpter, B., Engram, J., Moanna, A., Paiardini, M., Mandl, J.N., Lawson, B., Garg, S., et al.

(2006). The AIDS-resistance of naturally SIV-infected sooty mangabeys is independent of cellular immunity to the virus. Blood.

Duvall, M.G., Jaye, A., Dong, T., Brenchley, J.M., Alabi, A.S., Jeffries, D.J., van der Sande, M., Togun, T.O., McConkey, S.J., Douek, D.C., et al. (2006). Maintenance of HIV-Specific CD4+ T cell help distinguishes HIV-2 from HIV-1 infection. J. Immunol. 176, 6973–6981.

Eyeson, J., King, D., Boaz, M.J., Sefia, E., Tomkins, S., Waters, A., Easterbrook, P.J., and Vyakarnam, A. (2003). Evidence for Gag p24-specific CD4 T cells with reduced susceptibility to R5 HIV-1 infection in a UK cohort of HIV-exposed-seronegative subjects. AIDS 17, 2299–2311.

Fowke, K., Nagelkerke, N., Kimani, J., Simonsen, J.N., Anzala, A.O., Bwayo, J.J., MacDonald, K.S., Ngugi, E.N., and Plummer, F.A. (1996). Resistance to HIV-1 infection amongst persistently seronegative prostitutes in Nairobi, Kenya. Lancet 348, 1347–1351.

Frenkel, L.M., Mullins, J.I., Learn, G.H., Manns-Arcuino, L., Herring, B.L., Kalish, M.L., Steketee, R.W., Thea, D.M., Nichols, J.E., Liu, S.L., et al. (1998). Genetic evaluation of suspected cases of transient HIV-1 infection of infants. Science 280, 1073–1077.

Fu, T.M., Friedman, A., Ulmer, J.B., Liu, M.A., and Donnelly, J.J. (1997). Protective cellular immunity: cytotoxic T-lymphocyte responses against dominant and recessive epitopes of influenza virus nucleoprotein induced by DNA immunization. J. Virol. 71, 2715–2721.

Gao, F., Bailes, E., Robertson, D.L., Chen, Y., Rodenburg, C.M., Michael, S.F., Cummins, L.B., Arthur, L.O., Peeters, M., Shaw, G.M., et al. (1999). Origin of HIV-1 in the chimpanzee Pan troglodytes troglodytes. Nature 397, 436–441.

Gardner, M.B. (1996). The history of simian AIDS. J. Med. Primatol. 25, 148–157.

Gauduin, M.C., Parren, P.W., Weir, R., Barbas, C.F., Burton, D.R., and Koup, R.A. (1997). Passive immunization with a human monoclonal antibody protects hu-PBL-SCID mice against challenge by primary isolates of HIV-1. Nature Med 3, 1389–1393.

Gray, R.H., Wawer, M.J., Brookmeyer, R., Sewankambo, N.K., Serwadda, D., Wabwire-Mangen, F., Lutalo, T., Li, X., vanCott, T., and Quinn, T.C. (2001). Probability of HIV-1 transmission per coital act in monogamous, heterosexual, HIV-1-discordant couples in Rakai, Uganda. Lancet 357, 1149–1153.

Hanke, T., and McMichael, A.J. (2000). Design and construction of an experimental HIV-1 vaccine for a year- (2000) clinical trial in Kenya. Nat Med 6, 951–955.

Hanke, T., Samuel, R. V., Blanchard, T.J., Neumann, V.C., Allen, T.M., Boyson, J.E., Sharpe, S.A., Cook, N., Smith, G.L., Watkins, D.I., et al. (1999). Effective induction of simian immunodeficiency virus-specific cytotoxic T lymphocytes in macaques by using a multiepitope gene and DNA prime-modified vaccinia virus Ankara boost vaccination regimen. J. Virol. 73, 7524–7532.

Henchal, E.A., Henchal, L.S., and Schlesinger, J.J. (1988). Synergistic interactions of anti-NS1 monoclonal antibodies protect passively immunized mice from lethal challenge with dengue 2 virus. J. Gen. Virol. 69 (Pt 8), 2101–2107.

Hirsch, V.M., Fuerst, T.R., Sutter, G., Carroll, M.W., Yang, L.C., Goldstein, S., Piatak, M., Jr., Elkins, W.R., Alvord, W.G., Montefiori, D.C., et al. (1996). Patterns of viral replication correlate with outcome in simian immunodeficiency virus (SIV)-infected macaques: effect of prior immunization with a trivalent SIV vaccine in modified vaccinia virus Ankara. J. Virol. 70, 3741–3752.

Hladik, F., Desbien, A., Lang, J., Wang, L., Ding, Y., Holte, S., Wilson, A., Xu, Y., Moerbe, M., Schmechel, S., and McElrath, M.J. (2003). Most highly exposed seronegative men lack HIV-1-specific, IFN-gamma-secreting T cells. J. Immunol. 171, 2671–2683.

Hsu, S.C., Obeid, O.E., Collins, M., Iqbal, M., Chargelegue, D., and Steward, M.W. (1998). Protective cytotoxic T lymphocyte responses against paramyxoviruses induced by epitope-based DNA vaccines: involvement of IFN-gamma. Int. Immunol. 10, 1441–1447.

Hu, J., Gardner, M.B., and Miller, C.J. (2000). Simian immunodeficiency virus rapidly penetrates the cervicovaginal mucosa after intravaginal inoculation and infects intraepithelial dendritic cells. J.Virol. 74, 6087–6095.

Iqbal, S.M., Ball, T.B., Kimani, J., Kiama, P., Thottingal, P., Embree, J.E., Fowke, K.R., and Plummer, F.A. (2005). Elevated T cell counts and RANTES expression in the genital mucosa of HIV-1-resistant Kenyan commercial sex workers. J. Infect. Dis. *192*, 728–738.

Jin, X., Bauer, D.E., Tuttleton, S.E., Lewin, S., Gettie, A., Blanchard, J., Irwin, C.E., Safrit, J. T., Mittler, J., Weinberger, L., *et al.* (1999). Dramatic rise in plasma viremia after CD8(+) T cell depletion in simian immunodeficiency virus-infected macaques. J. Exp. Med. *189*, 991–998.

Kagi, D., and Hengartner, H. (1996). Different roles for cytotoxic T cells in the control of infections with cytopathic versus noncytopathic viruses. Curr. Opin. Immunol. *8*, 472–477.

Kagi, D., Ledermann, B., Burki, K., Seiler, P., Odermatt, B., Olsen, K.J., Podack, E.R., Zinkernagel, R.M., and Hengartner, H. (1994). Cytotoxicity mediated by T cells and natural killer cells is greatly impaired in perforin-deficient mice. Nature *369*, 31–37.

Kato, H., Kato, R., Fujihashi, K., and McGhee, J.R. (2001). Role of mucosal antibodies in viral infections. Curr. Top. Microbiol. Immunol. *260*, 201–228.

Kaul, R., Dong, T., Plummer, F.A., Kimani, J., Rostron, T., Kiama, P., Njagi, E., Irungu, E., Farah, B., Oyugi, J., *et al.* (2001a). CD8(+) lymphocytes respond to different HIV epitopes in seronegative and infected subjects. J. Clin. Invest. *107*, 1303–1310.

Kaul, R., Plummer, F.A., Kimani, J., Dong, T., Kiama, P., Rostron, T., Njagi, E., MacDonald, K.S., Bwayo, J.J., McMichael, A.J., and Rowland-Jones, S.L. (2000). HIV-1-Specific mucosal CD8[+] lymphocyte responses in the cervix of HIV-1- resistant prostitutes in Nairobi [In Process Citation]. J. Immunol. *164*, 1602–1611.

Kaul, R., and Rowland-Jones, S.L., eds. (1999). Methods of detection of HIV-specific CTL and their role in protection against HIV infection (Los Alamos National Laboratory, Theoretical Biology and Biophysics, Los Alamos, New Mexico).

Kaul, R., Rowland-Jones, S.L., Kimani, J., Dong, T., Yang, H.B., Kiama, P., Rostron, T., Njagi, E., Bwayo, J.J., MacDonald, K.S., *et al.* (2001). Late seroconversion in HIV-resistant Nairobi prostitutes despite pre- existing HIV-specific CD8[+] responses. J. Clin. Invest. *107*, 341–349.

Kaul, R., Rutherford, J., Rowland-Jones, S.L., Kimani, J., Onyango, J.I., Fowke, K., MacDonald, K., Bwayo, J.J., McMichael, A.J., and Plummer, F. A. (2004). HIV-1 Env-specific cytotoxic T-lymphocyte responses in exposed, uninfected Kenyan sex workers: a prospective analysis. AIDS *18*, 2087–2089.

Klenerman, P., Phillips, R.E., Rinaldo, C.R., Wahl, L.M., Ogg, G., May, R.M., McMichael, A.J., and Nowak, M. A. (1996). Cytotoxic T lymphocytes and viral turnover in HIV type 1 infection. Proc. Natl. Acad. Sci. USA *93*, 15323–15328.

Klenerman, P., and Zinkernagel, R.M. (1997). What can we learn about human immunodeficiency virus infection from a study of lymphocytic choriomeningitis virus? Immunol. Rev. *159*, 5–16.

Koff, W.C., Johnson, P.R., Watkins, D.I., Burton, D.R., Lifson, J.D., Hasenkrug, K.J., McDermott, A. B., Schultz, A., Zamb, T.J., Boyle, R., and Desrosiers, R.C. (2006). HIV vaccine design: insights from live attenuated SIV vaccines. Nature Immunol. *7*, 19–23.

Lifson, J.D., Rossio, J.L., Arnaout, R., Li, L., Parks, T.L., Schneider, D.K., Kiser, R.F., Coalter, V.J., Walsh, G., Imming, R.J., *et al.* (2000). Containment of simian immunodeficiency virus infection: cellular immune responses and protection from rechallenge following transient postinoculation antiretroviral treatment. J. Virol. *74*, 2584–2593.

Liu, R., Paxton, W.A., Choe, S., Ceradini, D., Martin, S.R., Horuk, R., MacDonald, M.E., Stuhlman, H., Koup, R.A., and Landau, N.R. (1996). Homozygous defect in HIV-1 coreceptor accounts for resistance of some multiply-exposed individuals to HIV-1 infection. Cell *88*, 7–20.

MacDonald, K.S., Fowke, K.R., Kimani, J., Dunand, V.A., Nagelkerke, N.J., Ball, T.B., Oyugi, J., Njagi, E., Gaur, L.K., Brunham, R.C., *et al.* (2000). Influence of HLA supertypes on susceptibility and resistance to human immunodeficiency virus type 1 infection. J. Infect. Dis. *181*, 1581–1589.

Makedonas, G., Bruneau, J., Alary, M., Tsoukas, C. M., Lowndes, C.M., Lamothe, F., and Bernard, N.F. (2005). Comparison of HIV-specific CD8 T-cell responses among uninfected individuals exposed to HIV parenterally and mucosally. AIDS *19*, 251–259.

Mattapallil, J.J., Douek, D.C., Hill, B., Nishimura, Y., Martin, M., and Roederer, M. (2005). Massive infection and loss of memory CD4[+] T cells in multiple tissues during acute SIV infection. Nature *434*, 1093–1097.

Mazzoli, S., Trabattoni, D., Lo Caputo, S., Piconi, S., Ble, C., Meacci, F., Ruzzante, S., Salvi, A., Semplici, F., Longhi, R., *et al.* (1997). HIV-specific mucosal and cellular immunity in HIV-seronegative partners of HIV-seropositive individuals. Nature Med. *3*, 1250–1257.

McMichael, A.J., and Phillips, R.E. (1997). Escape of human immunodeficiency virus from immune control. Annu. Rev. Immunol. *15*, 271–296.

Miller, C.J., McChesney, M.B., Lu, X., Dailey, P.J., Chutkowski, C., Lu, D., Brosio, P., Roberts, B., and Lu, Y. (1997). Rhesus macaques previously infected with simian/human immunodeficiency virus are protected from vaginal challenge with pathogenic SIVmac239. J. Virol. *71*, 1911–1921.

Murphey-Corb, M., Wilson, L.A., Trichel, A. M., Roberts, D.E., Xu, K., Ohkawa, S., Woodson, B., Bohm, R., and Blanchard, J. (1999). Selective induction of protective MHC class I-restricted CTL in the intestinal lamina propria of rhesus monkeys by transient SIV infection of the colonic mucosa. J. Immunol. *162*, 540–549.

Nishimura, Y., Igarashi, T., Haigwood, N., Sadjadpour, R., Plishka, R.J., Buckler-White, A., Shibata, R., and Martin, M.A. (2002). Determination of a statistically valid neutralization titer in plasma that confers protection against simian-human immunodeficiency virus challenge following passive transfer of high-titered neutralizing antibodies. J. Virol. *76*, 2123–2130.

Oehen, S., Waldner, H., Kundig, T.M., Hengartner, H., and Zinkernagel, R.M. (1992). Antivirally protective cytotoxic T cell memory to lymphocytic choriomeningitis virus is governed by persisting antigen. J. Exp. Med. *176*, 1273–1281.

Ogra, P. L., Faden, H., and Welliver, R.C. (2001). Vaccination strategies for mucosal immune responses. Clin. Microbiol. Rev. *14*, 430–445.

Ourmanov, I., Bilska, M., Hirsch, V.M., and Montefiori, D.C. (2000a). Recombinant modified vaccinia virus Ankara expressing the surface gp120 of simian immunodeficiency virus (SIV) primes for a rapid neutralizing antibody response to SIV infection in macaques. J. Virol. *74*, 2960–2965.

Ourmanov, I., Brown, C.R., Moss, B., Carroll, M., Wyatt, L., Pletneva, L., Goldstein, S., Venzon, D., and Hirsch, V.M. (2000b). Comparative efficacy of recombinant modified vaccinia virus Ankara expressing simian immunodeficiency virus (SIV) Gag-Pol and/or Env in macaques challenged with pathogenic SIV. J. Virol. *74*, 2740–2751.

Parren, P.W., Marx, P.A., Hessell, A.J., Luckay, A., Harouse, J., Cheng-Mayer, C., Moore, J.P., and Burton, D.R. (2001). Antibody protects macaques against vaginal challenge with a pathogenic R5 simian/human immunodeficiency virus at serum levels giving complete neutralization *in vitro*. J. Virol. *75*, 8340–8347.

Parren, P.W., Mondor, I., Naniche, D., Ditzel, H.J., Klasse, P.J., Burton, D.R., and Sattentau, Q.J. (1998). Neutralization of human immunodeficiency virus type 1 by antibody to gp120 is determined primarily by occupancy of sites on the virion irrespective of epitope specificity. J. Virol. *72*, 3512–3519.

Patterson, L.J., Malkevitch, N., Venzon, D., Pinczewski, J., Gomez-Roman, V.R., Wang, L., Kalyanaraman, V.S., Markham, P.D., Robey, F.A., and Robert-Guroff, M. (2004). Protection against mucosal simian immunodeficiency virus SIV(mac251) challenge by using replicating adenovirus-SIV multigene vaccine priming and subunit boosting. J. Virol. *78*, 2212–2221.

Pircher, H., Moskophidis, D., Rohrer, U., Burki, K., Hengartner, H., and Zinkernagel, R.M. (1990). Viral escape by selection of cytotoxic T cell-resistant virus variants *in vivo*. Nature *346*, 629–633.

Poignard, P., Sabbe, R., Picchio, G.R., Wang, M., Gulizia, R.J., Katinger, H., Parren, P.W., Mosier, D.E., and Burton, D.R. (1999). Neutralizing antibodies have limited effects on the control of established HIV-1 infection *in vivo*. Immunity *10*, 431–438.

Price, D.A., Sewell, A.K., Dong, T., Tan, R., Goulder, P.J., Rowland-Jones, S.L., and Phillips, R.E. (1998). Antigen-specific release of beta-chemokines by anti-HIV-1 cytotoxic T lymphocytes. Curr. Biol. *8*, 355–358.

Promadej, N., Costello, C., Wernett, M.M., Kulkarni, P.S., Robison, V.A., Nelson, K.E., Hodge, T.W., Suriyanon, V., Duerr, A., and McNicholl, J.M. (2003). Broad human immunodeficiency virus (HIV)-specific T cell responses to conserved HIV proteins in HIV-seronegative women highly exposed to a single HIV-infected partner. J. Infect. Dis. *187*, 1053–1063.

Putkonen, P., Makitalo, B., Bottiger, D., Biberfeld, G., and Thorstensson, R. (1997). Protection of human immunodeficiency virus type 2-exposed seronegative macaques from mucosal simian immunodeficiency virus transmission. J. Virol. *71*, 4981–4984.

Reynolds, M.R., Rakasz, E., Rudersdorf, R., McDermott A.B., O'Connor, D.H., Friedrich. T.C., Allison, D.B., Patki, A., Picker, L.J., Burton, D.R., Lin, J., Huang, L., Patel, D., Heindecker, G., Fan, J., Citron, M., Horton, M., Wang, F., Liang, X., Shiver, J.W., Casimiro, D.R., Watkins, D.I. (2006). Vaccine-induced cellular immune responses reduce plasma viral concentrations after repeated low-dose challenge with pathogenic simian immunodeficiency virus SIVmac 239. J Virol. *80*, 5875–5885.

Reynolds, M.R., Rakasz, E., Skinner, P.J., White, C., Abel, K., Ma, Z.M., Compton, L., Napoe, G., Wilson, N., Miller, C.J., et al. (2005). CD8+ T-lymphocyte response to major immunodominant epitopes after vaginal exposure to simian immunodeficiency virus: too late and too little. J. Virol. *79*, 9228–9235.

Rose, N.F., Marx, P.A., Luckay, A., Nixon, D.F., Moretto, W.J., Donahoe, S.M., Montefiori, D., Roberts, A., Buonocore, L., and Rose, J.K. (2001). An effective AIDS vaccine based on live attenuated vesicular stomatitis virus recombinants. Cell *106*, 539–549.

Rowland-Jones, S.L., Pinheiro, S., Kaul, R., Hansasuta, P., Gillespie, G., Dong, T., Plummer, F.A., Bwayo, J.B., Fidler, S., Weber, J., et al. (2001). How important is the "quality" of the cytotoxic T lymphocyte (CTL) response in protection against HIV infection? Immunol. Lett. *79*, 15–20.

Schlesinger, J.J., and Chapman, S. (1995). Neutralizing F(ab')2 fragments of protective monoclonal antibodies to yellow fever virus (YF) envelope protein fail to protect mice against lethal YF encephalitis. J. Gen. Virol. *76 (Pt 1)*, 217–220.

Schmitz, J.E., Kuroda, M.J., Santra, S., Sasseville, V.G., Simon, M.A., Lifton, M.A., Racz, P., Tenner-Racz, K., Dalesandro, M., Scallon, B.J., et al. (1999). Control of viremia in simian immunodeficiency virus infection by CD8+ lymphocytes. Science *283*, 857–860.

Shedlock, D.J., and Shen, H. (2003). Requirement for CD4 T cell help in generating functional CD8 T cell memory. Science *300*, 337–339.

Silvestri, G., Sodora, D.L., Koup, R. A., Paiardini, M., O'Neil, S.P., McClure, H.M., Staprans, S.I., and Feinberg, M.B. (2003). Nonpathogenic SIV infection of sooty mangabeys is characterized by limited bystander immunopathology despite chronic high-level viremia. Immunity *18*, 441–452.

Smith, S.M. (2002). HIV vaccine development in the nonhuman primate model of AIDS. J. Biomed. Sci. *9*, 100–111.

Spear, G.T., Hart, M., Olinger, G.G., Hashemi, F.B., and Saifuddin, M. (2001). The role of the complement system in virus infections. Curr. Top. Microbiol. Immunol. *260*, 229–245.

Spear, G.T., Sullivan, B.L., Landay, A.L., and Lint, T.F. (1990). Neutralization of human immunodeficiency virus type 1 by complement occurs by viral lysis. J. Virol. *64*, 5869–5873.

Spear, G.T., Sullivan, B.L., Takefman, D.M., Landay, A.L., and Lint, T.F. (1991). Human immunodeficiency virus (HIV)-infected cells and free virus directly activate the classical complement pathway in rabbit, mouse and guinea-pig sera; activation results in virus neutralization by virolysis. Immunology *73*, 377–382.

Stott, J., and Almond, N. (1995). Assessing animal models of AIDS. Nature Med. *1*, 295–297.

Sun, J.C., and Bevan, M.J. (2003). Defective CD8 T cell memory following acute infection without CD4 T cell help. Science *300*, 339–342.

Traub, E. (1935). A Filterable Virus recovered from white mice. Science, 298–299.

Ulmer, J.B., Donnelly, J.J., Parker, S.E., Rhodes, G.H., Felgner, P.L., Dwarki, V.J., Gromkowski, S.H., Deck, R.R., DeWitt, C.M., Friedman, A., et al. (1993). Heterologous protection against influenza by injection of DNA encoding a viral protein. Science *259*, 1745–1749.

Veazey, R.S., DeMaria, M., Chalifoux, L.V., Shvetz, D.E., Pauley, D.R., Knight, H.L., Rosenzweig, M., Johnson, R.P., Desrosiers, R.C., and Lackner, A.A. (1998). Gastrointestinal tract as a major site of CD4+ T cell depletion and viral replication in SIV infection. Science *280*, 427–431.

Whittle, H.C., Ariyoshi, K., and Rowland-Jones, S. (1998). HIV-2 and T cell recognition. Curr. Opin. Immunol. *10*, 382–387.

Yang, O.O., Kalams, S.A., Trocha, A., Cao, H., Luster, A., Johnson, R.P., and Walker, B.D. (1997). Suppression of human immunodeficiency virus type 1 replication by CD8+ cells: evidence for HLA class I-restricted triggering of cytolytic and noncytolytic mechanisms. J. Virol. *71*, 3120–3128.

Zajac, A.J., Blattman, J.N., Murali-Krishna, K., Sourdive, D.J., Suresh, M., Altman, J.D., and Ahmed, R. (1998). Viral immune evasion due to persistence of activated T cells without effector function. J. Exp. Med. *188*, 2205–2213.

Zhang, C., Cui, Y., Houston, S., and Chang, L.J. (1996). Protective immunity to HIV-1 in SCID/beige mice reconstituted with peripheral blood lymphocytes of exposed but uninfected individuals. Proc. Natl. Acad. Sci. USA 93, 14720–14725.

Zhang, Z., Schuler, T., Zupancic, M., Wietgrefe, S., Staskus, K.A., Reimann, K.A., Reinhart, T.A., Rogan, M., Cavert, W., Miller, C.J., et al. (1999). Sexual transmission and propagation of SIV and HIV in resting and activated CD4+ T cells. Science *286*, 1353–1357.

Zhu, T., Corey, L., Hwangbo, Y., Lee, J M., Learn, G.H., Mullins, J.I., and McElrath, M.J. (2003). Persistence of extraordinarily low levels of genetically homogeneous human immunodeficiency virus type 1 in exposed seronegative individuals. J. Virol. *77*, 6108–6116.

# Part III

# Preclinical Development: Design Challenges

# Antigen Selection and the Design of an AIDS Vaccine

John R. Mascola and Gary J. Nabel

Abstract

Among the many scientific hurdles and uncertainties facing AIDS vaccine development, we are still learning how to optimize immunogens and vaccination strategies to elicit protective HIV-specific immune responses in humans. Many vaccine prototypes have been studied in preclinical and phase I studies, most based on reasonable assumptions about the need to induce HIV-1-specific CD8 T-cell immunity and/or neutralizing antibodies. This chapter provides an overview of the rationale for the choice of immunogens to include in a candidate vaccine and of strategies to optimize their efficacy.

## Introduction

The choice of antigens for an HIV vaccine begins with the 12 or so gene products normally expressed by the virus. These viral gene products include both the major structural proteins and the potent viral regulatory genes that control the expression of HIV during infection. The structural proteins Env, Gag and Pol have long been considered the most relevant targets for HIV vaccine design. Exposure of Env on the surface of the viral envelope makes it the most accessible antigen for antibody neutralization, while the internal proteins Gag and Pol are relatively abundant and therefore logical targets for recognition by the cellular immune system.

However, while Env and Gag are the most abundant viral proteins and most likely to be exposed to the immune system during natural infection, there are good reasons to consider other viral proteins as additional vaccine components. The expression of HIV proteins in infected cells begins with the synthesis of the early, highly spliced RNA species that give rise to the Tat, Rev and Nef gene products. Although these regulatory proteins are synthesized at lower levels within the cell, their function—to regulate expression of the viral structural proteins made from unspliced messages later in the viral replication cycle—suggests that Tat, Rev and Nef offer reasonable "early" vaccine targets. However, further investigation is needed to help determine their relative contribution to protection against HIV.

In choosing specific gene products as immunogens, the character of the immune responses they induce is of paramount importance to HIV vaccine design strategies. It is likely that containment of HIV is more effective when multiple epitopes are presented to the immune system, providing greater selective pressure on viral replication. It is also desirable, at least in theory, to generate T-cell immunity to linear epitopes that span a large percentage of the viral open reading frames. In terms of humoral immunity, antibody responses can be generated to nearly all HIV proteins. However, finding strategies that induce relevant broadly neutralizing antibodies to the viral envelope and can deal with the enormous clade and strain diversity of Env remains the most important challenge in designing HIV vaccines (Chapters 7 and 10).

This chapter presents an overview of the rationale for various vaccine strategies and for the choice of immunogens to include in candidate vaccines, in light of these considerations.

## Vaccines designed to elicit HIV-specific CD8 T-cell responses

Several lines of evidence suggest that HIV-specific CD8[+] T-cells play an important role in controlling HIV replication in humans (Douek *et al.*, 2006; Pantaleo and Koup, 2004), while more direct proof comes from the SIV/SHIV macaque model (Chapters 4 and 5). Based on this evidence, a major goal of many HIV-1 vaccine strategies is to generate cellular immunity, particularly HIV-specific CD8[+] T-cells. These types of vaccines are often referred to as cytotoxic T-cell (CTL)-based vaccines. (Additional design considerations for CTL-based vaccines are discussed in Chapter 8, and the potential contribution of CD4[+] T-(helper) cells to protection is reviewed in Chapter 5.)

### Gene-based vaccine strategies

Safety concerns inherent in the traditional approaches of live attenuated and whole-inactivated virus vaccination have made these modalities impractical for HIV. These constraints have led to a plethora of novel vaccine strategies aimed at generating potent T-cellular immunity. These newer gene-based platforms include DNA plasmids and recombinant viral vectors, each encoding HIV immunogens under the control of potent eukaryotic promoters. DNA plasmid immunization can induce detectable immune responses in non-human primates, but more robust responses are generated after boosting with a viral vector (Letvin *et al.*, 2002). This bimodal strategy of DNA prime followed by viral vector boost has become a common approach for eliciting cellular responses. However, viral vectors, alone or in sequential combinations, may also induce robust immunity.

Vectors of the poxvirus family have been the most extensively studied for SIV and HIV vaccines. Initial studies were performed with the prototype replication-competent vaccinia virus; more recent work has used less pathogenic poxviruses such as modified vaccinia Ankara (MVA), NYVAC (New York vaccinia virus attenuated by gene deletions) and canarypox (ALVAC). Other replication-competent viral vectors in use include the adenovirus attenuated serotypes 4 and 7, vesicular stomatitis virus (VSV) and poliovirus, all of which can induce cellular responses in non-human primates.

Another group of viral vectors are those that have been engineered to produce a single cycle of infection and gene delivery, which may offer some inherent safety advantages. This category includes vectors of the alphavirus family (such as Venezuelan equine encephalitis virus, Semliki forest virus and Sindbis), recombinant serotype-5 adenovirus (rAd-5), adeno-associated virus (AAV) and herpes simplex virus (HSV). The details of these vectors are reviewed elsewhere (Barouch, 2006; Letvin *et al.*, 2002; Nabel, 2001). Among these vectors, the largest body of human clinical data exists for serotype 5 rAd, since these vectors have been used for both gene therapy and as candidate AIDS vaccines, having been tested in hundreds of volunteers. Immunization data from non-human primate studies with rAd vectors are promising, and two candidate vaccines using rAd5 vectors have advanced into phase II human trials. Of note, owing to the potential for decreased immunogenicity of these vaccines in people with pre-existing immunity to rAd-5 (a widespread virus that causes the common cold), novel rAd serotypes are also being evaluated preclinically.

## Choice of immunogens

HIV-1 vaccine design is complicated by the enormous genetic diversity of the virus, which adds greatly to its antigenic complexity in nature. A key vaccine design challenge is therefore to find strategies that induce coverage against the highly diverse range of circulating strains. It is also important to note that the extreme variability of the major histocompatibility (HLA) complex in humans, a genetic region which determines what epitopes the immune system can recognize, adds to the unpredictable nature of immune responsiveness to any given epitope.

Since gene-based vectors can be readily manipulated, investigators have considerable flexibility in choosing (and varying) the immunogens to include in these HIV vaccine candidates. While some insight comes from knowledge of HLA-restricted epitopes in natural HIV infection and from data on non-human primate models, there is unfortunately little direct scientific evidence to guide the choice of immunogens. Furthermore, the genetic diversity of HIV-1 does not necessarily translate into differences in immunogenicity among viral isolates, so it remains unknown how this genetic variability will affect the breadth of protective immunity. For now, these uncertainties mean that vaccine designers must make numerous empirical choices regarding immunogens. As more data accumulates from phase I studies of different vaccines, these choices will increasingly be guided by carefully derived data on the types and potencies of immune responses the different candidates generate.

Currently, there are various vaccine approaches under development, including those containing single or multiple conserved genes; genes genetically matched to the most common circulating strains in a given geographic region; "cocktails" with multiple genes derived from diverse HIV-1 strains; and consensus or ancestral sequences.

### Vaccines based on conserved genes

Because CTLs are more likely than antibodies to be effective against internal viral proteins, T-cell-based vaccine development has focused largely on using Gag and Pol, two of the most conserved HIV proteins, as immunogens. Gag proteins from HIV strains of different genetic subtypes differ by only about 15% in their amino acid sequences, and Pol proteins by roughly 10%—in contrast to the envelope protein, where inter-subtype diversity is as high as 35%, and up to 20% even within a single subtype (Gaschen *et al.*, 2002). Thus, one strategy for CTL-based vaccine design is to target proteins that are 85—90% conserved among diverse HIV strains. If the immune responses to Gag and Pol prove to be protective, an effective vaccine may not need to be multivalent.

Unfortunately, there are only very limited data to support or refute this approach (McMichael and Hanke, 2002). Non-human primate studies indicate that DNA and/or viral vectors containing Gag or Gag–Pol induce partial protection against a homologous SIV challenge (Amara *et al.*, 2002; Ourmanov *et al.*, 2000). These studies support the notion that Gag and Pol are useful in a vaccine, but they do not address the breadth of protective immunity against heterologous virus challenge. Recombinant rAd type 5 vectors expressing SIV Gag have also been shown to provide partial protection against homologous SHIV challenge (Shiver *et al.*, 2002).

However, vaccines of this type have a potential downside: the documented occurrence of CTL escape. In the SHIV-macaque model, the partial protection afforded by SIV Gag-specific CD8$^+$ T-cell responses can be overcome by a single mutation in the immunodominant Gag CTL epitope, which led to increased plasma viremia and disease progression in several Gag-vaccinated animals (Barouch *et al.*, 2002). In humans, CTL escape from a conserved HLA B27-restricted Gag CTL epitope leads to loss of immune recognition and to disease progression (Goulder *et al.*, 2001). These data provide a conceptual rationale for including multiple genes in a vaccine construct—that vaccine-induced responses to a diverse array of epitopes may, in the event of infection with HIV, prevent or limit viral escape from these responses.

Indeed, many research groups have developed gene-based constructs that express multiple HIV proteins, usually including Gag, Pol and Env, and in a few cases regulatory genes such as Tat, Rev and Nef. Among the latter genes, Tat has received the most attention because it is expressed very early after viral infection and may therefore be a useful initial target for vaccine-induced responses. While macaque challenge studies have yielded conflicting data about the effect of Tat vaccination (Allen *et al.*, 2002; Cafaro *et al.*, 1999), there remains interest in both protein and gene-based immunization strategies for Tat, and a phase I human study of a recombinant Tat protein is now under way in Italy.

## Multiclade "cocktail" vaccines

To address the question of how vaccine designers should tackle the issue of viral diversity, the Vaccine Research Center (VRC) of the US National Institutes of Allergy and Infectious Disease (within the National Institutes of Health) sponsored a meeting in July 2001, together with the World Health Organization and the Joint United Nations Program on HIV/AIDS, leading to a set of consensus recommendations (Nabel *et al.*, 2002). There was general agreement that HIV diversity may be an obstacle, but that there is little scientific rationale for matching vaccine immunogens directly to strains circulating in each country. Producing and testing multiclade vaccines was also suggested, but practical limitations on manufacturing and testing dictate that vaccine candidates should be representative of clades rather than country specific.

As a result of these recommendations, the VRC undertook efforts to develop a multigene, multiclade immunogen based on DNA plasmids and recombinant rAd vectors. This candidate vaccine contains six different DNA plasmid constructs: one each encoding Gag, Pol and Nef (based on the clade B HxB2 viral sequence), and the other three encoding the gp145 envelope sequence from clade A, B and C respectively. Four rAd vectors were also made, and will be used to boost the DNA immunization. One rAd virus encodes a Gag-Pol fusion protein and the other three encode secreted gp140 versions of the clade A, B and C Env glycoproteins. Phase I studies of the individual DNA and rAd vaccines have been completed, and further phase I studies are evaluating DNA prime, given as 3 immunizations, followed by a single boost with rAd. Phase II studies are ongoing.

## Immunogens matched to circulating clades/ geographic region

Another approach to vaccines and viral diversity is to match the vaccine immunogen to the predominant viral sequences circulating in the region where the vaccine will be tested. The first such candidate vaccine to be tested in the clinic was

a DNA/MVA combination containing a consensus clade A Gag gene fused to a string of partially overlapping clade A-derived CTL epitopes (Hanke and McMichael, 2000). The Gag protein contained both HLA class I- and II-restricted epitopes to induce CTLs as well as T-cell help, which is thought to be important in inducing potent immune responses. This candidate vaccine has been studied in phase I trials in Kenya (where clade A viruses predominate) and in the United Kingdom and initial data demonstrated a low level of immunogenicity. Whether this was due to the immunization platform, or gene inserts, or a combination of the two, is not yet clear.

## Vaccines based on consensus or ancestral sequences

As an alternative to clade-specific vaccine constructs, some investigators have suggested that evolutionary relationships may be more useful (Gaschen *et al.*, 2002). They propose using consensus or ancestral sequences that minimize the genetic differences between vaccine strains and circulating isolates. This is an intriguing approach to CTL-based immunization: rather than using genes from a single, arbitrarily chosen HIV-1 isolate, the hypothesis is that a consensus or ancestral sequence will induce an immune response which recognizes a greater proportion of circulating viruses than would responses induced by/vaccines based on any one isolate. Immunogens incorporating these types of designs are progressing through preclinical evaluation, and further studies should indicate if this approach does in fact expand the breadth of immunity.

## Vaccines designed to elicit neutralizing antibodies

Traditional viral vaccines, such as those for polio and influenza, elicit neutralizing antibodies that play a major role in conferring protective immunity. The success of the hepatitis B vaccine, which is based on recombinant protein expression of the viral surface antigen, led to optimism that the surface glycoprotein of HIV-1 could also be used as an effective vaccine. However, phase I studies of gp120 and gp160 vaccine products demonstrated that the neutralizing antibodies they elicited were active mainly against laboratory-adapted rather than primary HIV-1 isolates (Mascola *et al.*, 1996). The successful completion of two phase III trials of bivalent gp120 recombinant vaccines has provided clear evidence that the antibody response they induced was not protective (Graham and Mascola, 2005).

We now appreciate that this outcome reflects the ability of HIV-1 to employ a complex array of immune evasion mechanisms, thereby avoiding antibody-mediated neutralization. This complexity explains why monomeric gp120 vaccines can elicit high levels of anti-gp120 antibodies that are limited in their ability to bind and neutralize most primary HIV-1 strains (Burton *et al.*, 2004). Yet, there is strong evidence from animal models that appropriately potent neutralizing antibodies *can* protect: passive immunization of macaques with neutralizing monoclonal antibodies, followed by SHIV-challenge, either prevents the establishment of infection or mediates long-term reductions in plasma viremia (Mascola, 2003). Thus, newer antibody-based vaccines strategies are aimed at developing immunogens that generate antibodies of greater potency and breadth of reactivity.

## Design of improved antibody-based immunogens

One approach to improving antibody responses is based on the hypothesis that a protein immunogen should closely mimic the native structure of the HIV-1 envelope glycoprotein. Antibody mapping studies, and the more recent HIV-1 gp120 atomic structure analyses, suggest that many epitopes exposed on monomeric gp120 are hidden within the native trimeric glycoprotein (Burton *et al.*, 2004; Chen *et al.*, 2005). Thus, trimeric envelope proteins may focus antibodies onto viral epitopes that are exposed on the native virion, and may therefore be more effective immunogens than monomers for eliciting neutralizing antibodies. Several groups are pursuing this strategy (Binley *et al.*, 2000; Farzan *et al.*, 1998), and emerging data tend to support this view (Yang *et al.*, 2001). However, the antibody specificities elicited by these oligomeric protein vaccines have not yet been well characterized and further research is required to determine if such proteins can be designed to elicit potent neutralizing antibody responses. A related approach attempts to use specific epitopes of the well-known neutralizing monoclonal antibodies 2F5, 4E10, 2G12 and b12 as immunogens. These immunogens can be linear peptides, peptide mimetics or peptides exposed on phage display libraries. While there is substantial ongoing work in this area, no immunogens to date have been able to elicit antibodies matching the specificities of these neutralizing mAbs. Of the four mAbs noted above, two neutralize by binding to the membrane proximal region of gp41. The epitopes of this region of gp41 were initially thought to be linear in nature, but attempts to elicit 2F5 or 4E10 like antibodies using linear peptides have been unsuccessful and recent structural data demonstrates a more complex non-linear conformation of the ectodomain of gp41. Thus, recent work has focused on an understanding of the structural basis of gp41-mediated neutralization, in hopes that this will lead to novel strategies for immunogen design (Cardoso *et al.*, 2005; Ofek *et al.*, 2004).

A complementary strategy for designing antibody-based vaccines is to introduce specific modifications into the HIV-1 envelope structure to expose or stabilize key epitopes better. Since HIV-1 is a chronically replicating lentivirus, it must continually evade the host's antibody response (Richman *et al.*, 2003; Wei *et al.*, 2003). Our understanding of these immune evasion mechanisms is still emerging, but it appears that the virus uses variable loop structures, sugar moieties and the tertiary conformation of the trimeric envelope structure to shield neutralization epitopes (Burton *et al.*, 2004). It may therefore be possible to modify the envelope structure to better display neutralization epitopes that are otherwise cryptic or suboptimally immunogenic. It is known that the removal of specific glycosylation sites in the variable loop regions leads to better exposure of neutralization epitopes and renders the virus highly sensitive to neutralizing antibodies. Immunogens based on these modifications may therefore generate better neutralizing antibody responses (Barnett *et al.*, 2001; Kolchinsky *et al.*, 2001; Yang *et al.*, 2004). However, it is not yet clear if the antibodies will be able to bind the native envelope glycoprotein present on most primary viruses.

Other investigators have pursued a strategy of stabilizing envelope glycoprotein intermediates that arise during the process of virus–cell fusion. Such fusion intermediate epitopes (which include epitopes on the chemokine binding domain, induced after CD4 binding, and on the pre-hairpin intermediate that forms before the final steps of fusion) (He *et al.*, 2003) are highly conserved and thus are promising potential targets for neutralizing antibodies. While we have an improved understanding of the structure and function of these epitopes, they have so far been difficult targets for vaccine design. Antibody access to these fusion intermediate epitopes appears to be restricted by both kinetic and special constraints, i.e., there may be limited time and space for antibodies to successfully bind to these epitopes (Burton *et al.*, 2004). Our group at the VRC has designed a gene-based *env* immunogen with deletions in the gp120/41 cleavage site, the fusion domain and the gp41 heptad repeats. These mutations appear to stabilize the envelope conformation and improve antibody responses (Chakrabarti *et al.*, 2002). More recently, we have shown that selective modifications which stabilize the V3 loop and remove the V12 region can improve the potency of neutralizing antibodies directed against the V3 loop (Yang *et al.*, 2004). While current immunogens do not elicit broadly neutralizing antibodies, these data provide conceptual proof that the immunogenicity of neutralization epitopes can be improved by structural modifications to the envelope glycoprotein. Another recent approach uses a hyperglycosylated envelope glycoprotein that shields most non-neutralizing epitopes. This type of modified envelope is designed to preferentially bind antibodies directed against the CD4 binding site of gp120, particularly the potently neutralizing IgG1b12 (Pantophlet *et al.*, 2003).

## Breadth of the neutralizing antibody response

Many studies of antibody reactivity have demonstrated that HIV-1 displays a remarkable amount of antigenic diversity. While genetic subtype may not strictly correspond to neutralization serotype, there is ample evidence that the antibody response in natural infection is generally not broadly neutralizing: for example, sera from most clade B-infected patients have a limited breadth of activity against other clade B viruses and even less activity against viruses from different clades (Bures *et al.*, 2002). Even neutralizing mAbs such as 2F5 and b12 neutralize only 70–90% of clade B viruses, and an even lower percentage of non-clade B viruses (Binley *et al.*, 2004). Only a few sera appear to be broadly neutralizing, and the specificities of antibodies that collectively create this activity have not yet been well defined. Since most current vaccine immunogens appear to induce neutralizing antibodies of only modest potency and breadth, the antigenic diversity of HIV-1 is viewed as a major obstacle for antibody-based vaccines.

Given this diversity, it is possible that antibodies induced by a particular vaccine immunogen will react best (or only) with closely related viruses, and many groups are therefore constructing envelope immunogens from non-clade B subtypes (Hanke and McMichael, 2000; Seaman et al., 2005; Williamson et al., 2003). There have been few studies evaluating multivalent antibody-based immunogens (Cho et al., 2001; Seaman et al., 2005) but several research groups are pursing this approach, especially using DNA immunization followed by protein or viral vector boost (since they allow rapid construction and evaluation of multiple env gene candidates). This strategy can potentially be used to elicit both virus-specific CTL and neutralizing antibodies.

As multivalent envelope immunogens are developed, we will need more accurate means to compare the breadth of neutralization elicited by candidate vaccines. A consensus working group has recently recommended the use of standardized panels of clonal Env-pseudoviruses as suitable reagents to assess and compare neutralizing antibody response (Mascola et al., 2005). Env-pseudoviruses are made by co-transfection of a suitable cells line with an env-defective HIV-1 molecular clone and an Env expression plasmid encoding the Env of interest. Env pseudoviruses have been used by several groups of investigators (Binley et al., 2004; Richman et al., 2003; Wei et al., 2003) to measure HIV-1 neutralization and there are several advantages to this assay format. The precise amino acid sequence of the Env glycoprotein for each virus is known and exists as a stable DNA plasmid. This facilitates reagent transfer and standardization across laboratories. In addition, the neutralizing antibody response can potentially be mapped to regions of known Env sequence. Understanding the precise specificities of antibodies elicited by novel vaccine immunogens could provide valuable information for future vaccine design. The first standard virus panel, based on clade B viruses, has been constructed (Li et al., 2005) and virus panels based on other clades are in progress.

## References

Allen, T.M., Mortara, L., Mothe, B.R., Liebl, M., Jing, P., Calore, B., Piekarczyk, M., Ruddersdorf, R., O'Connor, D. H., Wang, X., et al. (2002). Tat-vaccinated macaques do not control simian immunodeficiency virus SIVmac239 replication. J. Virol. 76, 4108–4112.

Amara, R.R., Smith, J.M., Staprans, S.I., Montefiori, D.C., Villinger, F., Altman, J.D., O'Neil, S.P., Kozyr, N.L., Xu, Y., Wyatt, L.S., et al. (2002). Critical role for Env as well as Gag-Pol in control of a simian-human immunodeficiency virus 89.6P challenge by a DNA prime/recombinant modified vaccinia virus Ankara vaccine. J. Virol. 76, 6138–6146.

Barnett, S.W., Lu, S., Srivastava, I., Cherpelis, S., Gettie, A., Blanchard, J., Wang, S., Mboudjeka, I., Leung, L., Lian, Y., et al. (2001). The ability of an oligomeric human immunodeficiency virus type 1 (HIV-1) envelope antigen to elicit neutralizing antibodies against primary HIV-1 isolates is improved following partial deletion of the second hypervariable region. J. Virol. 75, 5526–5540.

Barouch, D.H. (2006). Rational design of gene-based vaccines. J. Pathol. 208, 283–289.

Barouch, D.H., Kunstman, J., Kuroda, M.J., Schmitz, J.E., Santra, S., Peyerl, F. W., Krivulka, G.R., Beaudry, K., Lifton, M.A., Gorgone, D.A., et al. (2002). Eventual AIDS vaccine failure in a rhesus monkey by viral escape from cytotoxic T lymphocytes. Nature 415, 335–339.

Binley, J.M., Sanders, R.W., Clas, B., Schuelke, N., Master, A., Guo, Y., Kajumo, F., Anselma, D.J., Maddon, P.J., Olson, W.C., and Moore, J.P. (2000). A recombinant human immunodeficiency virus type 1 envelope glycoprotein complex stabilized by an intermolecular disulfide bond between the gp120 and gp41 subunits is an antigenic mimic of the trimeric virion- associated structure. J. Virol. 74, 627–643.

Binley, J.M., Wrin, T., Korber, B., Zwick, M.B., Wang, M., Chappey, C., Stiegler, G., Kunert, R., Zolla-Pazner, S., Katinger, H., et al. (2004). Comprehensive cross-clade neutralization analysis of a panel of anti-human immunodeficiency virus type 1 monoclonal antibodies. J. Virol. 78, 13232–13252.

Bures, R., Morris, L., Williamson, C., Ramjee, G., Deers, M., Fiscus, S.A., Abdool-Karim, S., and Montefiori, D.C. (2002). Regional clustering of shared neutralization determinants on primary isolates of clade C human immunodeficiency virus type 1 from South Africa. J. Virol. 76, 2233–2244.

Burton, D.R., Desrosiers, R.C., Doms, R.W., Koff, W.C., Kwong, P.D., Moore, J.P., Nabel, G.J., Sodroski, J., Wilson, I.A., and Wyatt, R.T. (2004). HIV vaccine design and the neutralizing antibody problem. Nature Immunol. 5, 233–236.

Cafaro, A., Caputo, A., Fracasso, C., Maggiorella, M.T., Goletti, D., Baroncelli, S., Pace, M., Sernicola, L., Koanga-Mogtomo, M.L., Betti, M., et al. (1999). Control of SHIV-89.6P-infection of cynomolgus monkeys by HIV-1 Tat protein vaccine. Nature Med. 5, 643–650.

Cardoso, R.M., Zwick, M.B., Stanfield, R.L., Kunert, R., Binley, J.M., Katinger, H., Burton, D.R., and Wilson, I.A. (2005). Broadly neutralizing anti-HIV antibody 4E10 recognizes a helical conformation of a highly conserved fusion-associated motif in gp41. Immunity 22, 163–173.

Chakrabarti, B.K., Kong, W.P., Wu, B.Y., Yang, Z.Y., Friborg, J., Ling, X., King, S.R., Montefiori, D. C., and Nabel, G.J. (2002). Modifications of the human immunodeficiency virus envelope glycoprotein enhance immunogenicity for genetic immunization. J. Virol. 76, 5357–5368.

Chen, B., Vogan, E.M., Gong, H., Skehel, J.J., Wiley, D.C., and Harrison, S.C. (2005). Structure of an unliganded simian immunodeficiency virus gp120 core. Nature 433, 834–841.

Cho, M.W., Kim, Y.B., Lee, M.K., Gupta, K.C., Ross, W., Plishka, R., Buckler-White, A., Igarashi, T., Theodore, T., Byrum, R., et al. (2001). Polyvalent envelope glycoprotein vaccine elicits a broader neutralizing antibody response but is unable to provide sterilizing protection against heterologous simian/human immunodeficiency virus infection in pigtailed macaques. J. Virol. 75, 2224–2234.

Douek, D.C., Kwong, P.D., and Nabel, G.J. (2006). The rational design of an AIDS vaccine. Cell 124, 677–681.

Farzan, M., Choe, H., Desjardins, E., Sun, Y., Kuhn, J., Cao, J., Archambault, D., Kolchinsky, P., Koch, M., Wyatt, R., and Sodroski, J. (1998). Stabilization of human immunodeficiency virus type 1 envelope glycoprotein trimers by disulfide bonds introduced into the gp41 glycoprotein ectodomain. J. Virol. 72, 7620–7625.

Gaschen, B., Taylor, J., Yusim, K., Foley, B., Gao, F., Lang, D., Novitsky, V., Haynes, B., Hahn, B.H., Bhattacharya, T., and Korber, B. (2002). Diversity considerations in HIV-1 vaccine selection. Science 296, 2354–2360.

Goulder, P.J., Brander, C., Tang, Y., Tremblay, C., Colbert, R.A., Addo, M.M., Rosenberg, E.S., Nguyen, T., Allen, R., Trocha, A., et al. (2001). Evolution and transmission of stable CTL escape mutations in HIV infection. Nature 412, 334–338.

Graham, B.S., and Mascola, J.R. (2005). Lessons from Failure–Preparing for Future HIV-1 Vaccine Efficacy Trials. J. Infect. Dis. 191, 647–649.

Hanke, T., and McMichael, A.J. (2000). Design and construction of an experimental HIV-1 vaccine for a year-(2000) clinical trial in Kenya. Nature Med. 6, 951–955.

He, Y., Vassell, R., Zaitseva, M., Nguyen, N., Yang, Z., Weng, Y., and Weiss, C.D. (2003). Peptides trap the human immunodeficiency virus type 1 envelope glycoprotein fusion intermediate at two sites. J. Virol. *77*, 1666–1671.

Kolchinsky, P., Kiprilov, E., and Sodroski, J. (2001). Increased Neutralization Sensitivity of CD4-Independent Human Immunodeficiency Virus Variants. J. Virol. *75*, 2041–2050.

Letvin, N.L., Barouch, D.H., and Montefiori, D.C. (2002). Prospects for vaccine protection against HIV-1 infection and AIDS. Annu Rev Immunol *20*, 73–99.

Li, M., Gao, F., Mascola, J.R., Stamatatos, L., Polonis, V.R., Koutsoukos, M., Voss, G., Goepfert, P., Gilbert, P., Greene, K.M., *et al.* (2005). Human Immunodeficiency Virus type 1 env clones from acute and early subtype B Infections for standardized assessments of vaccine-elicited neutralizing antibodies. J. Virol. *79*, 10108–10125.

Mascola, J.R. (2003). Defining the protective antibody response for HIV-1. Curr. Mol. Med. *3*, 209–216.

Mascola, J.R., D'Souza, P., Gilbert, P., Hahn, B.H., Haigwood, N.L., Morris, L., Petropoulos, C.J., Polonis, V.R., Sarzotti, M., and Montefiori, D.C. (2005). Recommendations for the design and use of standard virus panels to assess neutralizing antibody responses elicited by candidate human immunodeficiency virus type 1 vaccines. J. Virol. *79*, 10103–10107.

Mascola, J.R., Snyder, S.W., Weislow, O.S., Belay, S.M., Belshe, R.B., Schwartz, D.H., Clements, M.L., Dolin, R., Graham, B.S., Gorse, G.J., *et al.* (1996). Immunization with envelope subunit vaccine products elicits neutralizing antibodies against laboratory-adapted but not primary isolates of human immunodeficiency virus type 1. The National Institute of Allergy and Infectious Diseases AIDS Vaccine Evaluation Group. J. Infect. Dis. *173*, 340–348.

McMichael, A., and Hanke, T. (2002). The quest for an AIDS vaccine: is the CD8+ T-cell approach feasible? Nature Rev. Immunol. *2*, 283–291.

Nabel, G., Makgoba, W., and Esparza, J. (2002). HIV-1 diversity and vaccine development. Science *296*, 2335.

Nabel, G.J. (2001). Challenges and opportunities for development of an AIDS vaccine. Nature *410*, 1002–1007.

Ofek, G., Tang, M., Sambor, A., Katinger, H., Mascola, J. R., Wyatt, R., and Kwong, P.D. (2004). Structure and mechanistic analysis of the anti-human immunodeficiency virus type 1 antibody 2F5 in complex with its gp41 epitope. J. Virol. *78*, 10724–10737.

Ourmanov, I., Brown, C. R., Moss, B., Carroll, M., Wyatt, L., Pletneva, L., Goldstein, S., Venzon, D., and Hirsch, V. M. (2000). Comparative efficacy of recombinant modified vaccinia virus Ankara expressing simian immunodeficiency virus (SIV) Gag-Pol and/or Env in macaques challenged with pathogenic SIV. J. Virol. *74*, 2740–2751.

Pantaleo, G., and Koup, R.A. (2004). Correlates of immune protection in HIV-1 infection: what we know, what we don't know, what we should know. Nat Med *10*, 806–810.

Pantophlet, R., Wilson, I.A., and Burton, D.R. (2003). Hyperglycosylated mutants of human immunodeficiency virus (HIV) type 1 monomeric gp120 as novel antigens for HIV vaccine design. J. Virol. *77*, 5889–5901.

Richman, D.D., Wrin, T., Little, S.J., and Petropoulos, C.J. (2003). Rapid evolution of the neutralizing antibody response to HIV type 1 infection. Proc. Natl. Acad. Sci. USA *100*, 4144–4149.

Seaman, M.S., Xu, L., Beaudry, K., Martin, K.L., Beddall, M.H., Miura, A., Sambor, A., Chakrabarti, B.K., Huang, Y., Bailer, R., *et al.* (2005). Multiclade human immunodeficiency virus type 1 envelope immunogens elicit broad cellular and humoral immunity in rhesus monkeys. J. Virol. *79*, 2956–2963.

Shiver, J.W., Fu, T.M., Chen, L., Casimiro, D. R., Davies, M.E., Evans, R.K., Zhang, Z. Q., Simon, A.J., Trigona, W.L., Dubey, S.A., *et al.* (2002). Replication-incompetent adenoviral vaccine vector elicits effective anti-immunodeficiency-virus immunity. Nature *415*, 331–335.

Wei, X., Decker, J.M., Wang, S., Hui, H., Kappes, J.C., Wu, X., Salazar-Gonzalez, J.F., Salazar, M.G., Kilby, J.M., Saag, M.S., *et al.* (2003). Antibody neutralization and escape by HIV-1. Nature *422*, 307–312.

Williamson, C., Morris, L., Maughan, M.F., Ping, L.H., Dryga, S.A., Thomas, R., Reap, E. A., Cilliers, T., van Harmelen, J., Pascual, A., *et al.* (2003). Characterization and selection of HIV-1 subtype C isolates for use in vaccine development. AIDS Res. Hum. Retroviruses *19*, 133–144.

Yang, X., Wyatt, R., and Sodroski, J. (2001). Improved elicitation of neutralizing antibodies against primary human immunodeficiency viruses by soluble stabilized envelope glycoprotein trimers. J. Virol. *75*, 1165–1171.

Yang, Z.Y., Chakrabarti, B.K., Xu, L., Welcher, B., Kong, W. P., Leung, K., Panet, A., Mascola, J.R., and Nabel, G.J. (2004). Selective modifications of variable loops alters tropism and enhances immunogenicity of HIV-1 envelope. J. Virol. *78*, 4029–4036.

# Broadly Neutralizing Antibodies and a Vaccine for HIV

7

Suganya Selvarajah and Dennis R. Burton

## Abstract

HIV vaccine developers increasingly believe that the best protection against HIV/AIDS will probably require both cellular immunity and antibodies that neutralize a broad range of viral strains. However, designing immunogens that elicit such antibodies has emerged as one of the most challenging problems facing the field. This article reviews these challenges, most of which pertain to the structural features of the HIV envelope (gp120 and gp41). It also describes several strategies being pursued to overcome them by favorably presenting conserved epitopes that have been identified as targets for broadly neutralizing antibodies. However, success will require considerable progress in understanding the structure of Env and its interaction with neutralizing antibodies, in identifying new neutralizing monoclonal antibodies that can fuel this research, and in immunogen design.

## Introduction

Over the past few years, a growing body of data suggests that an effective HIV vaccine needs to elicit both broadly effective neutralizing antibodies and vigorous cell-mediated immunity (CMI) (Letvin and Walker, 2003). Much of this evidence comes from studies that highlight the limitations of CMI alone (Chapter 4), and from the failure of vaccines based on gp120 monomers to prevent infection or mitigate the course of disease in two recent phase III efficacy trials (Chapter 14). At the same time, neutralizing antibodies have been shown to be protective in several animal models, most convincingly in macaques challenged either intravenously or vaginally with SHIV (Mascola, 2003). This emerging picture has rekindled efforts to design immunogens that elicit neutralizing antibodies (NAbs) to the broadest possible range of HIV strains, so that protection extends to the extensive (and continuously increasing) diversity of HIV strains circulating globally (Chapter 10).

## Challenges in designing immunogens that elicit broadly neutralizing antibodies to HIV

Monomeric gp120, the target for the first generation of candidate HIV vaccines, elicits NAbs against HIV strains adapted to grow in laboratory tissue culture, but not against primary isolates of HIV circulating in populations. This observation, initially made more than a decade ago, began to focus attention on the structural biology of gp120 and gp41 (the HIV envelope spike) (Env) and on understanding the interaction of HIV with the few known antibodies that *can* neutralize a broad range of strains. Such antibodies have been detected both in sera from HIV-infected people and as *broadly* neutralizing monoclonal antibodies (mAbs).

Analysis of these broadly neutralizing antibodies has shown that they recognize conserved gp120 and gp41 regions exposed (intrinsically or during the fusion process) on the surface of the viral envelope (Fig. 7.1) (Sattentau and Moore, 1995; Golding et al., 2002). Studies of the broadly neutralizing mAbs suggest that their neutralizing capacity is associated with the ability to bind to functional Env on the virus, but does *not* correlate with binding to isolated gp120 or gp41 subunits (Sattentau and Moore, 1995). Therefore, failure of an immunogen to elicit broad NAbs is interpreted as a failure to elicit antibodies with reasonable binding affinities for conserved parts of the Env protein, either before or during fusion.

The structure of the monomeric gp120 core (Kwong et al., 1998, 2000; Wyatt et al., 1998) (Fig. 7.2) and the mod-

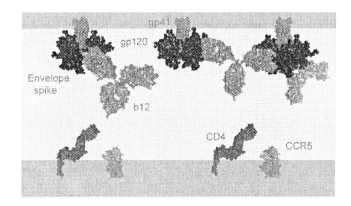

**Figure 7.1** Model of neutralization of HIV-1 by anti-gp120 antibodies. Gp120-specific antibodies such as b12 bind to envelope spikes and probably prevent interaction with viral receptors by steric obstruction (adapted from Poignard et al., Annual Reviews of Immunology, 2001).

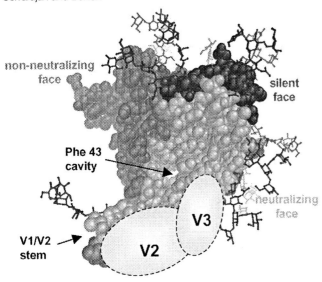

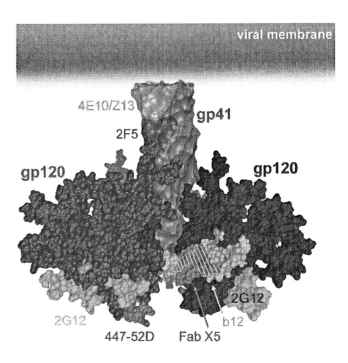

**Figure 7.2** The structure of the gp120 core. The faces of the gp120 molecule were defined by the interactions between gp120 and antibodies (Wyatt *et al.*, 1998). The neutralizing face encompasses the CD4 binding site; the location of the cavity into which Phe43 of the CD4 binds is indicated. The non-neutralizing face is inaccessible to antibody on trimeric Env because of interaction with gp41 and/or close approach of other gp120 protomers. The silent face is covered with carbohydrate chains. The approximate locations of the V1/V2 and V3 loops are shown schematically.

**Figure 7.3** Cartoon model of HIV-1 trimeric envelope spike representing epitopes of broadly neutralizing antibodies. The antibodies b12, Fab X5, 447–52D and 2G12 recognize relatively conserved epitopes on gp120. The antibodies 2F5, 4E10 and Z13 recognize conserved epitopes on gp41. The trimer structure is based on the structure proposed by Kwong *et al.* (2000). The image was made using PMV and msms programs by E. Ollman Saphire.

eled structure of the native Env trimer (which consists of three gp120-gp41 heterodimers) (Fig. 7.3) suggest explanations for this failure. A large region of the gp120 surface is covered by carbohydrate molecules that mask potential epitopes (hence its designation as the "silent face"). Much of the remaining surface is involved in interaction with gp41 or neighboring gp120 protomers and is therefore not accessible to antibodies (the "non-neutralizing face"). The conserved CD4 binding site (CD4bs), an important potential target for NAbs (since the binding of gp120 to CD4 on target T-cells is a crucial early step in the HIV replicative cycle) is somewhat recessed within the core of gp120, where it is readily available to the long, thin CD4 molecule but not to more bulky antibody molecules. Access to the CD4bs is also further restricted by the immuno-dominant variable loops. Another potential target for NAbs, gp120's conserved co-receptor binding site, only becomes reasonably accessible once CD4 has bound to gp120; it then becomes accessible to antibody fragments but not to whole antibody molecules. Moreover, a degree of structural disorder within the gp120 molecule may also reduce antibody recognition, a phenomenon known as "entropic masking" (Kwong *et al.*, 2002). Lastly, except possibly for a region close to the membrane, gp41 on Env trimers appears to be largely inaccessible to antibodies.

However, on the more promising side, a small panel of broadly neutralizing mAbs (Fig. 7.3) isolated from HIV-infected people has helped identify conserved regions of the Env trimer that *can* be targeted by a next-generation HIV vaccine. These mAbs include b12, which recognizes an epitope overlap-

ping the CD4 binding site (CD4bs) of gp120 (Saphire *et al.*, 2001); 2G12, recognizing a conserved cluster of oligomannose chains on gp120 (Scanlan *et al.*, 2002; Sanders *et al.*, 2002a; Calarese *et al.*, 2003); 447–52D, recognizing a conserved motif at the tip of the V3 loop (Gorny *et al.*, 2002; Stanfield *et al.*, 2004); Fab X5, recognizing the CD4-induced site (Moulard *et al.*, 2002; Darbha *et al.*, 2004); and 2F5 (Ofek *et al.*, 2004) and 4E10/Z13 (Zwick *et al.*, 2001; Cardoso *et al.*, 2005), recognizing a conserved region of gp41 peptide proximal to the viral membrane. Most evidence suggests that those mAbs which recognize epitopes in gp120 (the b12, 2G12 and 447–52D mAbs) neutralize by binding to virus *before* it attaches to CD4 on target T-cells, whereas the anti-gp41 mAbs (2F5 and 4E10/Z13) may have neutralizing activity *after* CD4 binding.

The rarity of neutralizing mAbs like these suggests that their cognate epitopes, at least as presented during natural infection, are poorly immunogenic. This, in turn, means that significantly more effort will be needed to identify broadly neutralizing mAbs recognizing other epitopes with potential as the basis for new immunogens.

## Approaches to designing vaccines that elicit broadly neutralizing antibodies

The failure of monomeric gp120 to prevent HIV infection in human efficacy trials has fueled the pursuit of new approaches for eliciting broadly neutralizing antibodies. A short-term goal is to design immunogens capable of eliciting NAbs comparable to those represented in Fig. 7.3. The long-term goal is to improve upon these immunogens, both in terms of neutralization breadth and strength, for example by combining immunogens and/or the use of more potent immunologic adjuvants. Here we discuss three approaches being investigated to address the short-term goal. (Another strategy, which uses immunogens based on consensus and ancestral HIV sequences, is discussed in the chapter by Korber et al.)

## Modified Env molecules presenting neutralizing epitopes more favorably

This approach focuses on the use of modified gp120, gp140 or gp160 glycoproteins. For example, several laboratories have generated envelope molecules in which the variable loops are deleted, with the aim of better exposing neutralizing epitopes in the CD4bs and CD4-induced site. Unfortunately thus far, this method has generally failed to elicit the desired level of NAbs that recognize their cognate epitopes on wild-type (non-deleted) virus. However, one recent study found that gp140 oligomers with a partially deleted V2 loop induced antibodies that neutralize the homologous wild-type virus but fail to neutralize heterologous virus (Barnett et al., 2001, Xu et al., 2006). Other studies have generated partially deglycosylated recombinant gp160 or recombinant viruses expressing glycosylation-deficient gp120 mutants, but these have so far also failed to generate antibodies that efficiently recognize wild-type virus.

Another type of modification is hyperglycosylation, where undesired epitopes (i.e., those that induce non-neutralizing antibodies) are masked using the selective incorporation of N-linked glycans (Pantophlet et al., 2003)—a mechanism similar to that used by HIV itself, in which glycans shield antigenic determinants from NAb recognition. An earlier report had shown that the addition of an N-glycan to the V3 loop could reduce the antibody response to part of the loop. Therefore, it is hoped that this method will decrease the induction of antibodies against the immunodominant variable loops and instead target responses to the conserved CD4bs. A recent immunization study with the first generation gp120 mutants showed that antibody response to multiple epitopes can be dampened by this strategy. However, more precise focusing to a neutralizing epitope will likely require several iterations comparing antigenicity and immunogenicity of engineered proteins (Selvarajah et al., 2005).

Other studies have used fusion intermediates made from gp120 or gp140 covalently cross-linked to CD4 as immunogens (Fouts et al., 2002). These molecules elicited antibodies that neutralized some primary viruses in macaque studies, but it is unclear whether these antibodies recognize gp120 or CD4. Moreover, antibodies against the CD4-induced site on Env have generally not proven successful so far in neutralizing primary HIV viruses.

Another report discussed an immunogen made by stabilizing the open conformation of monomeric gp120 to mimic its CD4-bound form, which might be achieved by introducing a mutation (such as S375W) that fills the Phe43 CD4 binding cavity (Fig. 7.2) (Xiang et al., 2002). A second possible strategy for stabilizing monomeric gp120 conformation is through the addition of inter-domain cysteines to form disulfide linkages (Dey and Wyatt, 2004; Chakraborty et al., 2005).

## Trimeric Env structures that mimic the native trimer on the virus surface

The second approach focuses on preserving or reconstructing the trimeric envelope spike, based on the hypothesis that immunizing with a close mimic of the functional trimer will improve the chances of eliciting neutralizing antibodies.

Soluble gp140 trimers are being used as the prototype immunogen for this strategy. For example, uncleaved gp140 (containing the ectodomain of gp41 covalently linked to gp120) has been expressed as trimers by fusing non-HIV trimerization motifs (such as yeast GCN4 and T4 bacteriophage fibritin-FT) to the C-terminus (Yang et al., 2002). These trimers have antigenic profiles that are similar but not identical (as determined by mAb reactivity) to Env expressed on HIV-infected cells. Immunization with gp140-GCN4/FT trimers was shown to be more efficient at eliciting NAbs than gp120 monomers (Yang et al., 2001, Bower et al., 2004, Grundner et al., 2005). These results are encouraging, since they indicate that soluble trimers are capable of presenting NAb-specific epitopes more effectively than are monomeric gp120.

Other modifications are also being tested for their ability to stabilize native trimers. For example, removal of the furin cleavage site between gp120 and the ectodomain of gp41 was found to be important for the stable expression and purification of Env trimers, while the incorporation of cysteine residues into gp120 and gp41 forms a disulfide bridge that prevents dissociation of the two subunits upon expression of cleaved gp140 (SOS gp140) (Binley et al., 2000). In addition, a mutation that destabilizes either the six-helix bundle formation (SOSIP gp140 trimers) (Sanders et al., 2002b) or its expression within membranes was needed to express this molecule in a stable trimeric form. A recent study showed that priming with DNA encoding membrane bound SOS gp140 protein followed by several immunizations with soluble SOSIP gp140 trimers results in eliciting antibodies capable of neutralizing sensitive strains at high titers and a few primary viruses at low titers (Beddows et al., 2005).

In order to present Env trimers to the immune system within a physiologic membrane setting, proteoliposomes containing native, trimeric uncleaved gp160ΔCT (cytoplasmic tail-deleted) glycoproteins have been generated (Grundner et al., 2002). In a comparative study, immune sera elicited following immunization with proteoliposomes expressing Env trimers had a slightly reduced breadth of neutralization potential compared to immune sera elicited following immunization with soluble gp140-GCN trimers (Grundner et al., 2005). Most attempts to mimic native Env trimers are currently being evaluated in small animal studies to determine whether these immunogens induce broad NAbs as well as means to further improve the efficiency of this process, such as, by the use of more potent immunologic adjuvants (Li *et al.*, 2006).

## Carbohydrate and peptide immunogens

A third strategy focuses on carbohydrate and peptide immunogens. While carbohydrates are rarely good immunogens, the broadly neutralizing mAb 2G12 recognizes terminal Manα1–2Man-linked moieties from oligomannose-type sugars that form a cluster on the silent face of gp120. A recent report on the crystal structure of 2G12 revealed that two Fabs assemble into an interlocked $V_H$ domain-swapped dimmer, providing an extended surface for high-affinity interaction of gp120 with multiple sugar moieties (Calarese *et al.*, 2003, 2005). These studies suggest a previously unrecognized template for HIV-1 vaccine design: immunogens that mimic the unique cluster of oligomannose sugars on gp120.

Another promising target for vaccine design is suggested by NAbs 2F5 and 4E10, both of which have considerable cross-isolate neutralizing ability directed at epitopes in the membrane-proximal external region (MPER) of gp41. The core epitope of 2F5 has been defined by a short linear peptide sequence, ELDKWA; and 4E10 by the sequence NWFDIT (Zwick *et al.*, 2001; Cardoso *et al.*, 2005), both located at the C-terminal end on the ectodomain of gp41. The 2F5 peptide has been tested for immunogenicity in many different contexts but has so far failed to elicit antibodies with similar neutralization ability. Nevertheless, the breadth of activity of 2F5 and 4E10 (Binley *et al.*, 2004) warrants much more effort at designing peptide-/protein- based immunogens against this region of the Env. There are suggestions that the recognition of ELDKWA by 2F5 is critically dependent on its environment within gp41 on native virus. This has been corroborated in a study where antibodies 2F5 and 4E10 recognized the respective epitopes better when presented in a membrane context (Ofek *et al.*, 2004). Therefore, several groups are currently expressing peptides based on MPER sequence on viral membranes and proteoliposomes in an attempt to improve immunogen design. The crystal structure of the Fab 4E10 in complex with a peptide containing the core epitope (NWFDIT) has provided insights into the helical nature of the epitope (Cardoso *et al.*, 2005). In order to mimic the helical nature of the 4E10 epitope, peptide immunogens are being designed with helix-promoting residues and helix-inducing tethers (Brunel *et al.*, 2006). These peptides also limit the conformational flexibility and can therefore be better templates for eliciting defined antibodies against peptide immunogens.

## Conclusions

Work on NAb-based vaccines is still in its infancy. Most of the novel antigens discussed above are in their early design stage, with few even tested yet in animal models. The need to accelerate work in this area is now widely recognized, and is under way in a growing number of labs and institutes. There are also efforts to expand the ongoing Neutralizing Antibody Consortium established by the International AIDS Vaccine Initiative (IAVI), which links some of the labs in this field with a series of projects to provide core reagents, high-speed robotic crystallization and the requisite infrastructure for immunogen design, testing and evaluation. More recently, the Global HIV Vaccine Enterprise, launched by the Bill and Melinda Gates Foundation as an alliance of stakeholders and endorsed by the G8 countries, has identified this problem as a key issue to be tackled under a broadened, more coordinated global effort (Klausner *et al.*, 2003).

Its solution will require considerable innovation in immunogen design, for which more molecular information on broadly NAbs and on Env is crucial. Once the first candidate immunogens capable of eliciting broadly effective NAbs are found, an iterative process of improving upon these immunogens will likely be required, examining combinations of candidates and using the most potent adjuvants to generate and maintain high antibody titers. Together with broadly effective CMI-based immunogens, this combination of anti-HIV responses appears at present to represent the best hope for an effective HIV vaccine.

## References

Barnett, S.W., Lu, S., Srivastava, I., Cherpelis, S., Gettie, A., Blanchard, J., Wang, S., Mboudjeka, I., Leung, L., Lian, Y., Fong, A., *et al.* (2001). The ability of an oligomeric human immunodeficiency virus type 1 (HIV-1) envelope antigen to elicit neutralizing antibodies against primary HIV-1 isolates is improved following partial deletion of the second hypervariable region. J. Virol. 75, 5526–5240.

Beddows, S., Schulke, N., Kirschner, M., Barnes, K., Franti, M., Michael, E., Ketas, T., Sanders, R.W., Maddon, P.J., Olson, W.C., and Moore, J.P. (2005). Evaluating the immunogenicity of a disulfide-stabilized, cleaved, trimeric form of the envelope glycoprotein complex of human immunodeficiency virus type 1. J Virol. 79, 8812–8827.

Binley, J.M., Sanders, R.W., Clas, B., Schuelke, N., Master, A., Guo, Y., Kajumo, F., Anselma, D.J., Maddon, P.J., Olson, W.C., and Moore J.P. (2000). A recombinant human immunodeficiency virus type 1 envelope glycoprotein complex stabilized by an intermolecular disulfide bond between the gp120 and gp41 subunits is an antigenic mimic of the trimeric virion-associated structure. J. Virol. 74, 627–643.

Binley, J.M, Wrin, T., Korber, B., Zwick, M.B., Wang, M., Chappey, C., Stiegler, G., Kunert, R., Zolla-Pazner, S., Katinger, H, Petropoulos, C.J, and Burton, D.R. (2004). A comprehensive cross-clade neutralization analysis of a panel of anti-HIV-1 monoclonal antibodies. J. Virol. 78, 13232–13252.

Bower, J.F., Yang, X., Sodroski, J., and Ross, T.M. (2004). Elicitation of neutralizing antibodies with DNA vaccines expressing soluble stabilized human immunodeficiency virus type 1 envelope glycoprotein trimers conjugated to C3d. J Virol. 78, 4710–4719.

Brunel, F.M., Zwick, M.B., Cardoso, R.M., Nelson, J.D., Wilson, I.A., Burton, D.R., and Dawson, P.E. (2006). Structure-function analysis of the epitope for 4E10, a broadly neutralizing human immunodeficiency virus type 1 antibody. J Virol. 80, 1680–1687.

Calarese, D.A., Scanlan, C.N., Zwick, M.B., Deechongkit, S., Mimura, Y., Kunert, R., Zhu, P., Wormald, M.R., Stanfield, R.L., *et al.* (2003). Antibody domain exchange is an immunological solution to carbohydrate cluster recognition. Science. 300, 2065–2071.

Calarese, D.A., Lee, H.K., Huang, C.Y., Best, M.D., Astronomo, R.D., Stanfield, R.L., Katinger, H., Burton, D.R., Wong, C.H., and Wilson, I.A. (2005). Dissection of the carbohydrate specificity of the broadly neutralizing anti-HIV-1 antibody 2G12. Proc. Natl. Acad. Sci. USA 20, 13372–13377.

Cardoso, R.M., Zwick, M.B., Stanfield, R.L., Kunert, R., Binley, J.M., Katinger, H., Burton, D.R., and Wilson, I.A. (2005). Broadly neutralizing anti-HIV antibody 4E10 recognizes a helical conformation of a highly conserved fusion-associated motif in gp41. Immunity 22, 163–173.

Chakraborty, K., Thakurela, S., Prajapati, R.S., Indu, S., Ali, P.S., Ramakrishnan, C., and Varadarajan, R. (2005). Protein stabilization by introduction of cross-strand disulfides. Biochemistry. 8, 14638–14646.

Coordinating Committee of the Global HIV/AIDS Vaccine Enterprise. (2005). The global HIV/AIDS vaccine enterprise: scientific strategic plan. PLoS Med. 2, 111–121.

Darbha, R., Phogat, S., Labrijn, A.F., Shu, Y., Gu, Y., Andrykovitch, M., Zhang, M.Y., Pantophlet, R., Martin, L., Vita, C., Burton, D.R., Dimitrov, D.S., and Ji, X. (2004). Crystal structure of the broadly cross-reactive HIV-1-neutralizing Fab X5 and fine mapping of its epitope. Biochemistry 17, 1410–1417.

Dey, B. and Wyatt, R. (2004). Characterization of Mutant HIV-1 Envelope Glycoproteins Stabilized in the CD4-Bound Conformation. Abstract 137. HIV Vaccine Development: Progress and Prospects (Keystone Symposium). Whistler, British Columbia.

Fouts, T., Godfrey, G., Bobb, K., Montefiori, D., Hanson, C.V., Kalyanaraman, V.S., DeVico, A., and Pal, R. (2002). Crosslinked HIV-1 envelope-CD4 receptor complexes elicit broadly cross-reactive neutralizing antibodies in Rhesus macaques. Proc. Natl. Acad. Sci. USA 99, 11842–11847.

Golding, H., Zaitseva, M., de Rosny, E., King, L.R., Manischewitz, J., Sidorov, I., Gorny, M.K., Zolla-Pazner, S., Dimitrov, D.S., and Weiss, C.D. (2002). Dissection of human immunodeficiency virus type 1 entry with neutralizing antibodies to gp41 fusion intermediates. J. Virol. 76, 6780–6790.

Gorny, M.K., Williams, C., Volsky, B., Revesz, K., Cohen, S., Polonis, V.R., Honnen, W.J., Kayman, S.C., Krachmarov, C., Pinter, A., and Zolla-Pazner, S. (2002). Human monoclonal antibodies specific for conformation-sensitive epitopes of V3 neutralize human immunodeficiency virus type 1 primary isolates from various clades. J. Virol. 7, 9035–9045.

Grundner, C., Mirzabekov, T., Sodroski, J., and Wyatt, R. (2002). Solid-phase proteoliposomes containing human immunodeficiency virus envelope glycoproteins. J. Virol. 76, 3511–3521.

Grundner, C., Li, Y., Louder, M., Mascola, J., Yang, X., Sodroski, J., and Wyatt, R. (2005). Analysis of the neutralizing antibody response elicited in rabbits by repeated inoculation with trimeric HIV-1 envelope glycoproteins. Virology 5, 33–46.

Klausner, R.D., Fauci, A.S., Corey, L., Nabel, G.J., Gayle, H., Berkley, S., Haynes, B.F., Baltimore, D., Collins, C., Douglas, R.G., et al. (2003). Medicine. The Need for a Global HIV Vaccine Enterprise. Science 300, 2036–2039.

Kwong, P.D., Wyatt, R., Robinson, J., Sweet, R.W., Sodroski, J., and Hendrickson, W.A. (1998). Structure of an HIV gp120 envelope glycoprotein in complex with the CD4 receptor and a neutralizing human antibody. Nature 393, 648–659.

Kwong, P.D., Wyatt, R., Sattentau, Q.J., Sodroski, J., and Hendrickson, W.A. (2000). Oligomeric modeling and electrostatic analysis of the gp120 envelope glycoprotein of human immunodeficiency virus. J. Virol. 74, 1961–1972.

Kwong, P.D., Doyle, M.L., Casper, D.J., Cicala, C., Leavitt, S.A., Majeed, S., Steenbeke, T.D., Venturi, M., Chaiken, I., Fung, M., et al. (2002). HIV-1 evades antibody-mediated neutralization through conformational masking of receptor-binding sites. Nature 420, 678–82.

Letvin, N.L. and Walker, B.D. (2003). Immunopathogenesis and immunotherapy in AIDS virus infections. Nature Med. 9, 861–866.

Li, Y., Svehla, K., Mathy, N.L., Voss, G., Mascola, J.R., and Wyatt, R. (2006). Characterization of antibody responses elicited by human immunodeficiency virus type 1 primary isolate trimeric and monomeric envelope glycoproteins in selected adjuvants. J. Virol. 80, 1414–1426.

Mascola, J.R. (2003). Defining the protective antibody response for HIV-1. Curr. Mol. Med. 3, 209–216.

Moulard, M., Phogat, S.K., Shu, Y., Labrijn, A.F., Xiao, X., Binley, J.M., Zhang, M.Y., Sidorov, I.A., Broder, C.C., Robinson, J., Parren, P.W., Burton, D.R., and Dimitrov, D.S. (2002). Broadly cross-reactive HIV-1-neutralizing human monoclonal Fab selected for binding

to gp120-CD4-CCR5 complexes. Proc. Natl. Acad. Sci. USA 14, 6913–6918.

Ofek, G., Tang, M., Sambor, A., Katinger, H., Mascola, J.R., Wyatt, R., and Kwong, P.D. (2004). Structure and mechanistic analysis of the anti-human immunodeficiency virus Type 1 antibody 2F5 in complex with its gp41 epitope. J. Virol. 78, 10724–10737.

Pantophlet, R., Wilson, I.A., and Burton, D.R. (2003). Hyperglycosylated mutants of human immunodeficiency virus (HIV) type 1 monomeric gp120 as novel antigens for HIV vaccine design. J. Virol. 77, 5889–5901.

Poignard, P., Saphire, E.O., Parren, P.W., and Burton, D.R. (2001). gp120: Biologic aspects of structural features. Annu. Rev. Immunol. 19, 253–274.

Sattentau, Q.J. and Moore, J.P. (1995). Human immunodeficiency virus type 1 neutralization is determined by epitope exposure on the gp120 oligomer. J. Exp. Med. 182, 185–196.

Sanders, R.W., Venturi, M., Schiffner, L., Kalyanaraman, R., Katinger, H., Lloyd, K.O., Kwong, P.D., and Moore, J.P. (2002a). The mannose-dependent epitope for neutralizing antibody 2G12 on human immunodeficiency virus type 1 glycoprotein gp120. J. Virol. 76, 7293–7305.

Sanders, R.W., Vesanen, M., Schuelke, N., Master, A., Schiffner, L., Kalyanaraman, R., Paluch, M., Berkhout, B., Maddon, P.J., Olson, W.C., Lu, M., and Moore, J.P. (2002b). Stabilization of the soluble, cleaved, trimeric form of the envelope glycoprotein complex of human immunodeficiency virus type 1. J Virol. 76, 8875–8889.

Saphire, E.O., Parren, P.W., Pantophlet, R., Zwick, M.B., Morris, G.M., Rudd, P.M., Dwek, R.A., Stanfield, R.L., Burton, D.R. and Wilson, I.A. (2001). Crystal structure of a neutralizing human IGG against HIV-1: a template for vaccine design. Science 293, 1155–1159.

Scanlan, C.N., Pantophlet, R., Wormwald, M.R., Saphire, E.O., Stanfield, R., Wilson, I.A., Katinger, H., Dwek, R.A., Rudd, P.M., and Burton, D.R. (2002). The broadly neutralizing anti-human immunodeficiency virus type 1 antibody 2G12 recognizes a cluster of alpha1−>2 mannose residues on the outer face of gp120. J. Virol. 76, 7306–7321.

Selvarajah, S., Puffer, B., Pantophlet, R., Law, M., Doms, R.W., and Burton, D.R. (2005). Comparing antigenicity and immunogenicity of engineered gp120. J. Virol. 79, 12148–12163.

Stanfield, R.L, Gorny, M.K, Williams, C., Zolla-Pazner, S., and Wilson, I.A. (2004). Structural rationale for the broad neutralization of HIV-1 by human monoclonal antibody 447–52D. Structure (Camb.) 12, 193–204.

Wyatt, R., Kwong, P.D., Desjardins, E., Sweet, R.W., Robinson, J., Hendrickson, W.A., and Sodroski, J. (1998). The antigenic structure of the HIV gp120 envelope glycoprotein. Nature 393, 705–711.

Xiang, S.H, Kwong, P.D, Gupta, R, Rizzuto, C.D, Casper, D.J, Wyatt, R, Wang, L., Hendrickson, W.A, Doyle, M.L, and Sodroski, J. (2002). Mutagenic stabilization and/or disruption of a CD4-bound state reveals distinct conformations of the human immunodeficiency virus type 1 gp120 envelope glycoprotein. J. Virol. 76, 9888–9899.

Xu, R., Srivastava, I.K., Kuller, L., Zarkikh, I., Kraft, Z., Fagrouch, Z., Letvin, N.L., Heeney, J.L., Barnett, S.W., and Stamatatos, L. (2006). Immunization with HIV-1 SF162-derived Envelope gp140 proteins does not protect macaques from heterologous simian-human immunodeficiency virus SHIV89.6P infection. Virology 349, 276–289.

Yang, X., Lee, J., Mahony, E.M., Kwong, P.D., Wyatt, R., and Sodroski, J. (2002). Highly stable trimers formed by human immunodeficiency virus type 1 envelope glycoproteins fused with the trimeric motif of T4 bacteriophage fibritin. J. Virol. 76, 4634–4642.

Yang, X., Wyatt, R., and Sodroski, J. (2001). Improved elicitation of neutralizing antibodies against primary human immunodeficiency viruses by soluble stabilized envelope glycoprotein trimers. J. Virol. 75, 1165–1171.

Zwick, M.B., Labrijn, A.F., Wang, M., Spenlehauer, C., Ollmann Saphire, E., Binley, J.M., Moore, J.P., Stiegler, G., Katinger, H., Burton, D.R., and Parren, P.W.H.I. (2001). Broadly neutralizing antibodies targeted to the membrane-proximal external region of human immunodeficiency virus type 1 glycoprotein gp41. J. Virol. 75, 10892–10905.

# Vaccines that Induce Cellular Immunity

Britta Wahren and Margaret A. Liu

## Abstract

The ability to induce cell-mediated immunity (CMI) is widely thought to be an important property of any potential AIDS vaccine or immunotherapy. The rationale is based on many observations, including: (1) a demonstrated role for CMI in containing HIV after infection; and (2) the ability of T-cells to target viral epitopes that may be more highly conserved amongst different strains (both intra-clade and cross-clade) than the Env structures that have been evaluated clinically as potential vaccine immunogens. This chapter examines the design issues specific for vaccines intended to induce cellular immunity against HIV/AIDS, discusses characteristics of these approaches (most of which are gene-based) and gives an overview of the different candidates under development.

## Introduction

Most recent efforts to make an AIDS vaccine have been directed towards developing technologies that specifically induce cellular immunity. Extensive animal models and human data provide the scientific rationale for this strategy and are described elsewhere in this volume (Chapters 4 and 5) and summarized briefly below. However, these efforts are complicated by several factors—in particular, the technological challenge of delivering antigens in a manner that effectively induces robust T-cellular immunity; and uncertainties regarding both the type of cellular immune response(s) needed for protection against HIV/AIDS and the best preclinical and clinical measurements, or correlates, of this immunity.

## Why CMI-based vaccines?

The impetus for making a vaccine that generates T-cell responses came from the accumulation of data showing that T-cellular immunity plays a key role in controlling viral replication (by killing virally infected cells which produce more virus). Efforts have therefore focused on exploiting the ability of CD4[+] and CD8[+] T-cells to target virally infected cells, based upon conserved epitopes in predominantly internal HIV proteins (but also conserved epitopes of the envelope protein).

Antibodies have an advantage over cellular responses in terms of their potential to prevent infection, since they can bind to the viral envelope and directly neutralize virus or prevent it from infecting a cell. Since HIV integrates its genome into the host's DNA following infection, thereby establishing a persistent infection, the ability of antibodies to kill virus extracellularly or to block infection is obviously beneficial. On the other hand, although T-cells play a role only *after* virus has infected a cell, they recognize epitopes on internal (as well as external) HIV proteins, which are more highly conserved than some regions of Env. This suggests that T-cell based vaccines might induce broader immune responses, and recognize more diverse viral strains, than vaccines based on antibodies which often target variable epitopes of Env. They may also help reduce the likelihood of immune escape by HIV, which can occur via mutation within viral epitopes targeted by immune responses. While such mutations have been demonstrated in both CTL epitopes (reviewed by Letvin and Walker, 2003) and antibody epitopes, the rationale for targeting non-surface HIV proteins includes the greater degree of conservation of proteins such as Gag and Pol compared with Env, and the virus need to conserve regions that serve a basic viral function or structure. The hypervariability of prominently accessible regions of Env (vs. the more cryptic location of key regions such as that involved in fusion of the virus with the cell) further supports the rationale for targeting cellular as well as antibody responses against the more conserved regions or proteins of HIV.

The enormous genetic diversity of HIV and its tremendous ability to mutate and recombine, plus the high degree of strain specificity demonstrated by many Env-directed antibodies, underscore the potentially critical need for cellular immune responses that are effective against multiple strains (within or across clades). Additional support for the potential of cellular immunity to provide cross-strain protection comes from the initial demonstration that a DNA vaccine can protect against an infectious challenge in an influenza model (Ulmer *et al.*, 1993). In that study, a DNA vaccine encoding the conserved nucleoprotein of influenza virus was able to protect mice that were subsequently challenged with influenza virus of a different subtype (analogous to a different HIV clade), which arose 34 years after the strain from which the nucleoprotein gene was cloned. The ability of CTL to mediate cross-strain protection has served as a paradigm for the type of cross-clade protection that an ideal HIV vaccine would generate.

## Key attributes of CMI-based vaccines

The two components of cellular immunity that are considered critical for an HIV vaccine are the cytotoxic T-lymphocyte response, or CTL (primarily CD8$^+$ cells) and the T-helper responses, primarily a Th1 phenotype (Letvin and Walker, 2003; Ulmer et al., 2006). Both interdependent and independent rationales for a role of these two responses exist, since the Th1 type of helper response is needed to generate a CTL (vs. antibody) response and because Th1 responses play a role in the development of the more benign long-term non-progressor phenotype rather than a more rapid disease progression. From a technological standpoint the focus has been on designing vaccines that deliver antigen into the cytosol of cells (primarily via introduction of the gene encoding the antigen) in order to induce MHC Class I-restricted CTL responses. Yet the readouts used as indicators of immunogenicity typically include the production of Th1-type cytokines such as gamma-interferon (IFN), which can be produced by both CD4$^+$ and CD8$^+$ T-cells. Thus some of the immunogenicity measures in widespread use do not always define which sort of CMI is induced, an approach justified by the fact that both CD4$^+$ and CD8$^+$ responses are thought to be important.

Alongside the need for CD4$^+$ and CD8$^+$ cells of adequate potency—a significant hurdle for gene-based vaccines—there are other critical design issues for CMI-based vaccines, which include the duration and location of immunity and the induction of memory vs. effector cells. While some licensed vaccines successfully confer long-term protection, the challenge of making a vaccine that protects against a disease with the transmission modality and epidemiology of HIV (where an individual can be exposed literally hundreds of times a year throughout adult life) is quite different from the situation of a disease such as influenza that has a seasonal incidence.

Two distinct patient populations offer insight into the role and duration of clinically induced CMI and provide evidence that despite its inability to prevent infection at a cellular level, it may still be adequate in a clinical setting involving real-life frequencies and multi-strain exposures. Certain seronegative individuals who appear to be uninfected despite multiple repeated exposure to HIV (Zhu et al., 2003), including a well-studied group of sex workers who likewise are uninfected despite frequent exposure (Kaul et al., 2001; Chapter 5) show HIV-specific cellular immune responses. Extremely low levels of virus have been demonstrated in the former group, suggesting that CMI helps prevent progression of HIV infection or disease. In the latter group, some of the women with CD8$^+$ T-cell responses to HIV returned to commercial sex work after a hiatus, and a small proportion of them then seroconverted. This provided a sobering hint of the potential limits of the CMI response in terms of duration, breadth or potency, at least without boosting.

Among the many implications of these observations for vaccine development is that it may be important to determine how best to induce memory vs. effector cells (and in what proportion), and how to best quantify each type. Memory T-cells have been categorized as either effector memory or central memory cells based upon differences in their phenotype, function and location in peripheral tissue vs. lymphoid organs. (reviewed by Kaech et al., 2002). This information may be important because of what it says about the kinetics of an immune response that cannot prevent infection but kills infected cells, and especially because it helps ensure the relevance of the immune readouts used to guide vaccine design. While many immune assays of peripheral blood lymphocytes or splenocytes are often viewed generically as representing the potency of a CMI-based vaccine, they may actually measure different subpopulations. For example, certain assays rely upon re-stimulation of T-cells in vitro prior to measurement of function (resulting in a measure of memory cells), whereas other assays assess function (such as cytokine production or cell killing) more immediately.

A fourth issue for CMI-based vaccines, besides potency, duration, and memory vs. effector responses, is the location of the response. While mucosal administration of vaccines has primarily been seen as important in protection against mucosal pathogens (where secretory IgA is believed to play a predominant role), the site of administration of all vaccines is now being considered more carefully. As the mechanisms that induce immune responses in different immune sites become better understood, it has become clear that a vaccine's route of administration may determine the types and potency of the resultant responses as well as their efficacy against infection via particular transmission routes (Otten et al., 2005; Brave et al. 2005). Moreover, from a purely logistical standpoint, the route and technology used to administer a vaccine will also greatly impact the feasibility and speed of widespread global usage in low-resource settings.

However, the main importance of a vaccine's properties and route of administration is that its ability to stimulate T-cells depends upon delivering antigen (or a gene encoding the antigen) to key antigen-presenting cells. Since activated mature dendritic cells (DCs) are the most effective cells for activating T-cells, the tropism of several vaccine vectors for dendritic cells (or their ability to induce cross-priming of DCs) and routes of administration will clearly affect the efficacy of different vaccines. The challenge has been that differences between humans and the various preclinical animal models mean that the intermediate steps in generating cellular responses are not evaluated, but rather only the net immune response.

For a vaccine to be capable of generating CTL responses, it has generally been deemed necessary to introduce the antigen into the cytosol of the cell (reviewed by Melief, 2003); moreover, the cell must either be a professional antigen presenting cell or it must be capable of transferring antigen in the proper form to a professional antigen presenting cell, a process known as cross-priming (reviewed by Gromme and Neefjes, 2002). Certain proteins, especially when presented within virus-like-particles, can directly transport proteins into the cytosol of cells. Another approach has been to deliver peptides directly to the MHC Class I molecules, although this strategy would obviously present only a limited number of epitopes restricted to specific MHC haplotypes. The more widely used approach for CMI-based vaccines under development is to deliver genes encoding the desired antigens into the target antigen-presenting or antigen-processing cell, rather than delivering the protein antigen directly. An antigen endogenously produced in the cell can then directly enter the correct antigen processing pathway for presentation on MHC-Class I molecules, which in turn stimulates CTLs. Alternatively, the transfected cell may serve as the producer of antigen which then is transferred in some format to the professional antigen presenting cell.

## Vector-based gene delivery systems

A variety of vectors for gene delivery have been developed, each with their own advantages and disadvantages. The simplest vector is plasmid DNA, consisting of just a bacterial plasmid containing a promoter that can function in mammalian cells (usually a strong viral promoter), the gene encoding the antigen of interest, a terminator and perhaps a selection marker for plasmid production (reviewed by Srivastava and Liu, 2003). The plasmid is taken up by cells (either APCs or myocytes), albeit very inefficiently, following direct intramuscular injection, or propelled from a jet injector, with subsequent expression of the encoded protein and, in the case of myocyte expression, followed by transfer of the antigen in some form into professional antigen presenting cells for cross-priming. Alternatively, the DNA can be precipitated onto gold beads which are then propelled into the epidermis.

Even simple vectors like plasmids are not simply an inert gene delivery system. The immune responses generated by DNA vaccines result from not only the cognate immune response against the antigen, but also from stimulation of innate immune responses provoked by the nature of the bacterial DNA and by the mode and route of inoculation. DNA vaccines have shown relatively poor immunogenicity in primate and human trials when given alone, although they have been able to generate both antibody and T-cell responses. Interestingly, in HIV-infected patients who had high viral titers (and hence significant quantities of HIV antigens present), DNA vaccines stimulated CTL responses that had not previously been present in the HIV-infected patients (Hejdeman et al., 2004). Nevertheless, next-generation delivery systems for DNA vaccines are under development and evaluation in order to increase the potency of these vaccines. An example of these second generation vaccines is the formulation of the DNA as a microparticle with PLG (polylactide co-glycolide) (O'Hagan et al., 2004), an approach now in a clinical trial. And as described below, a promising development has been the combination of DNA vaccines with other gene-based vector systems in mixed-modality vaccines.

Viral vectors have been extensively developed for vaccines in order to take advantage of the ability of viruses to infect various cells, including professional antigen-presenting cells, in some cases, and then to utilize the cell's transcription machin-

ery to express viral genes. These viruses have been modified by the alteration or removal of some of their own genes, rendering them non-pathogenic and usually also replication-defective and also making sufficient room in the vector for inserting heterologous genes encoding the desired antigens. A number of viral vectors are being developed (Chapter 11): mammalian pox viruses (modified vaccinia Ankara-MVA and NYVAC), avian poxvirus, adenovirus type 5 (and more recently other serotypes, chimpanzee strains, and replication-competent human adenoviruses), Venezuelan encephalitis virus, Semliki forest virus, measles virus or adeno-associated virus.

While the different viral vectors have unique characteristics such as their tissue tropism and insert capacity, they all share the property that immune responses are generated not just against the encoded antigen of interest (i.e., hepatitis C or HIV proteins), but also against the viral vector itself and any proteins that it still encodes. For certain vectors this may potentially limit the usefulness of the vaccine due to pre-existing immunity to the viral vector in people who have either been immunized with a related virus (for example, to vaccinia for patients immunized previously against smallpox) or infected with the wild type virus (as in the case of adenovirus infection). Additionally, following immunization, an immune response against the viral antigens will be raised (or boosted, if one existed previously), potentially limiting further use of the vector. It is not clear that this will be a significant hindrance to the efficacy of the vectors, if boosts are given with adequate time intervals. However, a murine study revealed that pre-existing immunity at a level comparable to that in humans previously infected with Ad5 decreased the immune response to an Ad5 vector encoding gag but not to an Ad35-Gag vector (Barouch et al., 2004). And as described below, the use of heterologous priming and boosting (e.g., DNA followed by MVA or VSV, or adeno followed by poxvirus) has been more potent in a number of preclinical models than repeat immunization with a single vector system.

Another vector system that is less advanced but may have advantages is the use of attenuated bacteria which either deliver plasmid DNA encoding HIV antigens or heterologously express HIV antigens (Xu et al., 2003). *Salmonella* and *Shigella* are bacteria that specifically invade mucosal cells in the intestine as part of their pathology. Thus they may be useful because of their ability to induce mucosal immune responses and their potential ease of oral administration. Of course these bacterial vectors share a safety concern with the attenuated viral vectors regarding the potential for reversion to virulence (although these vectors all have significant gene deletions) and for potential recombination with existing gut flora.

It is worth highlighting some of the specific tropisms of different vectors which may provide them with potential advantages. The bacterial vectors noted above provide a clear-cut advantage of mucosal administration. Poxviruses and adenoviruses have broad tissue tropisms, and both they and alpha viruses (such as VEE) also have tropism for dendritic cells, the most important class of antigen presenting cells. DNA injected intramuscularly appears to be best taken up by myocytes that then cross-prime antigen presenting cells, although some lymphocytes are apparently directly transfected as well. DNA has also been injected mucosally by using a dental device that avoids the need for a needle (Lundholm *et al.*, 2002). DNA on gold beads injected with the gene gun non-specifically transfects any cell in its pathway, but these include epidermal Langerhans cells, which are antigen-presenting cells.

Immunization with a combination of different gene delivery systems results in more potent immune responses (Hanke *et al.*, 1998, Casimiro *et al.*, 2004, Bråve *et al.*, 2005) and better protection against pathogen challenge than repeat immunizations with the same vectors. In some cases the reason for this may be that certain vectors also encode genes for proteins from the vectors themselves so that repeat administration of the vector might be limited by immune responses against the vectors as well as the encoded viral proteins (Mwau *et al.*, 2004). However, the potency of mixed modality vaccination seems to extend beyond circumvention of anti-vector immune responses. It is generally true that the presence of more antigen results in the stimulation of greater numbers of T (and B) cells. First-generation DNA vaccines transfect fewer cells and hence produce less antigen than other vector systems, yet have been shown in general to be the most effective prime compared to other viral vectors when used in a mixed modality vaccine. It is possible that this is because of the known ability of DNA vaccines to bias the T-helper response towards predominantly a Th1 type of response. It may also be that the expression of single genes in the absence of vector focuses the important primary response to the desired gene product. Priming with one vector and boosting with another vector can present the same/similar antigen in various contexts, thus permitting both boosting of a primary response and further broadening of the total epitope response (Sandström *et al.*, 2006). Further clinical studies of mixed modality prime-boost regimens will need to evaluate specific immune parameters in man, such as the type and extent of T-cell help and the breadth and flexibility of the T-cells responses against a variety of epitopes, to determine which combinations generate the most effective immune responses.

Predicted clinical efficacy of different vaccines and different prime-boost regimens has relied upon preclinical challenge models or immunotherapeutic studies in man (MacGregor *et al.*, 2005). Various regimens including DNA (Barouch *et al.*, 2000), adenovirus (Shiver *et al.*, 2002), and DNA followed by MVA (Amara *et al.*, 2001; Sandström *et al.*, 2006) have demonstrated an ability to elicit CMI (both C8+ and CD4[+] T-cells), and/or to protect against challenge or decrease viral loads. Although vaccination did not prevent the animals from becoming infected, their viral loads were significantly lower than those of control monkeys. Barouch *et al.* (2002), also detected immune escape of the challenge virus based upon a single amino acid mutation for the dominant T-cell response, underlining the need for broad and flexible responses even for cellular immunity.

In summary, significant progress has been made in developing a variety of technologies to induce and measure cell-mediated immunity. But significant challenges remain in determining which responses will correlate with protection or therapy; in turn this understanding will provide better guidance about how to increase the potency, duration, and localization of the total immune response, particularly key CD8[+] and CD4[+] T-cell responses.

## References

Amara, R.R., Villinger, F., Altman, J.D., Lydy, S.L., O'Neil, S.P., Staprans, S.I., Montefiori, D.C., Xu, Y., Herndon, J.G., Wyatt, L.S., *et al.* (2001). Control of a mucosal challenge and prevention of AIDS by a multiprotein DNA/MVA vaccine. Science 292, 69–74.

Barouch, D.H., Santra, S., Schmitz, J.E., Kuroda, M.J., Fu, T.M., Wagner, W., Bilska, M., Craiu, A., Zheng, X.X., Krivulka, G.R., *et al.* (2000). Control of viremia and prevention of clinical AIDS in Rhesus monkeys by cytokine-augmented DNA vaccination. Science 290, 486–492.

Barouch, D.H., Kunstman, J., Kuroda, M.J., Schmitz, J.E., Santra, S., Peyerl, F.W., Krivulka, G.R., Beaudry, K., Lifton, M.A., Gorgone, D.A., *et al.* (2002). Eventual AIDS vaccine failure in a Rhesus monkey by viral escape from CTL. Nature 415, 335–9.

Barouch, D.H., Pau, M.G., Custers, J.H., Koudstaal, W., Kostense, S., Havenga, M.J., Truitt, D.M., Sumida S.M., Kishko, M.G., Arthur, J.C., Korioth-Schmitz, B., Newberg, M.H., Gorgone, D.A., Lifton, M.A., Panicali, D.L., Nabel, G.J., Letvin, N.L., Goudsmit, J. (2004). Immunogenicity of recombinant adenovirus serotype 35 vaccine in the presence of pre-existing anti-Ad5 immunity. J. Immunol. 172:(6290)–7.

Brave, A.., Ljungberg, K., Boberg, A., Rollman, E., Isaguliants, M., Lundgren, B., Blomberg, P., Hinkula, J., and Wahren, B. (2005). Multigene/multisubtype HIV-1 vaccine induces potent cellular and humoral responses by needle-free intradermal delivery. Mol. Ther. 12, 1197–1205.

Casimiro, D.R., Bett, A.J., Fu, T.M., Davies, M.E., Tang, A., Wilson, K.A., Chen, M., Long, R., McKelvey, T., Chastain, M., *et al.* (2004). Heterologous human immunodeficiency virus type 1 priming-boosting immunization strategies involving replication-defective adenovirus and poxvirus vaccine vectors. J. Virol. 78, 11434–11438.

Gromme, M. and Neefjes, J. (2002). Antigen degradation or presentation by MHC Class I molecules via classical and non-classical pathways. Mol. Immunol. 39, 181–202.

Hanke, T., Blanchard, T.J., Schneider, J., Hannan, C.M., Becker, M., Gilbert, S.C., Hill, A.V., Smith, G.L., and McMichael, A.J. (1998). Enhancement of MHC Class I-restricted peptide-specific T-cell induction by a DNA prime/MVA boost vaccination regime. Vaccine 16, 439–445.

Hejdeman, B., Boström, A.C., Matsuda, R., Calarota, S., Lenkei, R., Fredriksson, E. L., Sandström, E., Bratt, G., and Wahren, B. (2004). DNA immunization with HIV early genes in HIV type-1 infected patients on highly active antiretroviral therapy. AIDS Res. Human Retroviruses 20, 860–870.

Kaul, R., Rowland-Jones, S.L., Kimani, J., Dong, T., Yang, H.B., Kiama, P., Rostron, T., Njagi, E., Bwayo, J.J., MacDonald, K.S., McMichael, A.J., and Plummer, F.A. (2001). Late seroconversion in HIV-resistant Nairobi prostitutes despite pre-existing HIV-specific CD8[+] responses. J. Clin. Invest. 107, 341–349.

Kaech, S.M., Wherry, E.J., and Ahmed, R. (2002). Effector and memory T-cell differentiation: implications for vaccine development. Nature Rev. Immun. 2, 251–262.

Letvin, N.L. and Walker B.D. (2003). Immunopathogenesis and immunotherapy in AIDS virus infections. Nature Med. 9, 861–866.

Lundholm, P. Leandersson, A.C., Christensson, B., Bratt, G., Sandstrom, E., and Wahren, B. (2002). DNA mucosal HIV vaccine in humans. Virus. Res. 82, 141–145.

MacGregor, R.R., Boyer, J.D., Ugen, K.E., Tebas, P., Higgins, T.J., Baine, Y., Ciccarelli, R.B., Ginsberg, R.S., Weiner, D.B. (2005). Plasmid vaccination of stable HIV-positive subjects of antiviral treatment results in enhanced CD8 T-cell immunity and increased control of virus "blips." Vaccine 23, 2066–2073.

McMichael, A. and Hanke, T. (2003). HIV. Vaccines. (1983)–2003. Nature Med. 9, 874–880.

Melief, C.J. (2003). Mini-review: Regulation of cytotoxic T-lymphocyte responses by dendritic cells: peaceful coexistence of cross-priming and direct priming? Eur. J. Immunol. 33, 2645–2654.

Mwau, M., Cebere, I., Sutton, J., Chikoti, P., Winstone, N., Wee, E.G., Beattie, T., Chen, Y.H., Dorrell, L., McShane, H. et al. (2004). An HIV-1 clade A vaccine in clinical trials: stimulation of HIV-specific T cell responses by DNA and recombinant modified vaccinia virus Ankara (MVA) vaccines in humans. J. Gen. Virol. 85, 911–919.

O'Hagan, D.T., Singh, M., Dong, C., Ugozzoli, M., Berger, K., Glazer, E., Selby, M., Wininger, M., Ng, P., Crawford, K., et al. (2004). Paliard X, Coates S, Houghton M. Cationic microparticles are a potent delivery system for a HCV DNA vaccine. Vaccine 23, 672–680.

Otten, G., Schaefer, M., Doe, B., Liu, H., Megede, J.Z., Donnelly, J., Rabussay, D., Barnett, S., Ulmer, J.B. (2005). Potent immunogenicity of an HIV-1 gag-pol fusion DNA vaccine delivered by in vivo electroporation. Vaccine Potent immunogenicity of an HIV-1 gag-pol fusion DNA vaccine delivered by in vivo electroporation. Vaccine (Epub ahead of print).

Sandstrom, E., Wahren, B., Hejdeman, B., Nilsson, C., Bråve, A., Bratt, G., Robb, M., Cox, J., VanCott, T., Marovich, M., et al. (2006). Multigene, multiclade HIV-1 plasmid DNA prime and MVA boost is safe and highly immunogenic in healthy human volunteers. Abstract 4th Conference of HIV and AIDS, Amsterdam.

Shiver, J.W., Fu, T.M., Chen, L., Casimiro, D.R., Davies, M.E., Evans, R.K., Zhang, Z.Q., Simon, A.J., Trigona, W.L., Dubey, S.A., et al. (2002). Replication-incompetent adenoviral vaccine vector elicits effective anti-immunodeficiency-virus immunity. Nature 415, 331–335.

Srivastava, I.K., and Liu, M.A. (2003). Gene vaccines. Ann. Int. Med. 138, 550–559.

Ulmer, J.B., Donnelly, J.J., Parker, S.E., Rhodes, G.H., Felgner, P.L., Dwarki, V.J., Gromkowski, S.H., Deck, R.R., DeWitt, C.M., Friedman, A., et al. (1993). Heterologous protective immunity to influenza by intramuscular injection of DNA encoding a conserved viral protein. Science. 259, 1745–1749.

Ulmer, J., Wahren, B. and Liu, M. (2006). Gene-based vaccines: recent technical and clinical advances. Trends Mol. Med. (in press).

Xu, F., Hong, M., and Ulmer, J.B. (2003). Immunogenicity of an HIV-1 gag DNA vaccine carried by attenuated Shigella. Vaccine 21, 644–648.

Zhu, T., Corey, L., Hwangbo, Y., Lee, J.M., Learn, G.H., Mullins, J.I., and McElrath, M.J. (2003). Persistence of extraordinarily low levels of genetically homogeneous human immunodeficiency virus type 1 in exposed seronegative individuals. J. Virol. 77, 6108–6116.

# Alternate Routes on the Roadmap to an HIV Vaccine: Importance of Innate and Adaptive Mucosal Immunity

9

Kenneth L. Rosenthal

## Abstract

HIV is a mucosally transmitted virus that rapidly targets and dramatically depletes activated CD4$^+$ CCR5$^+$ T-cells in mucosal tissues and establishes a major reservoir for viral persistence in gut-associated lymphoid tissues. Several lines of evidence implicate mucosal responses in immune protection against HIV (and SIV), which argues that HIV vaccine development should be re-oriented to emphasize mucosal immunization routes that induce long-term innate and adaptive mucosal responses.

A growing body of knowledge and methods can accelerate progress towards this goal. Recent advances in our understanding of innate immunity have ushered in a new era of studies on vaccine adjuvants that promote mucosal responses when used with a variety of candidate vaccines (including some based on recombinant vectors that target the mucosa) and are proving effective at inducing durable mucosal immunity in mouse models. At the same time, advances in immunogenomics and proteomics are providing opportunities to discover novel genes and molecules involved in vaccine-induced mucosal immunity, while new assays that permit simultaneous measurement of multiple immune responses will greatly facilitate the assessment of mucosal immunity in the context of HIV vaccine trials.

## Introduction

Twenty-five years after the discovery of HIV-1 it is clear that the road to an effective vaccine will be a long and winding one, with many bumps; indeed, as many chapters in this volume highlight, the scientific challenges confronting HIV vaccine development are substantial. Currently great emphasis is being placed on strategies that induce CD8$^+$ cytotoxic T-lymphocytes (CTLs). But there are also concerns about the possible limitations of this approach. These include the potential for viral escape and the recognition that overall frequencies of HIV-specific T-cells are not the sole determinant of immune-mediated protection (Chapters 4 and 5). Additionally, superinfection with closely related strains of HIV in the face of strong and broad CTL responses raises questions about the role of CTL in protection (Altfeld et al., 2002).

In light of these questions, it is important to consider alternate routes for preventing the establishment of lifelong HIV infection. Several lines of evidence argue strongly for vaccine approaches that emphasize induction of mucosal immune responses and enhancement of innate immunity. Beyond the fact that HIV is transmitted primarily by mucosal routes, there is growing appreciation that, regardless of transmission route, acute HIV infection is a disease of the mucosal immune system. Further rationale for considering alternative approaches comes from recent advances in our understanding of innate immunity, and from dramatic demonstrations that passive transfer of neutralizing monoclonal antibodies can prevent mucosal infection.

## Acute HIV infection: targeting the mucosal immune system

The major transmission mode of HIV is through exposure of mucosal surfaces to cell-free virus and HIV-infected cells (Cromwell et al., 2000; Shattock, 2003; Margolis and Shattock, 2006). Although entry of virus across mucosal barriers is greatly facilitated when the epithelium is damaged (by physical abrasion or trauma, ulcerative sexually transmitted disease or cervical ectopy), studies of SIV transmission in monkeys have shown that T-cell-free virus can infect undamaged cervico-vaginal mucosa in females, foreskin and urethral epithelium in males, and rectal, oro-pharyngeal and upper gastrointestinal tract mucosa. These findings are consistent with old observations from artificial insemination in humans (made before HIV screening of donor semen was done in the US) that insemination, which causes minimal trauma compared to sexual intercourse, resulted in transmission of HIV in up to 141 women.

Several mechanisms have been proposed to account for HIV transmission across undamaged mucosa in vitro but it is still unclear whether these mechanisms explain transmission in vivo (Shattock, 2003; Margolis and Shattock, 2006). Furthermore, infection at different mucosal sites may involve distinct mechanisms. Thus, while HIV does not directly infect and replicate in mucosal epithelial cells, it can bind to galactosyl ceramide on intestinal epithelial cells and then undergo transcytosis to the underlying lymphoid cells. Several types of cells, including Langerhans cells (LC) and dendritic cells (DCs) present in human cervico-vaginal, foreskin and oral mucosa (and expressing CD4 and CCR5), as well as DCs found beneath rectal or vaginal mucosa (and expressing DC-SIGN) can play a key role in binding HIV and transporting it to local lymph nodes. Indeed, it was recently shown that DCs in the gut sample antigens in the lumen by extending their dendrites between epithelial cells without disrupting the tight junction barrier (Rescigno et al., 2001). In contrast to the multilayered stratified squamous epithelium in the vagina, single-layered rectal epithelium provides little protection against HIV entry and has organized lymphoid follicles containing specialized microfold or M-cells that bind and present HIV to underlying lymphoid tissues.

An important feature of mucosal HIV infection is its rapid speed of transmission. This is illustrated by the finding that SIV given via direct intravaginal (IVAG) inoculation was detectable in DCs or LCs and macrophages in the lamina propria within 4 hours, and in draining iliac lymph nodes within 2 days. Once HIV crosses the mucosal epithelium, it finds many CD4$^+$ T-cells, DCs and macrophages in the lamina propria to infect.

Recent studies have shown that—regardless of the route of transmission—the acute phase of infection with SIV and HIV leads to rapid, massive depletion of mucosal CD4$^+$ T-cells in the gastrointestinal and respiratory tracts, occurring well before significant depletion in peripheral blood and lymph nodes (Douek et al., 2003; Brenchley et al., 2006). In other words, acute infection targets the mucosal immune system. This is not surprising, since a large fraction of the body's CD4$^+$ T-cells are found in mucosal tissues (with over 60% in the gut), and these cells express CCR5 and an activated phenotype. Consequently, the mucosa provides a rich source of prime targets for CCR5-tropic HIV, which is almost always the co-receptor for naturally transmitted virus. Following infection, the gut serves as a major reservoir for HIV-1 (Veazey and Lackner, 1998).

## Role of mucosal immunity in protection against HIV

Most infections are initiated at mucosal surfaces of the body, which are estimated to be about the size of a basketball court in surface area. Protection of mucosal surfaces is mediated by a combination of local innate and adaptive mucosal immune responses (Lehner, 2003).

The major antibody at mucosal surfaces is secretory IgA (sIgA), which is composed of two monomeric IgA molecules covalently linked through the J chain and joined to secretory component (SC). The IgA and J chains are produced by plasma cells, whereas SC is derived from the polymeric Ig receptor (pIgR) that is produced by epithelial cells and ensures selective transcytosis of IgA across the epithelial layer.

SIgA antibodies are protease-resistant immunoglobulins that survive well in external secretions and plays multiple roles in mucosal defense—roles that are markedly distinct from

those of IgG. By serving as an external barrier, sIgA helps protect mucosal surfaces against colonization, entry and invasion by pathogens (Phalipon and Corthesy, 2003; Neutra and Kozlowski, 2006). Intracellular IgA also contributes to protection by neutralizing virus replication inside cells or by blocking transcytosis of viruses from the apical to basolateral cell surface (that is, from the outside-facing surface towards the body's interior). An IgA-mediated excretory pathway also serves to eliminate antigens present in the tissues via binding to IgA and subsequent pIgR-mediated transport of the resulting immune complex to the lumen. Recently, it was shown that secretory component improves the immune exclusion ability of sIgA by targeting the antibody to mucus (Phalipon and Corthesy, 2003). Additionally, microfold or M-cells that cover Peyer's patches and help transport antigens from the intestinal lumen to underlying gut-associated lymphoid tissues express an IgA receptor (Mantis et al., 2002).

All effective vaccines that have been analyzed induce sufficient levels of long-lasting neutralizing antibodies (Zinkernagel, 2003). For HIV—which rapidly establishes persistent infection, has a high mutation rate and can escape from immune control—preventing infection must be a goal of an effective HIV vaccine strategy. Although protective antibodies to HIV have generally been viewed as serum neutralizing antibodies, at mucosal sites even non-neutralizing anti-HIV antibodies, especially IgA, may prevent virus from contacting mucosal surfaces, adhering or crossing epithelial cells or neutralizing virus replication intracellularly. Indeed, non-neutralizing sIgA antibodies have been shown to protect against mucosal infections with rotavirus (Burns et al., 1996).

Other lines of evidence bolster the case for including induction of mucosal IgA in immunization strategies. One is the demonstration in the SHIV-macaque model that passively transferred neutralizing monoclonal antibodies (nmAbs) against HIV-1 confer sterilizing immunity against *mucosal* challenge. In one series of studies, high titer combinations of anti-HIV nmAbs were passively transferred to newborn monkeys, and completely protected them against oral challenge (Ruprecht et al., 2003). In separate experiments, adult female macaques pretreated with progesterone received similar nmAb combinations and were protected against intravaginal SHIV challenge (Mascola, 2003).

Although these findings clearly indicate the importance of neutralizing antibodies in protection against HIV infection, the difficulty in inducing and maintaining adequate levels of these nAbs remains a major obstacle to HIV vaccine development. Passive transfer protection is dependent on IgG transudation from the serum to the mucosal surface. In contrast, locally produced mucosal antibodies were found at markedly enhanced levels. Thus, induction of mucosal IgA as well as IgG antibodies that neutralize HIV-1 should be a goal of mucosal HIV vaccine development.

Individuals who are highly exposed to HIV-1 but remain uninfected (highly exposed, persistently seronegative, or HEPS), provide an important "experiment of nature" that can help identify the correlates of immune protection against mucosal HIV transmission (Chapter 5). In several cohorts of HEPS individuals, resistance to infection was associated with anti-HIV envelope IgA in urogenital tract secretions and with local HIV-specific T-cells detected in cervical scrapings. IgA purified from HEPS individuals was able to neutralize HIV-1 and to block the transcytosis of HIV across a model of mucosal epithelium (Belec et al., 2001). Anti-envelope IgA in these women was directed against the gp41 protein, and the epitope was mapped to a conserved gp41 neutralization determinant rarely recognized by IgA in HIV-infected individuals. More recently, it was shown that IgA purified from the genital tract and saliva of most HEPS sex workers mediated significant cross-clade neutralization of HIV-1 (Devito et al., 2002). This activity, together with local HIV-specific T-cell responses and other factors, may contribute to the protection against HIV infection seen in these individuals.

## Novel mucosal adjuvants and microbicides: take the Toll way

Most vaccines (except those made with replicating viruses) require an adjuvant to induce effective immune responses. Adjuvants, sometimes called "the immunologist's dirty little secret," are defined as substances and formulations that increase immune responses to an antigen. They can also control the type of immune response elicited and, from a practical standpoint, can reduce the amount of antigen needed in a vaccine. Until recently, adjuvant research has been mostly empirical and without simplifying concepts of how these compounds work.

Recently, though, new insights into innate immunity have revolutionized our understanding of immune activation and the mechanisms underlying adjuvant activity. Innate immunity is evolutionarily ancient, highly conserved in animals as well as plants, and serves as our first line of defense against pathogens. In the last few years we have become aware that the innate immune system detects infection through germ line-encoded pattern recognition receptors (PRRs) which recognize highly conserved structures called pathogen-associated molecular patterns (PAMPs), present in large groups of microorganisms but not in the host. Examples of PAMPs include lipopolysaccharide (LPS), peptidoglycan, flagellin, double-stranded RNA (dsRNA) and bacterial CpG DNA. Activation of innate immunity through PRRs such as the Toll-like receptors (TLRs) induces a diverse array of antimicrobial molecules and effector cells which attack microorganisms at multiple levels. Activation of innate immunity also leads to the release of cytokines and chemokines that recruit and activate many types of cells important for the transition from innate to adaptive responses. Thus, activation of the innate immune system through PRRs using their respective ligands or agonists represents a strategy to enhance immune responses against pathogens, making PRRs excellent adjuvants.

We and others demonstrated that a ligand for TLR9 (called CpG oligodeoxynucleotides, or ODN) could serve as an effective mucosal adjuvant (Ashkar and Rosenthal, 2002). Our studies showed that intranasal (i.n.) administration of purified envelope glycoprotein (gB) from HSV-2 plus CpG

ODN as an adjuvant induced strong gB-specific IgA and IgG in the vaginal tract (persisting throughout the estrous cycle) as well as systemic and genital gB-specific CTL, and protected against lethal IVAG HSV-2 infection (Gallichan et al., 2001). Subsequently, we showed that i.n. immunization with inactivated gp120-depleted HIV-1 plus CpG ODN induced anti-HIV IgA in the genital tract and HIV-specific T-cell-mediated immune responses, including production of IFNγ and β-chemokines (Dumais et al., 2002). Further, mice immunized i.n. with HIV-1 plus CpG induced CD8[+] T-cells in the genital tract, providing cross-clade protection against IVAG challenge with recombinant vaccinia viruses expressing HIV-1 *gag* from different clades (Jiang et al., 2005).

Similarly, TLR4 agonists, such as monophosphoryl lipid A (MLA, a chemically modified LPS that retains many of LPS's immunostimulatory properties without its toxic effects), is also an effective mucosal adjuvant (Persing et al., 2002). Mice immunized i.n. with influenza hemagglutinin plus MPL (clinical grade formulation of MLA) generated mucosal immune responses, including IgA in vaginal washes, and enhanced protection against i.n. challenge with influenza virus. Novel approaches to vaccine development could exploit the effects of TLR-activating compounds on innate and adaptive immune responses, especially at mucosal surfaces.

More recent studies from our laboratory and others (Ashkar et al., 2003) demonstrated that a single dose of CpG ODN delivered to the vaginal mucosa, in the absence of any viral antigen, protected against genital infection with HSV-2. This protection was mediated by the innate immune system, since it occurred even in knockout mice lacking B and T-cells. Local IVAG delivery of CpG ODN resulted in rapid proliferation and thickening of the vaginal epithelium and induction of a TLR-9-dependent antiviral state that did not block virus entry but inhibited viral replication in vaginal epithelial cells (Ashkar et al., 2003). More recently, we showed that mucosal delivery of dsRNA, the ligand for TLR3, protected against genital HSV-2 infection without the local or systemic inflammation seen with CpG ODN (Ashkar et al., 2004). Therefore, local delivery of TLR3 ligand may be a safer means of protecting against genital viral infection. We believe it highly likely that this innate immune-mediated antiviral state will protect against a variety of sexually transmitted viral infections (STIs), including HIV-1. Thus, in addition to the use of TLR ligands/agonists as novel adjuvants with mucosal vaccines against HIV and other STIs, a complementary approach may be topical application of these "innate immunologicals" that rapidly induce a local antiviral state which protects mucosal surfaces against infection. Indeed, these may represent "natural microbicides."

## Designing vaccines that elicit mucosal immunity

Delivery of vaccines to mucosal sites is important for induction and long-term maintenance of mucosal immune responses (Kozlowski and Neutra, 2003; Neutra and Kozlowski, 2006). In contrast, parenteral immunization does not effectively induce mucosal sIgA or durable mucosal T-cell-mediated immunity. This dichotomy likely reflects preferential homing of activated lymphocytes and compartmentalization of immune responses to sites of induction. A variety of approaches to inducing mucosal responses have been evaluated. These include co-administration of non-replicating or subunit immunogens with adjuvants active at mucosal surfaces; coupling immunogens to carrier molecules that promote their uptake at mucosal inductive sites; expression of antigens in live-attenuated bacterial or viral vectors that colonize or are tropic for mucosal tissues; and incorporation of antigens into microparticles or adhesive vehicles that are taken up in mucosal inductive sites.

Live recombinant vectors provide a safe method for eliciting both neutralizing antibodies and T-cell immunity (Chapter 8). Since some are based on agents that are naturally transmitted mucosally, this feature can be exploited for induction of local mucosal immunity (Voltan and Robert-Guroff, 2003). Additional advantages include relative ease of production and growth, and the opportunity to include cytokines, chemokines and/or co-stimulatory molecules that enhance and target the immunogenicity of these vectors.

A number of recombinant vectors have undergone extensive preclinical studies in animal models and several have moved into human clinical trials. However, no single vector system will be optimal in all respects, which argues for parallel development of multiple vaccine vectors. Ultimately, decisions about which candidate vectors to advance should rely on head-to-head comparative studies.

Since most vaccination strategies require booster immunizations to achieve maximal efficacy but live vectors usually cannot be used to boost themselves (due to induced immunity and/or pre-existing immunity in to the vector), many heterologous prime-boost strategies are being evaluated. Recent interest in enhancing T-cell-mediated immunity has largely focused on the use of plasmid DNA to prime and recombinant vectors to boost. In an impressive study, monkeys primed with DNA encoding several SIV gene products and boosted with recombinant modified vaccinia Ankara (rMVA) controlled an intrarectal challenge with highly pathogenic SHIV-89.6P given 7 months later (Amara *et al.*, 2002). Protection was associated with a burst of antiviral T-cells.

Over a dozen human clinical trials of HIV vaccines based on DNA prime-heterologous boost are under way in the United States, Europe and Africa (www.iavi.org/trialsdb).

These vaccines are being delivered via parenteral immunization. In light of our growing understanding of mucosal immune responses, it will be important that future trials incorporate mucosal delivery. Indeed, evidence suggests that the rules governing optimal prime-boost strategies may differ in seeking to optimize mucosal versus systemic immunity (Eo *et al.*, 2001).

## Assessing mucosal immune responses in vaccine trials

Understanding both innate and virus-specific immune responses at mucosal surfaces will be critical for HIV vaccine development. Our lack of knowledge is partly due to difficul-

ties in accessing mucosal compartments and collecting adequate amounts of mucosal secretions and cells. To adequately evaluate and compare mucosal-based vaccines, the field needs reliable, sensitive, reproducible and standardized methods of assessing innate and virus-specific mucosal responses. Further, these procedures will have to provide adequate numbers of viable lymphocytes without significant clinical risk and with minimal laboratory manipulation.

Methods such as MHC Class I and II tetramer staining, cytokine flow cytometry (CFC) or intracellular cytokine staining (ICS), and enzyme-linked immunospot (ELISPOT) provide faster, more sensitive techniques for characterizing lymphocyte phenotype and functions (Shacklett, 2002, 2003). Tetramer staining provides an elegant and sensitive means of quantifying CD8+ and CD4+ T-cells specific for a known immunodominant peptide epitope. CFC/ICS are based on stimulating lymphocytes with specific antigen, followed by inhibition of protein secretion and measurement of accumulated intracellular cytokines using multi-color flow cytometry. Recently, CFC was used to simultaneously assess CD4+ and CD8+ T-cell responses to peptides encompassing the entire HIV genome (Betts *et al.*, 2001). Flow cytometry-based assays have been developed to measure CTL killing and cytokine/chemokine production by CD8+ effector cells. The use of fluorescence-based T-cell killing assays in combination with MHC Class I tetramer binding and immunophenotypic staining should allow simultaneous assessment of CTL killer and target T-cell populations.

Advances in flow cytometry-based assays can also be extended to examine innate mucosal immune responses. Thus, innate effector cells such as NK, NKT, γδ T-cells, and dendritic cells, as well as important innate cytokines and chemokines such as IL-15, RANTES, SDF-1, interferons and β-defensins, can be quantitated following mucosal immunization.

More recently, new developments in cytometry hardware, fluorochrome dyes and software have made it possible to measure over 10 simultaneous parameters by flow cytometry. This method, called multi-parameter flow cytometry, holds enormous promise for the characterization of novel and rare antigen-specific cell populations, such as those involved in mucosal immune responses. Using 8-colour staining, γδ T-cell subsets in HIV-infected patients were recently characterized (De Rosa *et al.*, 2001). This method also provides an important opportunity to maximize the information gained from a single experiment, especially from small (and precious) mucosal samples. Thus, it is ideal for obtaining a broader and clearer picture of mucosal immune responses.

To assess mucosal immune responses in large clinical trials, there is great interest in developing peripheral blood-based assays that correlate with mucosal immune responses. One approach would be to develop assays that detect specific mucosal homing T-cells in peripheral blood following vaccination. For example, lymphocytes expressing α4β7 bind to the mucosal addressin MAdCAM-1, which is selectively expressed on high endothelial venules in the intestine. It was recently shown that rhesus macaques immunized intravenously with attenuated

SIV, which replicates in mucosal tissue, generated SIV-specific CD8[+] T-cells expressing $\alpha 4\beta 7$ in peripheral blood, whereas monkeys immunized cutaneously by a combined DNA-MVA regimen did not (Cromwell *et al.*, 2000). These results suggest that induction of virus-specific lymphocytes that home to mucosal sites may be an important characteristic of a successful AIDS vaccine. Although mucosal homing receptors for the small intestine have been characterized, genital tract homing receptors remain unidentified.

Another novel technology with great promise for discovering and assessing vaccine-induced mucosal immune responses is the use of immunogenomics. DNA microarray makes it possible to assess the expression of thousands of genes from cells or tissues under different conditions, and should help reveal broad vaccine-induced changes in the expression of large classes of innate and adaptive immune-related genes. The ability to correlate altered expression patterns with protective mucosal immunity can serve as indicators of effective mucosal immunity and contribute to our understanding of mechanisms of protection.

## Conclusions: challenges and opportunities

Mucosal tissues serve as a major entry site for HIV, an important site for early, rapid, and profound CD4 T-cell loss and a major reservoir for virus replication. The road to an effective vaccine strategy against HIV must therefore take advantage of mucosal innate and adaptive immune responses. Given the compartmentalization of our immune system and the selective homing of lymphocytes, mucosal delivery of vaccines will be important for triggering and maintaining durable mucosal responses. The challenges ahead include the identification of safe and effective mucosal adjuvants, understanding correlates of mucosal immune protection and how best to induce and sustain these responses, and the development of suitable methods for assessing mucosal responses. It will also be important to move a number of mucosal vaccines that are successful in animal and primate studies into clinical trials.

## References

Altfeld, M., Allen, T.M., Yu, X.G., Johnston, M.N., Agrawal, D., Korber, B.T., Montefiori, D.C., O'Connor, D.H., Davis, B.T., Lee, P.K., *et al.* (2002). HIV-1 superinfection despite broad CD8[+] T-cell responses containing replication of the primary virus. Nature *420*, 434–439.

Amara, R.R., Villinger, F., Altman, J.D., Lydy, S.L., O'Neil, S.P., Staprans, S.I., Montefiori, D.C., Xu, Y., Herndon, J.G., Wyatt, L.S., *et al.* (2002). Control of a mucosal challenge and prevention of AIDS by a multiprotein DNA/MVA vaccine. Vaccine *20*, 1949–1955.

Ashkar, A.A., Bauer, S., Mitchell, W.J., Vieira, J., and Rosenthal, K.L. (2003). Local delivery of CpG oligodeoxynucleotides induces rapid changes in the genital mucosa and inhibits replication, but not entry, of herpes simplex virus type 2. J. Virol. *77*, 8948–8956.

Ashkar, A.A., and Rosenthal, K.L. (2002). Toll-like receptor 9, CpG DNA and innate immunity. Curr. Mol. Med. *2*, 545–556.

Ashkar, A.A., Yao, X.D., Gill, N., Sajic, D., Patrick, A. J., and Rosenthal, K.L. (2004). Toll-like receptor (TLR)-3, but not TLR4, agonist protects against genital herpes infection in the absence of inflammation seen with CpG DNA. J. Infect. Dis. *190*, 1841–1849.

Belec, L., Ghys, P.D., Hocini, H., Nkengasong, J.N., Tranchot-Diallo, J., Diallo, M.O., Ettiegne-Traore, V., Maurice, C., Becquart, P., Matta, M., *et al.* (2001). Cervicovaginal secretory antibodies to human immunodeficiency virus type 1 (HIV-1) that block viral transcytosis through tight epithelial barriers in highly exposed HIV-1-seronegative African women. J. Infect. Dis. *184*, 1412–1422.

Betts, M.R., Ambrozak, D.R., Douek, D.C., Bonhoeffer, S., Brenchley, J.M., Casazza, J.P., Koup, R.A., and Picker, L.J. (2001). Analysis of total human immunodeficiency virus (HIV)-specific CD4(+) and CD8(+) T-cell responses: relationship to viral load in untreated HIV infection. J. Virol. 75, 11983–11991.

Brenchley, J.M., Price, D.A., Douek, D.C. (2006). HIV disease: fallout from a mucosal catastrophe? Nature Immunol. 7, 235–239.

Burns, J.W., Siadat-Pajouh, M., Krishnaney, A.A., and Greenberg, H.B. (1996). Protective effect of rotavirus VP6-specific IgA monoclonal antibodies that lack neutralizing activity. Science 272, 104–107.

Cromwell, M.A., Veazey, R.S., Altman, J.D., Mansfield, K.G., Glickman, R., Allen, T.M., Watkins, D.I., Lackner, A.A., and Johnson, R.P. (2000). Induction of mucosal homing virus-specific CD8(+) T lymphocytes by attenuated simian immunodeficiency virus. J. Virol. 74, 8762–8766.

De Rosa, S.C., Mitra, D.K., Watanabe, N., Herzenberg, L.A. and Roederer, M. (2001). Vdelta1 and Vdelta2 gammadelta T-cells express distinct surface markers and might be developmentally distinct lineages. J. Leukoc. Biol. 70, 518–526.

Devito, C., Hinkula, J., Kaul, R., Kimani, J., Kiama, P., Lopalco, L., Barass, C., Piconi, S., Trabattoni, D., Bwayo, J. J., *et al.* (2002). Crossclade HIV-1-specific neutralizing IgA in mucosal and systemic compartments of HIV-1-exposed, persistently seronegative subjects. J. Acquir. Immune. Defic. Syndr. 30, 413–420.

Douek, D.C., Picker, L.J., and Koup, R.A. (2003). T-cell dynamics in HIV-1 infection. Annu. Rev. Immunol. 21, 265–304.

Dumais, N., Patrick, A., Moss, R.B., Davis, H.L., and Rosenthal, K.L. (2002). Mucosal immunization with inactivated human immunodeficiency virus plus CpG oligodeoxynucleotides induces genital immune responses and protection against intravaginal challenge. J. Infect. Dis. 186, 1098–1105.

Eo, S.K., Gierynska, M., Kamar, A.A., and Rouse, B.T. (2001). Primeboost immunization with DNA vaccine: mucosal route of administration changes the rules. J. Immunol. 166, 5473–5479.

Gallichan, W.S., Woolstencroft, R.N., Guarasci, T., McCluskie, M.J., Davis, H.L., and Rosenthal, K.L. (2001). Intranasal immunization with CpG oligodeoxynucleotides as an adjuvant dramatically increases IgA and protection against herpes simplex virus-2 in the genital tract. J. Immunol. 166, 3451–3457.

Jiang, J.Q., Patrick, A., Moss, R.B., and Rosenthal, K.L. (2005). CD8[+] T-cell-mediated cross-clade protection in the genital tract following intranasal immunization with inactivated human immunodeficiency virus antigen plus CpG oligodeoxynucleotides. J. Virol. 79, 393–400.

Kozlowski, P.A. and Neutra, M.R. (2003). The role of mucosal immunity in prevention of HIV transmission. Curr. Mol. Med. 3, 217–228.

Lehner, T. (2003). Innate and adaptive mucosal immunity in protection against HIV infection. Vaccine 21, Suppl. 2, S68–S76.

Mantis, N.J., Cheung, M.C., Chintalacharuvu, K.R., Rey, J., Corthesy, B., and Neutra, M.R. (2002). Selective adherence of IgA to murine Peyer's patch M-cells: evidence for a novel IgA receptor. J. Immunol. 169, 1844–1851.

Margolis, L. and Shattock, R. (2006). Selective transmission of CCR5-utilizing HIV-1: the "gatekeeper" problem resolved? Nature Rev. Microbiol. 4, 312–317.

Mascola, J.R. (2003). Defining the protective antibody response for HIV-1. Curr. Mol. Med. 3, 209–216.

Neutra, M.R. and Kozlowski, P.A. (2006). Mucosal vaccines: the promise and the challenge. Nature Rev. Immunol. 6, 148–158.

Persing, D.H., Coler, R.N., Lacy, M.J., Johnson, D.A., Baldridge, J.R., Hershberg, R.M., and Reed, S.G. (2002). Taking toll: lipid A mimetics as adjuvants and immunomodulators. Trends Microbiol. 10, S32–S37.

Phalipon, A., and Corthesy, B. (2003). Novel functions of the polymeric Ig receptor: well beyond transport of immunoglobulins. Trends. Immunol. *24*, 55–58.

Rescigno, M., Urbano, M., Valzasina, B., Francolini, M., Rotta, G., Bonasio, R., Granucci, F., Kraehenbuhl, J.P., and Ricciardi-Castagnoli, P. (2001). Dendritic cells express tight junction proteins and penetrate gut epithelial monolayers to sample bacteria. Nature Immunol. *2*, 361–367.

Ruprecht, R.M., Ferrantelli, F., Kitabwalla, M., Xu, W., and McClure, H.M. (2003). Antibody protection: passive immunization of neonates against oral AIDS virus challenge. Vaccine *21*, 3370–3373.

Shacklett, B.L. (2002). Beyond 51Cr release: New methods for assessing HIV-1-specific CD8⁺ T-cell responses in peripheral blood and mucosal tissues. Clin. Exp. Immunol. *130*, 172–182.

Shacklett, B.L., Yang, O., Hausner, M.A., Elliott, J., Hultin, L., Price, C., Fuerst, M., Matud, J., Hultin, P., Cox, C., *et al.* (2003). Optimization of methods to assess human mucosal T-cell responses to HIV infection. J. Immunol. Methods *279*, 17–31.

Shattock, R.J. and Moore, J.P. (2003). Inhibiting sexual transmission of HIV-1 infection. Nature Rev. Microbiol. *1*, 25–34.

Veazey, R.S. and Lackner, A.A. (1998). The gastrointestinal tract and the pathogenesis of AIDS. AIDS 12 Suppl. A, S35–42.

Voltan, R. and Robert-Guroff, M. (2003). Live recombinant vectors for AIDS vaccine development. Curr. Mol. Med. *3*, 273–284.

Zinkernagel, R.M. (2003). On natural and artificial vaccinations. Annu. Rev. Immunol. *21*, 515–546.

# HIV Subtypes, Antigenic Diversity, and Vaccine Design

# 10

Bette T. Korber, Catherine C. Miller, and Thomas K. Leitner

## Abstract

The variation of HIV-1 on the individual level, between individuals, and between different subtypes is considered one major obstacle in HIV-1 vaccine design. HIV-1 subtypes, or clades, are clearly distinguishable genetic classifications of HIV. Recombination is an inherent aspect of HIV evolution, and inter-subtype recombinant forms are frequently found in regions of the world where multiple forms are co-circulating. Vaccine reagents, to be useful, must elicit immune responses that are cross-reactive in the context of this complex backdrop of diverse strains. There are limited genotype–serotype relationships between sequences and neutralizing antibodies. T-lymphocyte responses to HIV cover the spectrum from subtype specific, to diminished but detectable inter-clade responses, to broadly cross-reactive. While the relative merits of developing HIV-1 subtype-specific vaccines for different proteins are as yet unresolved, given the polyclonal and host-specific nature of the immune response, regional subtype appropriate vaccines may be a helpful for maximizing the set of potential cross-reactive responses between vaccine strains and the circulating population. Different strategies for vaccine design that attempt to contend with diversity are discussed.

## HIV-1 subtype definitions

### Subtypes

HIV-1 displays extensive genetic diversity. Based on the phylogenetic relationships between DNA sequences, HIV-1 has been divided into three groups of distant genetic variants: M, N, and O (Fig. 10.1A). Because these groups are interspersed by sequences from Chimpanzees, it is believed that they each represent a cross-species transmission (Bailes *et al.*, 2002). Group M (for main, as most infections in the pandemic fall in this group) is further divided into subtypes, also commonly referred to as clades, and sub-subtypes (Robertson *et al.*, 2000). The subtypes are approximately equidistant from each other, and currently eleven subtypes and sub-subtypes have been characterized throughout the complete genome (Kuiken *et al.*, 2002).

### Recombination

In addition to subtypes, HIV-1 is also frequently found as mosaic forms of the subtypes, believed to be the consequence of superinfection and recombination. There are numerous examples in the literature of such forms, and some of these have had great impact on the HIV pandemic. Once a recombinant form is detected, and fully described, in at least three individuals, who are not directly epidemiologically linked, they are called circulating recombinant forms (CRFs). Currently, there are over 30 CRFs described in the world (Leitner, 2004).

A full length HIV-1 genome for at least one subtype (E), has not been identified. This lineage was designated based on distinctive envelope sequences embedded in a background of a subtype A virus. The lineage that contains subtype E envelope has been designated CRF01, as an A-E recombinant (Robertson *et al.*, 2000). It has also been suggested that CRF01 may not be a product of recombination between A and a parental subtype E strain, rather that it is a distinctive off shoot of the subtype A lineage (Anderson *et al.*, 2000). In either case, it forms a distinct lineage that may be useful for vaccine design in parts of Asia, where CRF01 is prevalent.

Furthermore, in addition to subtypes and recombinant forms there are many HIV-1 M group sequences that do not fall into these classes because their origin has not been possible to establish. These sequences may be representatives of rare subtypes, recombinants of extinct subtypes or multiple recombinations making it difficult to characterize their origin. Note that a phylogenetic analysis with recombinant sequences present will not give an accurate representation of the evolutionary history of the data set.

### Origins

It is still not clear why and how the subtypes were formed. For several reasons, most likely they are the result of genetic drift and founder effects rather than selective mechanisms. First, for example, when sequences from specific subtypes are transmitted between African populations to Europeans or Asians, there is no indication that the virus sequence changes in unique characteristic ways that dominate phylogenetic patterns, de-

**A.**

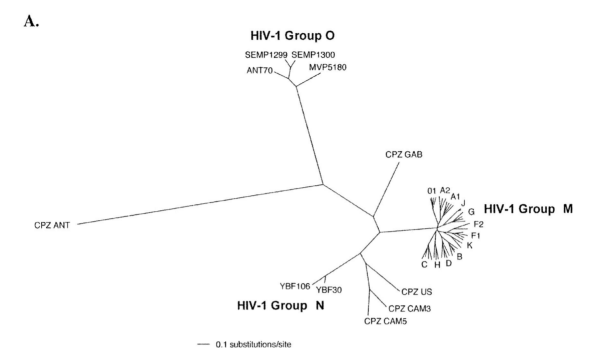

**B.** **C.**

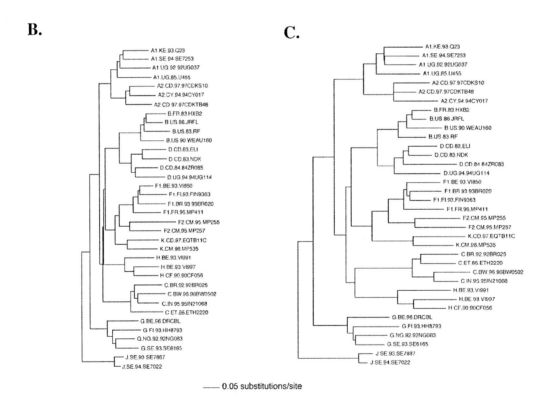

**Figure 10.1** Unrooted phylogenetic reconstructions of HIV-1 evolution. (A) The *env* phylogeny of HIV-1 in relation to SIV CPZ. HIV-1 groups M, N and O are interspersed by SIV CPZ sequences. HIV-1 group is divided into subtypes and sub-subtypes (A–K). CRF01 is also shown because it consists of subtype E in *env*. (B) Group M phylogeny based on first and second codon position. (C) Group M phylogeny based on third codon position. Note that the third codon position tree is longer than the tree from first and second position, i.e., there is more information about the subtype division in the third position ($P < 0.00001$). The topology of all trees was calculated under the F84 model (transition/transversion rate bias 1.66, 1.52 and 2.18, for trees A, B and C, respectively) using the neighbor-joining (NJ) algorithm. The branch lengths were subsequently optimized under general-time-reversible models for each data set including invariable sites and Γ-distributed variable sites using maximum likelihood calculations. Scale bars are according to this model. All subtypes are supported by > 96% bootstrap values, calculated under the F84 model and NJ from 2000 replicates. All phylogenetic calculations were performed using PAUP*.

spite differences in frequencies in the immune response genes in the host population. Second, since selective mechanisms mainly operate on the protein level, if the distinguishing characteristics of the subtype pattern are driven by selection, they should be more obvious on amino acid changing DNA mutations while silent mutations (e.g., third codon positions, that usually do not alter amino acids) would show a random pattern. This is not the case. Third codon positions display the same subtype pattern as first and second (Fig. 10.1B and C). In fact, third codon positions have comparatively more phylogenetic signal ($P < 0.00001$).

Interestingly, among the variable sites in *env* the rate distribution for which substitutions occur is similar in all codon positions, with a $\Gamma$ shape parameter of about 0.72. $\Gamma$ distributions are often used to model the different levels of variation at different nucleotide positions in an alignment, so the fact that some positions vary rapidly, others are more conserved can be taken into account when building a phylogenetic tree. Considering rate variation at different sites is an important aspect of modeling the evolution of HIV (Leitner *et al.*, 1997), and defining relative rates of variation at different sites by assuming a $\Gamma$ distribution is a common way to do this, implemented in many tree building packages. The consistency among the codon position substitutions, supporting the phylogenetic relationships, is also similar (CI = 0.38). The difference is that the estimated invariable sites in amino acid changing positions (first + second) is 34%, compared to only 1.3% in the third position, where nucleotide changes are usually silent, and so the third positions are seldom completely conserved.

Finally, the occurrence of recombinant forms suggests that sequence space is not limited by selective mechanisms that could have formed the subtypes. Rather, numerous new mosaic genetic forms have been established throughout the expansion of HIV-1 in both Africa and other geographic locales. Furthermore, HIV-1 M, N and O, and HIV-2 while highly divergent, are all viable viruses that result in AIDS and have similar biological characteristics, reflecting the vast potential sequence space encompassed by the pathogenic HIV-related viral family.

## Superinfection, recombination, and implications for vaccines

### Intersubtype recombination

Intersubtype recombination cannot happen without two subtypes co-existing in the same individual, and both parental genomes co-existing in the same cell. By the mid-1990s it was established that intersubtype recombination occurs (Sabino, 1994), can be transmitted (Leitner *et al.*, 1995) and is frequently observed (Robertson *et al.*, 1995), making it abundantly clear that co-infections by two subtypes are not uncommon within individuals. In fact, in regions where multiple subtypes co-circulate with high prevalence, intersubtype recombinants are very common (Dowling *et al.*, 2002; Harris *et al.*, 2002). Although most of the more than 150,000 sequences currently

in the Los Alamos HIV database (www.hiv.lanl.gov) are only partial genomes, one can use the database to at least crudely ask if countries that have more diverse distributions of subtypes co-circulating tend to have more unique recombinants emerging. If simply the opportunity for exposure to more than one subtype results in an increased frequency of novel recombinants, this should be the case. If one calculates how common the most common subtype is in each country, as a measure of the complexity of the subtype distribution in the country, it turns out to be inversely correlated with the proportion of sequences that are unique recombinants (Fig. 10.2). Thus regional epidemics that are the result from a diverse admixture of different subtypes tend to give rise to novel recombinants more frequently.

Most samples for HIV sequencing are taken cross-sectionally from individuals well into their infections. When the primary evidence for multiple infections in one individual is the indirect observation of recombinants, it is unclear what fraction of these stemmed from multiple infections prior to developing a primary immune response, and what fraction were due to serial infections where a second infection occurs despite the immune response to the first infection. Thus, the relative frequency with which (i) the dual infection events both occur during primary infection, prior to the individual's mounting an immune response against HIV, compared to (ii) serial infections, in which a primary infection occurs, and immune responses are mounted, and a new virus is able to subsequently infect the individual, are unknown. Given that a natu-

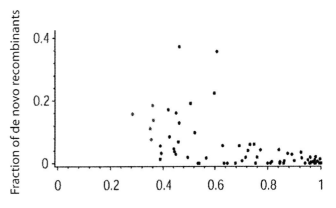

Fraction of the most common subtype or CRF

**Figure 10.2** This figure illustrates the inverse correlation between the frequency of the most common subtype or CRF, and the frequency of de novo recombinants. The frequency of the most common subtype in a country is a crude measure of the subtype diversity in that county; as the value approaches 1, the dominance of a single subtype in the population is greater. The frequency of de novo recombinants refers to the fraction of sequences from a country that are clearly a recombinant but are not one of the defined circulating recombinant forms. The data used for generating this figure comes from the Los Alamos database (www.hiv.lanl.gov). There were 110 countries included in the comparison, and 83 of these countries had sequences available from more than 25 individuals. The evidence for the correlation of these two values was very high, using a non-parametric rank correlation Spearman's test gave a $P$ value of $4 \times 10^{-10}$.

ral, persistent infection is a very potent immunogen compared to many vaccines give rise to a transient immune stimulus, if serial infections between subtypes are indeed frequent events in regions where exposures to different clades are commonplace, then one might imagine that vaccines would have little power to protect across-clades. Also, vaccines would be given to populations of people with healthy immune systems, while HIV infection begins to compromise the CD4$^+$ T-lymphocyte immune response early in infection (Altfeld *et al.*, 2001; Musey *et al.*, 1999), thus uninfected vaccinees could greet newly encountered virus with a healthy T-cell memory response and this might confer an advantage.

Finally, there is growing evidence that superinfection can occur with two distinct viruses from the same subtype, in spite of a strong immune response to the first infection (e.g., Altfeld *et al.*, 2002; Koelsch *et al.*, 2003). Such examples are infrequently observed (Gonzales *et al.*, 2003), although it is not clear whether this is due to their being very rare or being hard to detect. More recently it was shown that superinfection with another form (an ACD recombinant) of HIV-1 than the original infection (an AC recombinant) is possible (McCutcahn *et al.*, 2005), and that superinfection may lead to acquired drug resistance (Smith 2005a). Currently, controversy exists about the relative role of superinfection (Diaz *et al.*, 2005; Smith *et al.*, 2005b). Partly because it is difficult to study, it is still unclear how common it is and therefore how big its role may be on the global pandemic and in local epidemics. Differences in viral fitness may make sampling a less common variant virtually impossible, and the clear track left by easily defined inter-subtype recombination events would not be as readily discernable in a within-subtype context. Nonetheless, the relative infrequency of finding superinfections, given the large number of longitudinal studies that have been undertaken through the years suggests that it may not be very common.

In the absence of data that clearly resolves these issues, one can only speculate about possible outcomes. While these factors will no doubt contribute to the outcome of vaccine trials, the relative protection conferred by a vaccine between and within clades will have to be empirically determined. The lack of protection indicated by the reported superinfections is a serious concern, but if such infections are real but relatively rare, the implications for vaccines at the population level may not be that bad. On the other hand, the high frequency of inter-clade recombinants may reflect at least in part relatively high rates of serial infections, supporting the concept of designing subtype-specific vaccines.

## Antigenic cross-reactivity

### Antibodies and subtypes
At the global level, subtypes and CRFs are one of the few relatively stable anchors we have for delineating consistent patterns in the vast range of HIV diversity. However, while serotypes and antibodies that bind to linear epitopes often cor-

relate with genotypes as defined by subtypes, there is generally less correspondence between neutralizing antibodies and genetic subtypes, perhaps because of the extraordinary diversity even within a clade (Moore *et al.*, 2001). Some isolates tend to be neutralization sensitive, some neutralization resistant, and these tendencies can over-ride clade specificity and potentially confound clear genotype–serotype relationships (Bures *et al.*, 2002). Despite the general difficulties in defining clear genetic and antigenic relationships, some specific subtype–serotype relationships have been detected. Isolates of subtype B and CRF01, subtypes both common in Thailand and in other parts of Asia, have distinct neutralization susceptibility profiles that correspond to subtypes (Mascola *et al.*, 1996). The B and C subtypes, like B and CRF01, also been have a genetic subtype-neutralization antibody correspondence, where sera preferential neutralize isolates from the same clade as the infecting strain (with some exceptions, such as two sera from C clade infections that broadly neutralized both B and C clade isolates) (Bures *et al.*, 2002). This study also found geographic differences in neutralization patterns in countries where subtype C infections dominate. In addition, broadly neutralizing monoclonal antibodies do have some consistent patterns of subtype reactivity, in particular the antibodies 2G12 does not recognize viruses from clade C and CRF01, and 2F5 does not recognize envelopes derived from subtype C, in each case as a result of mutations in their core epitope (Binley *et al.*, 2004). In contrast, 4E10 neutralizes most M group viruses to some degree, and b12 can block infection of some strains from most clades (Binley *et al.*, 2004).

In a recent study, CRF01 non-syncytium-inducing strains were found to be more neutralization sensitive than syncytium-inducing strains, and this was a lineage specific characteristic not founding B subtype (Polonis *et al.*, 2003). Furthermore, there are clearly distinct subtype-specific selective pressures on different regions of B and C subtype Envelopes (Gaschen 2002a), and these differences may reflect generally distinct sensitivities to neutralizing antibodies through differential antigenic exposure on the protein surface. Such lineage-specific characteristics may be important for vaccine design in subtle ways. As scientists work to develop vaccines that can elicit neutralizing antibodies, the constructs they develop may turn out to have some clade specific properties, particularly if the constructs are designed to reveal a specific antigenic domain that is distinct in different subtypes. Furthermore, there are clearly subtype-specific selective pressures on regions of Envelope (Gaschen *et al.*, 2002a), and this may reflect generally distinct sensitivities to neutralizing antibodies through differential antigenic exposure on the protein surface of different subtype lineages.

HIV-1 rapidly evades neutralizing antibody responses during the course of the infection of an individual (Arendrup *et al.*, 1992; Richman *et al.*, 2003; Wei *et al.*, 2003), and such immune escape involves recurring evasion of polyclonal responses in the host. Infected people target a variety of epitopes; presumably the precise combination of epitopes is specific to the host and infecting HIV quasispecies. Escape from neutralizing antibodies within a host may confer varying degrees of resistance to sera collected from other infected individuals, and viruses with different levels of immune refractive properties will emerge during the cycles of escape. Thus it is reasonable that a broad range of neutralization resistance characteristics are found among different primary viral isolates. Some regions of Env, like the CD4 binding site, tend to elicit pan-reactive antibodies, while other have more sporadic cross-reactivity, like the variable loops (Moore et al., 1994). V3 loop antibodies with conformational binding characteristics tend to be more cross-reactive and more potent at neutralization than linear V3 epitopes (Gorny et al., 2002). In summary, antibodies may interact with epitopes which are: (i) well-preserved due to functional or structural constraints across-clades, (ii) essentially unique to the autologous virus that stimulated the response, (iii) sporadically cross-reactive with different isolates in a clade-independent manner, or (iv) preserved within a specific clade, or maybe several clades, but not in all clades (Nyambi et al., 2000; Moore et al., 1994). Even if the fourth class of subtype-specific epitopes occur reasonably frequently, but are not the most common or intense responses, it might be difficult to distinguish them when overlaid on a background of broadly cross-reactive or strain-specific responses. However, even when neutralization serotype–genotype correlations are not overtly evident, other more subtle clade-specific aspects of cross-reactivity may be important in a vaccine context, such as an inability of sera or antibodies to react with a particular clade or clades. For example, a set of antibodies that bind to the crown of the V3 loop with conformational dependency show cross-clade binding to virions of clades A, B, C, D, and F, but not CRF01isolates from subtype E (Gorny et al., 2002). Similarly the broadly neutralizing antibodies 2G12 and 2F5 neutralizes many primary isolates from multiple clades, but 2G12 and 2F5 fail to neutralize most clade C isolates (Bures et al., 2002).

### T-lymphocyte responses to HIV

Similarly, the importance of subtypes for T-cell responses are complicated and could be viewed as a glass half full or a glass half empty. While some specific CD8$^+$ Cytotoxic T-lymphocyte (CTL) responses have been shown to be broadly cross-reactive (Cao et al., 1997; Innwoley, 2005), others are cross-reactive but with diminished reactivity, or cross-reactive with a some subtypes but not others (Fukada et al., 2002; Yu et al., 2005), and still other changes in HIV can completely abrogate a particular T-cell response to sequences from other clades (Dorrell et al., 1999, 2001). The studies referenced above are the tip of the iceberg; there are dozens of responses to specific epitopes that had been characterized in the literature that show different patterns of inter-subtype cross-reactivity. Thus, there is a spectrum of cross-reactivity in terms cross-clade CTL responses, and most of these are summarized in the HIV immunology database (www.hiv.lanl.gov). CD4$^+$ T-cell

responses also show varying degrees of sensitivity to subtype differences (Norris et al., 2004).

Even escape from a single, specific CTL response in a SHIV vaccine-challenge study can allow virus to escape from the beneficial immunity conferred by the vaccine (Barouch et al., 2003). It is hard to extrapolate what this might mean in the context of a human population with diverse HLA backgrounds and infecting viral sequences. A priori it seems desirable to attempt to build vaccines that elicit responses to multiple, potent, cross-reactive epitopes. In this way, the probability is enhanced that a useful subset of the epitopes stimulated by a vaccine will be cross-reactive with the strains encountered and circulating in a human population. By analogy with the benefit of using multi-drug cocktails, if infections occur in a vaccinated population that are held in check as a result of encountering vaccine-stimulated immune responses, escape from any one epitope will be less likely to lead to expanded viral load and decline to AIDS if multiple specific responses are in place. One way to approach is adding additional proteins to the vaccine (Hel et al., 2006), another alternative is by adding variants of the same protein (Seaman, 2006), as discussed below.

## Vaccine strategies to contend with diversity

### Polyvalent HIV vaccines

Scientists are considering many strategies for expanding the potential for cross-reactivity immunity elicited by HIV vaccines. The first obvious choice is to make vaccines that focus the immune response on conserved epitopes that elicit broadly cross-reactive responses, such as the method proposed by Wilson and colleagues in the context of Helper T-cell epitopes (Wilson et al., 2001). Alternatively, based on the subtypes prevalent in the geographic region where the vaccine is intended for use, by using a subtype-appropriate vaccine one can narrowing the diversity field so the vaccine response primarily has to contend with within subtype-diversity. This option might help in countries like the United States, South Africa, or India, where a single subtype dominates the epidemic. A traditional approach that expands upon this is to use multivalent vaccines that comprise multiple HIV strains (Nabel et al., 2002). For example, one strain could be included to represent each of the major circulating subtypes in the region where the vaccine is intended for use, or alternatively multiple strains from the predominant epidemic subtype could be used to attempt to expand the within-subtype coverage. There will be a balance of between how many variants one could successfully include in such a vaccine and the potency of the immune response against specific variants. The optimum number of variants to reach a balance in breadth and strength of response would need to be determined empirically for different vaccine strategies, but experiments to date show that inclusion of a combination of one A, one B, and one C clade virus allow robust responses to each antigen in the cocktail (Seaman, 2006).

## Modifying envelope to expose conserved neutralizing epitopes

Another concept is to modify envelope to provide access to conserved neutralizing epitopes that otherwise might only be either transiently exposed or otherwise well protected on the natural protein surface of envelope. There are many such strategies currently being explored, here we will just describe a few of them. One concept is the deletion of the sections of hypervariable loop domains, to leave better exposed some of the more conserved domains that are normally masked (Srivastava *et al.*, 2003; Sanders *et al.*, 2000). Another idea is to chemically cross-link proteins to force exposure of potentially useful epitopes. The SOS-Env protein includes a disulfide bond joining the gp120 and gp41 protein. This locks the protein into an intermediate state, comparable to binding Envelope after binding to co-receptors, but prior to fusion, a stable conformation that may expose otherwise difficult to access epitopes (Abrahamyan *et al.*, 2003; Beddows *et al.*, 2005). Another cross-linking strategy uses CD4 bound to gp120 or gp140, and this protein construct also seems to expose novel neutralizing epitopes (Fouts *et al.*, 2002). Yet another concept is to try to force preferential exposure of the neutralizing determinants of the potent broadly neutralizing monoclonal antibodies. For example, the broadly neutralizing monoclonal IgG1b12 and its Fab b12 bind to gp120 by projecting deeply into CD4 binding pocket (Saphire *et al.*, 2001). Directed addition of glycosylation sites can force preferential binding of the IgG1b12 Fab b12, relative to non-neutralizing CD4 binding site antibodies, and might be useful for focusing the antibody response toward this epitope (Pantophlet *et al.*, 2003). Recent structural studies are providing insights that ultimately may facilitate antigen design to allow exposure of the membrane-proximal region of gp41 in a correct conformation to elicit neutralizing antibodies with properties like 4E10 and 2F5, but this remains a difficult problem despite accruing knowledge (Zwick *et al.*, 2005).

## Artificial central strains

A final option is considering incorporating "central strains" into strategies for HIV vaccine design (Gaschen *et al.*, 2002b; Korber *et al.*, 2001b; Nickle *et al.*, 2003). The simplest approach is to use a consensus sequence derived by concatenating the most common amino acid found in each position in an alignment of protein sequences from a clade of interest. Ties can be resolved by using what is most common in other subtypes (www.hiv.lanl. gov). A consensus sequence is far more similar to circulating forms than they are to each other, and so shares more identities with known epitopes (Korber *et al.*, 2001a). Immunogenicity can be negatively affected by a single amino acid substitution, and there are epitopes spanning most regions of viral proteins, thus reductions in the number of substitutions between a vaccine strains and circulating strains would presumably enhance cross-reactivity with multiple epitopes (Kuiken *et al.*, 1999). Initial studies with the B and C clade cetramas (Doria-Rose *et al.*, 2005) and M group consensus/ancestral strains (Gaschen *et al.*, 2002b; Gao *et al.*, 2005) are showing some promise. The

M group consensus/ancestral envelope protein folds correctly, binds CD4 and appropriate antibodies, and is immunogenic in small animal studies eliciting antibody and T-cell immune responses that react with some viruses from multiple clades.

HIV M group sequences evolve in such a way that phylogenies created from the sequences give rise to what is known as a star-phylogeny (Fig. 10.1A). In other words, when isolates are selected randomly from a population, there tends to be limited resolvable structure within phylogenetic reconstructions near the base of the clades, and sequences instead radiate out with very shallow branches near the root, expanding outward from a central point. Maximum likelihood phylogenetic methods allow one to estimate the most likely sequences at interior branch points within the tree, and reconstruct a model sequence of the most probable base at each position. This reconstructed sequence is at the root of a clade, and is generally is near the center of the clade. Like the consensus, it is much more similar to modern circulating forms than they are to each other. One can go back even further to the root of the entire M group tree, and derive a sequence which models the most recent common ancestor of the global strains; such a sequence is roughly equidistant to sequences from all subtypes. Rather than picking the ancestor, one can instead choose something called the COT, or center of tree, which is an ancestral point selected to minimize the branch length to the taxa of interest in a tree (say all sequences of a single clade; Nickle *et al.*, 2003). While all such central sequences are by definition artificial, the first M group envelope consensus (built as a consensus of all subtype consensus sequences, and which corresponded to the predicted the M group ancestor) (Korber *et al.*, 2000), showed good cross-reactive properties, and folded in a way that preserved antigenic characteristics of binding sites for key monoclonal antibodies (Gao *et al.*, 2005). The M group consensus is immunogenic in small animals studies, and shows some initial promise in terms of eliciting B call and T-cell responses that can react with viruses from multiple subtypes (Liao *et al.*, 2006; Weaver *et al.*, 2006). As the M group consensus is even farther from real sequences than the consensus or ancestor of a single clade, and Env, being the most variable protein, would be the most challenging to reconstruct, this is a hopeful result for such sequences in general. B clade and C clade central sequences have also been generated and are showing promise (Doria-Rose *et al.*, 2005; Kothe *et al.*, 2006).

Both consensus and ancestral sequences for reagent design are available at the HIV database (www.hiv.lanl.gov), as are extensive reference alignments of HIV sequences for people who prefer to build their own versions using database alignments. These sequences are updated periodically, and change slightly from year to year as more information is available for their derivation. Consensus, COT, and ancestral sequences are all very similar to each other, relative to differences between circulating strains. The differences are likely to be in the most variable positions, however, and may be in some of the most immunologically interesting sites in terms of immune response and escape.

# References

Abrahamyan, L.G., Markosyan, R.M., Moore, J.P., Cohen, F.S., and Melikyan, G.B. (2003). Human immunodeficiency virus type 1 Env with an intersubunit disulfide bond engages coreceptors but requires bond reduction after engagement to induce fusion. J. Virol. 77, 5829–5836.

Altfeld, M., Allen, T.M., Yu, X.G., Johnston, M.N., Agrawal, D., Korber, B.T., Montefiori, D.C., O'Connor, D.H., Davis, B.T., Lee, P.K., Maier, E.L., Harlow, J., Goulder, P.J., Brander, C., Rosenberg, E.S., and Walker, B.D. (2002). HIV-1 superinfection despite broad CD8$^+$ T-cell responses containing replication of the primary virus. Nature 420, 434–439.

Altfeld, M., Rosenberg, E.S., Shankarappa, R., Mukherjee, J.S., Hecht, F.M., Eldridge, R.L., Addo, M.M., Poon, S.H., Phillips, M.N., Robbins, G.K., Sax, P.E., Boswell, S., Kahn, J.O., Brander, C., Goulder, P.J., Levy, J.A., Mullins, J.I., and Walker, B.D. (2001). Cellular immune responses and viral diversity in individuals treated during acute and early HIV-1 infection. J. Exp. Med. 193, 169–180.

Anderson, J.P., Rodrigo, A.G., Learn, G.H., Madan, A., Delahunty, C., Coon, M., Girard, M., Osmanov, S., Hood, L., and Mullins, J.I. (2000). Testing the hypothesis of a recombinant origin of human immunodeficiency virus type 1 subtype E. J. Virol. 74, 10752–10765.

Arendrup, M., Nielsen, C., Hansen, J.E., Pedersen, C., Mathiesen, L., and Nielsen, J.O. (1992). Autologous HIV-1 neutralizing antibodies, emergence of neutralization-resistant escape virus and subsequent development of escape virus neutralizing antibodies. J. Acquir. Immune. Defic. Syndr. 5, 303–307.

Bailes, E., Chaudhuri, R., Santiago, M.L., Bibollet-Ruche, F., Hahn, B., and Sharp, P.M. (2002). The evolution of primate lentiviruses and the origins of AIDS. Leitner, T. The molecular epidemiology of human viruses. Boston, Kluwer Academic Publishers.

Barouch, D.H., Kunstman, J., Glowczwskie, J., Kunstman, K.J., Egan, M.A., Peyerl, F.W., Santra, S., Kuroda, M J., Schmitz, J.E., Beaudry, K., Krivulka, G.R., Lifton, M.A., Gorgone, D.A., Wolinsky, S.M., and Letvin, N.L. (2003). Viral escape from dominant simian immunodeficiency virus epitope-specific cytotoxic T lymphocytes in DNA-vaccinated rhesus monkeys. J. Virol. 77, 7367–7375.

Beddows, S., Schulke, N., Kirschner, M., Barnes, K., Franti, M., Michael, E., Ketas, T., Sanders, R., Maddon, P., Olson, W., and Moore, J. (2005). Evaluating the immunogenicity of a disulfide-stabilized, cleaved, trimeric form of the envelope glycoprotein complex of human immunodeficiency virus type 1. J. Virol. 79, 8812–8827.

Binley, J., Wrin, T., Korber, B., Zwick, M., Wang, M., Chappey, C., Stiegler, G., Kunert, R., Zolla-Pazner, S., Katinger, H., Petropoulos, C., and Burton, D. (2004). Comprehensive cross-clade neutralization analysis of a panel of anti-human immunodeficiency virus type 1 monoclonal antibodies. J. Virol., 78, 13232–13252.

Bures, R., Morris, L., Williamson, C., Ramjee, G., Deers, M., Fiscus, S.A., Abdool-Karim, S., and Montefiori, D.C. (2002). Regional clustering of shared neutralization determinants on primary isolates of clade C human immunodeficiency virus type 1 from South Africa. J. Virol. 76, 2233–2244.

Cao, H., Kanki, P., Sankale, J.L., Dieng-Sarr, A., Mazzara, G.P., Kalams, S.A., Korber, B., Mboup, S. and Walker, B.D. (1997). Cytotoxic T-lymphocyte cross-reactivity among different human immunodeficiency virus type 1 clades, implications for vaccine development. J. Virol. 71, 8615–8623.

Diaz, R., Pardini R., Catroxo, M., Operskalski, E., Mosley, J., and Busch, M. (2005). HIV-1 superinfection is not a common event. J. Clin. Virol. 33, 328–330.

Doria-Rose, N., Learn, G., Rodrigo, A., Nickle, D., Li, F., Mahalanabis, M., Hensel, M., McLaughlin, S., Edmonson, P., Montefiori, D., Barnett, S., Haigwood, N., and Mullins, J. (2005). Human immunodeficiency virus type 1 subtype B ancestral envelope protein is functional and elicits neutralizing antibodies in rabbits similar to those elicited by a circulating subtype B envelope. J. Virol. 79, 11214–11224.

Dorrell, L., Dong, T., Ogg, G.S., Lister, S., McAdam, S., Rostron, T., Conlon, C., McMichael, A.J., and Rowland-Jones, S.L. (1999). Distinct recognition of non-clade B human immunodeficiency virus type 1 epitopes by cytotoxic T lymphocytes generated from donors infected in Africa. J. Virol. 73, 1708–1714.

Dorrell, L., Willcox, B.E., Jones, E.Y., Gillespie, G., Njai, H., Sabally, S., Jaye, A., DeGleria, K., Rostron, T., Lepin, E., McMichael, A., Whittle, H., and Rowland-Jones, S. (2001). Cytotoxic T lymphocytes recognize structurally diverse, clade-specific and cross-reactive peptides in human immunodeficiency virus type-1 gag through HLA-B53. Eur. J. Immunol. 31, 1747–1756.

Dowling, W.E., Kim, B., Mason, C.J., Wasunna, K.M., Alam, U., Elson, L., Birx, D.L., Robb, M.L., McCutchan, F.E., and Carr, J.K. (2002). Forty-one near full-length HIV-1 sequences from Kenya reveal an epidemic of subtype A and A-containing recombinants. AIDS 16, 1809–1820.

Fouts, T., Godfrey, K., Bobb, K., Montefiori, D., Hanson, C.V., Kalyanaraman, V.S., DeVico, A. and Pal, R. (2002). Crosslinked HIV-1 envelope-CD4 receptor complexes elicit broadly cross-reactive neutralizing antibodies in rhesus macaques. Proc. Natl. Acad. Sci. USA 99, 11842–11847.

Fukada, K., Tomiyama, H., Wasi, C., Matsuda, T., Kusagawa, S., Sato, H., Oka, S., Takebe, Y., and Takiguchi, M. (2002). Cytotoxic T-cell recognition of HIV-1 cross-clade and clade-specific epitopes in HIV-1-infected Thai and Japanese patients. AIDS 16, 701–711.

Gao, F., Bhattacharya, T, Gaschen, B., Taylor J., Moore, J.P., Novitsky, V., Yusim, K., Lang, D., Foley, B., Beddows, S., Alam, M., Haynes, B., Hahn, B. and Korber, B. (2003). Diversity considerations in HIV-1 vaccine selection; correspondence. Science 299, 1515–1518.

Gao, F., Weaver, E., Lu, Z., Li, Y., Liao, H.X., Ma, B., Alam, S., Scearce, R., Sutherland, L., Yu, J., Decker, J., Shaw, G., Montefiori, D., Korber, B., Hahn, B., and Haynes, B. (2005). Antigenicity and immunogenicity of a synthetic human immunodeficiency virus type 1 group M consensus envelope glycoprotein. J. Virol. 79, 1154–1163.

Gaschen, B., Taylor, J., Yusim, K., Foley, B., Gao, F., Lang, D., Novitsky, V., Haynes, B., Hahn, B.H., Bhattacharya, T. and Korber, B. (2002a). Diversity considerations in HIV-1 vaccine selection. Science 296, 2354–2360.

Gaschen, B., Taylor, J., Yusim, K., Foley, B., Gao, F., Lang, D., Novitsky, V., Haynes, B., Hahn, B.H., Bhattacharya, T., and Korber, B. (2002b). Diversity considerations in HIV-1 vaccine selection. Science 296, 2354–2360.

Gonzales, M.J., Delwart, E., Rhee, S.Y., Tsui, R., Zolopa, A.R., Taylor, J. and Shafer, R.W. (2003). Lack of detectable human immunodeficiency virus type 1 superinfection during (1072) person-years of observation. J. Infect. Dis. 188, 397–405.

Gorny, M.K., Williams, C., Volsky, B., Revesz, K., Cohen, S., Polonis, V.R., Honnen, W.J., Kayman, S.C., Krachmarov, C., Pinter, A., and Zolla-Pazner, S. (2002). Human monoclonal antibodies specific for conformation-sensitive epitopes of V3 neutralize human immunodeficiency virus type 1 primary isolates from various clades. J. Virol. 76, 9035–9045.

Harris, M.E., Serwadda, D., Sewankambo, N., Kim, B., Kigozi, G., Kiwanuka, N., Phillips, J.B., Wabwire, F., Meehen, M., Lutalo, T., Lane, J.R., Merling, R., Gray, R., Wawer, M., Birx, D.L., Robb, M.L., and McCutchan, F.E. (2002). Among 46 near full length HIV type 1 genome sequences from Rakai District, Uganda, subtype D and AD recombinants predominate. AIDS Res. Hum. Retroviruses 18, 1281–1290.

Hel, Z., Tsai, W., Tryniszewska, E., Nacsa, J., Markham, P.D., Lewis, M.G., Pavlakis, G.N., Felber, B.K., Tartaglia, J., and Franchini, G. (2006). Improved vaccine protection from simian AIDS by the addition of nonstructural simian immunodeficiency virus genes. J. Immunol. 176(1), 85–96.

Koelsch, K.K., Smith, D.M., Little, S.J., Ignacio, C.C., Macaranas, T.R., Brown, A.J., Petropoulos, C.J., Richman, D.D., and Wong, J.K. (2003). Clade B HIV-1 superinfection with wild-type virus after primary infection with drug-resistant clade B virus. AIDS 17, F11–F16.

Korber, B., Foley, B., Gaschen B and Kuiken C. (2001a). Epidemiological and immunological implications of the global variability of HIV-1. Pantaleo, G and Walker, B. Humana Press, Totowa, NJ.

Korber, B., Gaschen, B., Yusim, K., Thakallapally, R., Kesmir, C., and Detours, V. (2001b). Evolutionary and immunological implications of contemporary HIV-1 variation. Br. Med. Bull. *58*, 19–42.

Korber, B., Muldoon, M., Theiler, J., Gao, F., Gupta, R., Lapedes, A., Hahn, B. H., Wolinsky, S., and Bhattacharya, T. (2000). Timing the ancestor of the HIV-1 pandemic strains. Science *288*, 1789–1796.

Kothe, D., Li, Y., Decker, J., Bibollet-Ruche, F., Zammit, K., Salazar, M., Chen, Y., Weng, Z., Weaver, E., Gao, F., Haynes, B., Shaw, G., Korber, B., and Hahn, B. (2006). Ancestral and consensus envelope immunogens for HIV-1 subtype C. Virology.

Kuiken, C.L., Foley, B.T., Guzman, E., and Korber, B.T. (1999). Determinants of HIV protein evolution. In: Molecular evolution of HIV. Edited by Keith Crandall, Baltimore, MD, Johns Hopkins University Press.

Kuiken C.L., Foley, B., Hahn, B., Korber, B., Marx, P.A., McCutchan F., Mellors J.W., and Wolinksy S. (2002). HIV sequence database. Los Alamos, NM,, Los Alamos National Laboratory.

Leitner, T., Escanilla D., Marquina S., Wahlberg J., Brostrom C., Hansson H.B., Uhlen M., and Albert J. (1995). Biological and molecular characterization of subtype D, G, and A/D recombinant HIV-1 transmissions in Sweden. Virology *209*, 136–146.

Leitner, T., Kumar, S., and Albert, J. (1997). Tempo and mode of nucleotide substitutions in gag and env gene fragments in human immunodeficiency virus type 1 populations with a known transmission history. J. Virol. *71*, 4761–4770.

Leitner, T., Korber, B., Daniels, M., Calef, C., and Foley, B. (2005). HIV-1 subtype and circulating recombinant form (CRF) reference sequences, p. 41–48. In T. Leitner *et al* (eds.), HIV Sequence Compendium 2005. Theoretical Biology and Biophysics, Los Alamos National Laboratory, Los Alamos, NM.

Liao, H., Sutherland, L., Xia, S., Brock, M., Scearce, R., Vanleeuwen, S., Munir Alam, S., McAdams, M., Weaver, E., Camacho, Z., Ma, B., Li, Y., Decker, J., Nabel, G., Montefiori, D., Hahn, B., Korber, B., Gao, F., and Haynes, B. (2006). A Group M consensus envelope glycoprotein induces antibodies that neutralize subsets of subtype B and C HIV-1 primary viruses. Virology (in press).

McCutchan, F., Hoelscher, M., Tovanabutra, S., Piyasirisilp, S., Sanders-Buell E., Ramos, G., Jagodzinski, L., Polonis, V., Maboko L., Mmbando, D., Hoffmann, O., Riedner, G., von Sonnenburg, F., Robb, M., and Birx, D. (2005). In-depth analysis of a heterosexuallly aquired human immunodeficiency virur type 1 superinfection, evolution, temporal fluctuation, and intercompartment dynamics from the seronegative window period through 30 months postinfection. J. Virol. *79*, 11693–11704.

Mascola, J.R., Louder, M.K., Surman, S.R., Vancott, T.C., Yu, X.F., Bradac, J., Porter, K.R., Nelson, K.E., Girard, M., McNeil, J.G., McCutchan, F.E., Birx, D.L., and Burke, D.S. (1996). Human immunodeficiency virus type 1 neutralizing antibody serotyping using serum pools and an infectivity reduction assay. AIDS Res. Hum. Retroviruses *12*, 1319–1328.

Moore, J.P., McCutchan, F.E., Poon, S.W., Mascola, J., Liu, J., Cao, Y. and Ho, D.D. (1994). Exploration of antigenic variation in gp120 from clades A through F of human immunodeficiency virus type 1 by using monoclonal antibodies. J. Virol. *68*, 8350–8364.

Moore, J.P., Parren, P.W. and Burton, D.R. (2001). Genetic subtypes, humoral immunity, and human immunodeficiency virus type 1 vaccine development. J. Virol. *75*, 5721–5729.

Musey, L.K., Krieger, J.N., Hughes, J.P., Schacker, T.W., Corey, L. and McElrath, M.J. (1999). Early and persistent human immunodeficiency virus type 1 (HIV-1)-specific T helper dysfunction in blood and lymph nodes following acute HIV-1 infection. J. Infect. Dis. *180*, 278–284.

Nabel, G., Makgoba, W., and Esparza, J. (2002). HIV-1 diversity and vaccine development. Science *296*, 2335.

Nickle, D.C., Jensen, M.A., Gottlieb, G.S., Shriner, D., Learn, G.H., Rodrigo, A.G., and Mullins, J.I. (2003). Consensus and ancestral state HIV vaccines. Science *299*, 1515–1518.

Nyambi, P.N., Mbah, H.A., Burda, S., Williams, C., Gorny, M.K., Nadas, A., and Zolla-Pazner, S. (2000). Conserved and exposed epitopes on intact, native, primary human immunodeficiency virus type 1 virions of group M. J. Virol. *74*, 7096–7107.

Norris, P., Moffett, H., Brander, C., Allen, T., O'Sullivan, K., Cosimi, L., Kaufmann, D., Walker, B., and Rosenberg, E. (2004). Fine specificity and cross-clade reactivity of HIV type 1 Gag-specific CD4[+] T cells. AIDS Res. Hum. Retroviruses *20*, 315–325.

Pantophlet, R., Wilson, I.A., and Burton, D.R. (2003). Hyperglycosylated mutants of human immunodeficiency virus (HIV) type 1 monomeric gp120 as novel antigens for HIV vaccine design. J. Virol. *77*, 5889–5901.

Polonis, V.R., de Souza, M.S., Darden, J.M., Chantakulkij, S., Chuenchitra, T., Nitayaphan, S., Brown, A.E., Robb, M.L., and Birx, D.L. (2003). Human immunodeficiency virus type 1 primary isolate neutralization resistance is associated with the syncytium-inducing phenotype and lower CD4 cell counts in subtype CRF01_AE-infected patients. J. Virol. *77*, 8570–8576.

Richman, D.D., Wrin, T., Little, S.J., and Petropoulos, C.J. (2003). Rapid evolution of the neutralizing antibody response to HIV type 1 infection. Proc. Natl. Acad. Sci. USA *100*, 4144–4149.

Robertson, D.L., Anderson, J.P., Bradac, J.A., Carr, J.K., Foley, B., Funkhouser, R.K., Gao, F., Hahn, B.H., Kalish, M.L., Kuiken, C., Learn, G.H., Leitner, T., McCutchan, F., Osmanov, S., Peeters, M., Pieniazek, D., Salminen, M., Sharp, P.M., Wolinsky, S., and Korber, B. (2000). HIV-1 nomenclature proposal. Science *288*, 55–56.

Robertson, D.L., Sharp, P.M., McCutchan, F.E. and Hahn, B.H. (1995). Recombination in HIV-1. Nature *374*, 124–126.

Sabino, E.C., Shpaer, E.G., Morgado, M.G., Korber, B.T., Diaz, R.S., Bongertz, V., Cavalcante, S., Galvao-Castro, B., Mullins, J.I., and Mayer, A. (1994). Identification of human immunodeficiency virus type 1 envelope genes recombinant between subtypes B and F in two epidemiologically linked individuals from Brazil. J. Virol. *68*, 6340–6346.

Sanders, R.W., Schiffner, L., Master, A., Kajumo, F., Guo, Y., Dragic, T., Moore, J.P., and Binley, J.M. (2000). Variable-loop-deleted variants of the human immunodeficiency virus type 1 envelope glycoprotein can be stabilized by an intermolecular disulfide bond between the gp120 and gp41 subunits. J. Virol. *74*, 5091–5100.

Saphire, E.O., Parren, P.W., Barbas, C.F., III, Burton, D.R., and Wilson, I.A. (2001). Crystallization and preliminary structure determination of an intact human immunoglobulin, b12, an antibody that broadly neutralizes primary isolates of HIV-1. Acta Crystallogr. D. Biol. Crystallogr. *57*, 168–171.

Seaman, M., Xu, L., Beaudry, K., Martin, K., Beddall, M., Miura, A., Sambor, A., Chakrabarti, B., Huang, Y., Bailer, R., Koup, R., Mascola, J., Nabel, G., and Letvin, N. (2005). Multiclade human immunodeficiency virus type 1 envelope immunogens elicit broad cellular and humoral immunity in rhesus monkeys. J. Virol. *79*, 2956–2963.

Smith, D., Wong, J., Hightower, G., Ignacio, C., Koelsch, K., Petropoulos, C., Richman, D., and Little, S. (2005a). HIV drug resistance acquired through superinfection. AIDS *19*, 1251–1256.

Smith, D., Richman, D., and Little, S. (2005b). HIV superinfection. J. Inf. Dis. *192*, 438–444.

Srivastava, I.K., Stamatatos, L., Kan, E., Vajdy, M., Lian, Y., Hilt, S., Martin, L., Vita, C., Zhu, P., Roux, K.H., Vojtech, L., Montefiori, C., Donnelly, J., Ulmer, J.B. and Barnett, S. W. (2003). Purification, characterization, and immunogenicity of a soluble trimeric envelope protein containing a partial deletion of the V2 loop derived from SF162, an R5-tropic human immunodeficiency virus type 1 isolate. J. Virol. *77*, 11244–11259.

Weaver, E,, Lu, Z., Camacho, Z., Moukdar, F., Liao, H.-X., Ma, B.-J., Kepler, T., Nabel, G., Letvin, N., Korber, B., Hahn, B., Haynes, B. and Gao, F. (2006). Cross-subtype T cell immune responses induced by an HIV-1 group M consensus Env immunogen. J. Virol. (in press).

Wei, X., Decker, J.M., Wang, S., Hui, H., Kappes, J.C., Wu, X., Salazar-Gonzalez, J.F., Salazar, M.G., Kilby, J.M., Saag, M.S., Komarova, N L., Nowak, M.A., Hahn, B.H., Kwong, P.D., and Shaw, G.M. (2003). Antibody neutralization and escape by HIV-1. Nature *422*, 307–312.

Wilson, C.C., Palmer, B., Southwood, S., Sidney, J., Higashimoto, Y., Appella, E., Chesnut, R., Sette, A., and Livingston, B.D. (2001).

Identification and antigenicity of broadly cross-reactive and conserved human immunodeficiency virus type 1-derived helper T-lymphocyte epitopes. J. Virol. 75, 4195–4207.

Yu, X., Lichterfeld, M., Perkins, B., Kalife, E., Mui, S., Chen, J., Cheng, M., Kang, W., Alter, G., Brander, C., Walker, B., Altfeld, M. (2005). High degree of inter-clade cross-reactivity of HIV-1-specific T cell responses at the single peptide level. AIDS 19, 1449–1456.

Zwick, M.B., Jensen, R., Church, S., Wang, M., Stiegler, G., Kunert, R., Katinger, H., and Burton, D.R. (2005). Anti-human immunodeficiency virus type 1 (HIV-1) antibodies 2F5 and 4E10 require surprisingly few crucial residues in the membrane-proximal external region of glycoprotein gp41 to neutralize HIV-1. J. Virol. 79, 1252–1261.

# Part IV

## Clinical Trials

# The HIV Vaccine Pipeline

José Esparza and Nina D. Russell

## 11

## Abstract

Since the first human trial of an HIV candidate vaccine was conducted in 1987, the HIV vaccine pipeline has experienced an important evolution. The first wave of candidate vaccines, based on the concept that neutralizing antibodies were capable of conferring protection against HIV/AIDS, led to the development of envelope vaccines based primarily on gp120. The second wave was guided by the paradigm that cytotoxic T-cells (CTL) were responsible for protection, and candidate vaccines were developed based on live recombinant viral vectors and naked DNA. The third wave is under way, with the recognition that a highly effective preventive vaccine may have to induce both broadly reactive antibodies capable of neutralizing primary isolates of HIV, as well as long-lasting cross-reactive CTL. Different candidate vaccines and combinations are advancing through the preclinical pipeline, and some are already generating preliminary data in clinical trials.

Innovative approaches, such as the use of structural biology, the development of novel viral vectors, or a more careful consideration of HLA-escape epitopes, promise a new era of more rational vaccine design. With the availability of larger numbers of candidate vaccines, a more systematic approach to expanding and evaluating the pipeline is needed. This will require the standardization of reagents, techniques and criteria to move candidate vaccines through the pipeline in a comparative fashion, including immunogenicity assays and animal protection experiments. It is also increasingly recognized that carefully designed efficacy trials (phase IIb or phase III) will be essential for the identification of immune correlates of protection, information that will accelerate the future development or improvement of HIV vaccines.

## Introduction

In the absence of information on potential immune correlates of protection against HIV/AIDS, the current strategy for the development of HIV preventive vaccines is a reasonable one and is based on an iterative process of conducting multiple clinical trials with different candidate vaccines, strongly supported by extensive laboratory research. This approach should produce incremental gains in our knowledge of the safety, immunogenicity and potential efficacy of successive generations of candidate vaccines. However, this strategy relies on the existence of a healthy pipeline of candidate vaccines based on different conceptual approaches which are simultaneously and systematically evaluated in the laboratory, in animal models, and in clinical trials in human volunteers (Esparza et al., 2006).

A robust HIV vaccine pipeline begins with an ample supply of novel or improved candidate vaccines based on different biological concepts. These candidate vaccines should include products aimed at inducing humoral, cell-mediated or mucosal immunity. They should be based on a variety of antigens, vectors and adjuvants, including prime-boost combinations of different products, as well as candidate vaccines based on different subtypes of HIV. The safety, immunogenicity and potential efficacy of the different candidate vaccines must be comparatively evaluated in the laboratory and in animal models using standardized assays, to ensure that the best products move through the pipeline into clinical evaluation in humans. The pipeline should also ensure that all selected candidate vaccines are manufactured in sufficient quantities and with the required quality for human testing (complying with good manufacturing practices).

The clinical trials component of the pipeline should be able to implement multiple phase I/II evaluations of various candidate vaccines to establish their safety and immunogenicity in healthy human volunteers (Moodie et al., 2006). Moreover, it should be able to systematically, together with well designed animal model studies, provide additional information to guide the design of efficacy trials of the most promising candidates. The end of the R&D pipeline should include several large-scale trials, to assess the protective efficacy of different types of candidate vaccines, against different HIV subtypes, and in different populations. These large-scale trials could be conducted as phase IIb proof-of-concept trials, and/or as full-sized phase III licensing trials. Ultimately, efficacy trials that show at least a low level of protection are the only way to identify immune correlates of protection, which in turn will serve as a powerful catalyst for further development (Esparza and Bhamarapravati, 2000).

As candidate vaccines progress through the pipeline, many will typically be discarded for a variety of reasons. They may fail to meet expectations regarding safety, immunogenicity or protective efficacy in animal models or in early clinical trials. They could also face unexpected product development obstacles which prevent their manufacturing in appropriate quantities for clinical trials. Or, they could simply be considered inferior to other products under development. In addition, non-scientific considerations could lead to the withdrawal of candidate vaccines from the pipeline, including financial considerations, lack of interest from investors, or intellectual property issues.

A healthy HIV vaccine pipeline should ensure a continuous supply of products, as well as strategies to avoid premature attrition of promising approaches to address scientific hypotheses. Excessive redundancy of products based on the same vaccine concept (usually following the paradigm of fashion) should be avoided; for example, the current plethora of DNA and poxvirus vector vaccines needs to be focused on the most promising strategies, so that adequate resources are available for other crucial steps/products. Advanced clinical development activities are necessary, including process development, manufacturing, and large-scale trials. Lastly, the pipeline must have sufficient capacity to ensure that all relevant products are tested, avoiding clogging due to uncertainty on how to proceed or, even worse, because of lack of facilities or infrastructure to proceed with the R&D process.

The current HIV vaccine pipeline was initiated soon after HIV was identified in 1983–84 as the cause of AIDS. The first phase I trial was conducted in 1987 with a candidate vaccine based on gp160, the precursor of the HIV envelope glycoprotein. Since then, over 50 candidate vaccines have entered phase I clinical trials, five have entered phase II trials, and only four candidate vaccines have entered phase IIb/III efficacy evaluation. Looking to the future, many products are presently at the early stages of conceptual development and, hopefully, a significant number will continue to move through the pipeline in the next few years. Greater coordination and systematic prioritization of the most promising candidates for testing is a concept that has now been embraced by the vast majority of global stakeholders in AIDS vaccine research and development (Klausner et al., 2003).

## Evolution of the vaccine pipeline

The current HIV vaccine pipeline has evolved through more than 18 years of clinical trials experience, with many lessons learned over the years (Johnston and Flores, 2001; Graham, 2002; Girard et al., 2006). A variety of HIV vaccine concepts have been tested in three successive overlapping "waves" of clinical trials which have been dominated by different vaccine development paradigms (Esparza and Osmanov, 2003). A summary of the candidate vaccines that have been tested in human trials since 1987 is provided in Table 11.1.

*First "wave" (1987 to mid-1990s): antibody-inducing vaccines*
The first "wave" of candidate HIV vaccines was based on the concept that antibodies were capable of conferring protection against HIV infection, a concept that received early support from chimpanzee protection experiments and, more recently, from protection in macaques using passively transferred antibodies (Berman et al., 1990, Putkonen et al., 1991, Emini et al., 1992; Mascola, 2003).

Several candidate vaccines based on the envelope proteins of HIV-1 (gp120 or gp160), or on synthetic peptides representing the V3 loop of gp120, have been tested in human trials (Pitisuttithum et al., 2003). In general, gp120 based envelope based candidate vaccines were found to be safe and immunogenic in diverse populations, inducing neutralizing antibodies in essentially 100% of the volunteers, although cell-mediated immunity was very rarely observed. The neutralizing antibodies induced by these candidate vaccines was, however, mostly directed against laboratory strains of HIV (X4 strains), with weak or no neutralizing activity against the more clinically relevant primary isolates of the virus (R5 strains) (Mascola et al., 1996). In addition, these antibodies were basically subtype-specific, with very little cross-reactivity.

The only phase III HIV vaccine efficacy trials completed thus far were done with two different versions of bivalent monomeric recombinant gp120 candidate vaccines (provided by VaxGen, Inc.) based on locally prevalent subtypes of HIV-1 (AIDSVAX B/B for a trial conducted in North America and Europe, and AIDSVAX B/E for a trial conducted in Thailand) (Francis et al., 2003; Flynn et al., 2005). The results from these two trials, which became available in 2003, conclusively showed that these candidate vaccines failed to significantly protect against HIV infection (primary endpoint), and had no impact on viral load in subjects who subsequently became HIV-infected post vaccination (secondary endpoint) (Gilbert et al., 2005).

These first two large-scale efficacy trials provided important information and lessons:

1 The quality and magnitude of immune responses elicited by gp120, including binding antibodies, neutralizing antibodies against laboratory adapted isolates of HIV, and by inference HIV-specific T helper immune responses measured in phase I/II trials of these immunogens, are not sufficient to confer effective protective immunity against HIV. This information will help guide the development of subsequent generations of envelope-based candidate vaccines (see Chapters 7 and 10).

2 HIV vaccine efficacy trials, once feared to be logistically impossible due to the challenges inherent in counseling subjects against high risk behavior for AIDS, the challenges of blinding subjects when readily available HIV diagnostics make it easy to determine one's status in an HIV vaccine trial, and the challenges of enrolling sufficient numbers of subjects to determine efficacy in the face

**Table 11.1** Summary of main candidate vaccines tested in clinical trials since 1987*

| Concept | Products |
|---|---|
| Envelope proteins | rgp160 produced in baculovirus/insect cell system |
| | rgp160 produced in mammalian cells |
| | rgp120 produced in mammalian cells (multiple products, B and E subtypes) |
| | rgp140 produced in Chinese hamster ovary cells (Clade B) |
| Non-envelope proteins | Matrix (p17) and core (p24) proteins in yeast transposons (Ty) |
| | p24 GAG protein produced in mammalian cells |
| | TAT protein produced in *E. coli* |
| | Multiepitope protein |
| Peptides | V3 loop of gp120 (multiple products) |
| | Matrix (p17) peptide (HGP-30) |
| | GAG lipopeptides |
| | C4-V3 gp120 peptides |
| | Lipopeptides (multiple products) |
| | Multiepitope peptides |
| DNA vaccines | *env/rev* in plasmid backbone |
| | *gag* in plasmid backbone |
| | *gag/pol* in plasmid backbone |
| | Multiple CTL epitopes in plasmid backbone (several constructs) |
| | Multiple genes in plasmid backbone (several constructs) |
| Poxvirus vectors | Recombinant vaccinia-gp160 |
| | Recombinant vaccinia-*env/gag/pol* |
| | Recombinant canarypox-HIV (multiple constructs) |
| | Recombinant modified vaccinia Ankara (MVA)-HIV (several constructs) |
| | Recombinant fowlpox (FPV)-HIV (multiple genes) |
| Other viral vectors | Recombinant adenovirus-HIV *gag* |
| | Recombinant adenovirus-HIV *gag, pol, nef* (Clade B) |
| | Recombinant adenovirus-HIV *gag, pol, env, nef* (multiclade) |
| | Venezuelan equine encephalitis (VEE) replicon-HIV-*gag* (Clade C) |
| | Adeno-associated virus (AAV)-gag (Clade C) |
| Bacterial vectors | *Salmonella typhi*-HIV |
| Combinations | rgp160 produced in mammalian cell boosted with V3 peptides |
| | Recombinant vaccinia-gp160 boosted with rgp160 or rgp120 |
| | Recombinant adenovirus-HIV boosted with recombinant canarypox-HIV |
| | Recombinant canarypox-HIV (several) boosted with rgp120 |
| | Recombinant canarypox-HIV boosted with lipopeptides |
| | DNA vaccines boosted with recombinant viral vectors |

*Adapted from www.iavi.org/trialsdb.

of the social stigmas associated with HIV/AIDS, have now been shown to be feasible on a scale that should enable multiple and parallel trials to be undertaken, including trials in developing countries.

3  Despite concentrated and extensive counseling regarding prevention of HIV over the 3-year course of an HIV vaccine efficacy trial, incidence rates of HIV infection in the trial population did not decrease significantly. While the capacity of the clinical vaccine trial design to determine the primary and secondary endpoints was preserved (Gilbert and Esparza, 2002), this sobering outcome reaffirmed the need for improved education and counseling methods for HIV prevention.

4  Efficacy trial designs need to establish in advance the greatest level of information to be gained from the study, including the validity of subanalyses that look at parameters such as gender, race and age of participants, as well as route of transmission and the genotype and phenotype of circulating HIV strains.

Thus, one of the conclusions from the VaxGen gp120 efficacy trials is that new and improved envelope-based immunogens are needed, particularly those capable of eliciting broadly effective neutralizing antibodies against circulating primary isolates of HIV. Several strategies are currently being implemented to address this challenge, including both immunogen and adjuvant design. From the perspective of immunogen design, new concepts include stabilized trimeric envelope constructs, envelope proteins with partial deletion of the dominant variable loops, the use of protein epitope scaffolds, molecular constructs containing CD4-bound gp120 or mimetics of such complexes, critical modifications of the glycosylation pattern of gp120, vaccines based on epitopes recognized by broadly neutralizing antibodies, and the use of consensus, ancestor, or optimized envelope sequences. Some of these immunogens have already been tested in preclinical models, and have elicited an improved neutralizing antibody profile, in terms of neutralization of primary isolates, as compared to monomeric gp120 (Srivistava et al., 2003; Beddows et al., 2005). These modest gains must be balanced by another challenge facing envelope-based vaccines i.e. the capacity to achieve biologically relevant titers of antibodies, and to maintain these titers at high levels and localized at/near the sites of HIV transmission to provide adequate defense against HIV. This has led to an increasing concentration on research aimed at development of effective adjuvants and delivery systems to improve humoral immune responses.

*Second "wave" (mid-1990s to early 2000s): CTL-inducing vaccines*

The second "wave" of HIV vaccine research and trials started in the mid-1990s with the recognition of the importance of CD8$^+$ T-cell responses in the control of HIV infection. This paradigm led to the design of DNA vaccines, and to the development or improvement of live recombinant vectors, including poxviral, alphaviral, adenoviral, and adeno-associated viral vectors, capable of delivering HIV-1 antigens in the context of the MHC class I pathway.

The first generation of viral vectors was based on replication defective canarypox–HIV recombinants (ALVAC) developed by Aventis-Pasteur. Canarypox vectors expressing different HIV genes from subtypes B (vCP205, vCP1452) and E (vCP1521) strains have undergone extensive phase I/II clinical evaluation, alone or in combination with envelope glycoprotein vaccines, including trials conducted in Thailand, Uganda, Brazil, Haiti, Peru, Trinidad and Tobago, France, and the US (Gupta et al., 2002; Cao et al., 2003; Ratto-Kim et al., 2003). A large body of data indicates that the ALVAC-HIV vectors are safe and well tolerated and that they are able to elicit detectable CTL responses, but only in a small proportion (approximately 25–30%) of immunized subjects (Goepfert et al., 2005). In some cases, cross-reactive CTL responses were observed, providing encouragement that improved CTL-based vaccines may be effective against a broad spectrum of circulating HIV strains. A phase III trial was initiated in Thailand at

the end of 2003, evaluating a vCP1521 prime with an rgp120 B/E boost, and efficacy data is expected in 2009.

More recently, viral vectors based on replication defective adenovirus type 5 (Ad5), modified vaccinia Ankara (MVA), Venezuelan equine encephalitis (VEE), and adeno-associated virus (AAV) have entered clinical trials, all of which offer promise of improvement over ALVAC for induction of cellular immune responses against HIV.

Merck and Co. has developed a clade B replication defective Ad5 vector, first as a prototype HIV *gag* recombinant and more recently as an HIV-*gag-pol-nef* candidate. In preclinical studies, this vaccine significantly suppressed viral loads in SHIV 89.6P challenged macaques (Shiver et al., 2002; Casimiro et al., 2003), and early clinical studies have demonstrated induction of cellular immune responses in approximately 60% of subjects immunized with the vaccine. This candidate has now advanced to phase IIB trials in collaboration with the NIH-funded HIV Vaccine Trials Network (HVTN), with data expected in 2008. The NIH-Vaccine Research Center (VRC) (Nabel et al., 2002) has also developed an Ad5 vector to include not only Clade B *gag-pol-nef* plasmid inserts, but also a multiclade (A, B, C) *env*. This candidate is currently in expanded international phase I and phase II trials in collaboration with the HVTN, the International AIDS Vaccine Initiative (IAVI), and the U.S. Military HIV Research Program. Both Merck and the VRC have evaluated adenovectors with and without DNA priming, but Merck is currently focusing on adenovectors as stand-alone candidates due to weak DNA priming observed in clinical trials, while the VRC studies are evaluating a matched combination DNA prime + Ad5 vector boost regimen.

One of the challenges facing the development of Ad5 as a vector for HIV vaccines is the large proportion of people worldwide who have already been naturally exposed to adenovirus serotype 5 and therefore have neutralizing antibodies against the virus which can potentially blunt the efficacy of Ad5 as a vaccine vector. As a result, several groups are evaluating other adenovirus subtypes as potential vectors, including low seroprevalent human adenovectors such as Ad35, Ad26, Ad41, chimp adenovectors, and chimeras of different adenovirus types (Nanda et al., 2005; Roberts et al., 2006).

IAVI, with its academic and industrial partners, has focused on the development of MVA vectors, with a prototype candidate MVA-*gag* (clade A), and a second generation multigenic MVA consisting of structural and regulatory genes (clade C), that have been tested in clinical trials.

Preclinical data in challenge studies with MVA alone and DNA + MVA (Amara et al., 2003) provided proof of concept for this vaccine strategy, with significant suppression of viral load in SHIV 89.6P challenged macaques. The prototype MVA strain has been engineered to vector the *gag* gene with approximately 25 CTL epitopes from HIV-1 subtype A (MVA.HIVA), and was tested alone or in combination with a similar DNA construct (DNA.HIVA), in the UK, Kenya, and Uganda (Hanke et al., 2002). Data from the first safety and immunogenicity trials of the prototype DNA and MVA determined that the vaccines are safe, but the immunogenicity levels failed to achieve IAVI's predetermined 60% response rate in validated ELISpot assays, and thus the candidate has not advanced to efficacy trials. Other groups, such as the US NIH, EuroVacc, Geovax Inc., Therion Corp., and the South African AIDS Initiative (SAAVI) are also developing MVA vectors as HIV vaccines, to be used alone and in combination with DNA and/or other vectors (Mulligan, *et al.*, 2006).

Other poxvirus-HIV vectors have entered phase I clinical trials in the past several years. A recombinant vaccinia-HIV (NYVAC-HIV C, vP2010) developed by EuroVacc and Aventis Pasteur expressing several genes from HIV clade C, is being evaluated in the UK and Switzerland. A recombinant fowlpox vector expressing several HIV clade B modified genes (*gag*, RT, *rev*, *tat*, *vpu*, *env*) was tested in Australia (Kent *et al.*, 1998) and shown to be poorly immunogenic. And, Therion Corp. is evaluating a heterologous MVA and fowlpox vector prime/boost regimen for which data should be available in 2006.

In addition, phase I trials are being completed for prototype VEE-*gag* replicon particle vaccines developed by AlphaVax, Inc. in collaboration with the HVTN, as well as a prototype AAV-*gag* vector developed by Targeted Genetics Corp., the Children's Research Institute, and IAVI. Analogous multigenic VEE and AAV candidates showed promising preclinical efficacy against a more robust monkey model challenge system (SIV-E660), and multigenic candidates for VEE and AAV vectors are currently in development.

The other primary approach for elicitation of CTL and other cell-mediated immune responses against HIV is the utilization of codon-optimized DNA vaccines, and several groups are developing such candidates either as stand-alone vaccines, or more commonly in prime-boost combinations. Although DNA vaccines have been promising in preclinical studies, clinical trials thus far suggest that DNA is less effective in humans, and it is unclear whether the less than robust responses observed in humans is due to dose, route, schedule of immunization, choice of HIV genes in the vaccine, use of adjuvants or some combination of these factors. Preliminary data presented by Merck has shown that less than 50% of subjects elicit IFN-gamma ELISPOT responses even at doses as high as 5 mg of DNA, and the addition of alum or CRL-1005 adjuvants, which was quite effective in monkeys, provided no significant improvement over naked DNA. Additionally, Merck's DNA was suboptimal as a priming vaccine, with a regimen of DNA + Ad5 demonstrating a quality and magnitude of cell-mediated immune responses that was no better than Ad5 alone.

In contrast, phase I studies with the NIH-VRC DNA vaccine have demonstrated that when HIV *env* is included in the vaccine, a higher percentage of human subjects respond than to *gag*-alone vaccines (CSH Meeting, December 2003). Additional DNA vaccines which have recently been assessed in clinical trials include the Geovax pGA2/JS2 that contains

several genes from HIV-1 subtype B (*gag*, RT, *env*, *tat*, *rev* and *vpu*) (Amara *et al.*, 2001). This DNA vaccine was not immunogenic as a stand alone vaccine, but is moving forward in a phase I study in combination with an MVA boost (Mulligan *et al.*, 2006). The EP HIV-1090 DNA vaccine from Epimmune, in which 21 CTL epitopes from several subtype B genes were carefully selected for their ability to bind multiple HLA types (Livingston *et al.*, 2002), has also been recently evaluated in phase I studies in the U.S. and Botswana with preliminary data showing it to be poorly immunogenic. Finally, FIT Biotech has initiated clinical trials with a DNA-*nef* prototype including a nuclear targeting element aimed at improving the immunogenicity of DNA vaccines.

Lastly, other approaches to elicit T-cell immune responses are focusing on novel adjuvants, such as cytokines, combined with DNA, subunit vaccines (Voss *et al.*, 2003), and lipopeptides (ANRS), where each of these approaches may be considered as boosts in prime-boost strategies, and potentially as stand-alone candidates.

*Third "wave" (from the early 2000s): systematic development of better immunogens*
The third "wave" of HIV vaccine immunogen design is just beginning, and it should bring to the pipeline novel candidate vaccines and combinations, aimed at optimizing immune responses of existing, or yet to be developed, vaccines. The primary emphasis of this third wave of immunogen design is: (1) to improve cellular immune responses beyond those elicited by current viral vector vaccines, such that they are capable of eliciting long-lasting cross-reactive CTL responses that can avoid immune escape, (2) to elicit neutralizing antibody responses capable of neutralizing the broad spectrum of circulating and globally diverse HIV strains, and (3) to determine if localization of anti-HIV immune responses to mucosal sites where transmission and initial amplification of HIV occurs provides improved efficacy.

## The state of the pipeline and future directions
As of this writing, many phase I/II trials are being conducted worldwide and, as indicated before, one prime-boost phase III trial (ALVAC + rgp120) is ongoing, as is one phase IIB efficacy trial (Merck-Ad5-*gag-pol-nef*). Comprehensive information on ongoing and planned HIV vaccine trials can be obtained on-line from the databases compiled by the International AIDS Vaccine Initiative (IAVI) (http://www.iavi.org/trials-db/basicsearchform.asp) and by the "The Pipeline Project" of the Center for HIV Information and the HIV Vaccine Trials Network (HVTN) (http://chi.ucsf.edu/vaccines/). Table 11.2 presents a non-exhaustive summary of current clinical trials.

The pipeline today is transitioning from the second "wave," focusing on first generation CTL-inducing vaccines, to the third "wave," with more complex CTL-inducing candidate vaccines and different prime-boost combinations. This has led

**Table 11.2** Ongoing trials of preventive HIV vaccines

| Trial no. | Sponsor/ manufacturer | Start date | Sites (no.) | Vaccine(s) | Antigen | Clade | Comment |
|---|---|---|---|---|---|---|---|
| *Phase III (large-size trials in high-risk populations; test vaccine efficacy)* | | | | | | | |
| RV144 | WRAIR, AFRIMS, MoH; Aventis, VaxGen | October 2003 | Thailand (several) | ALVAC vCP1521 AIDSVAX B/E | *env, gag, pol env* | B, E B/E | 16,000 healthy normal HIV negative adult volunteers |
| *Phase II or IIB (mid-size trials in low- and high-risk populations; test vaccine safety, immunogenicity or proof-of-concept)* | | | | | | | |
| IAVI A002 | IAVI; Targeted Genetics | November 2005 | South Africa (3), Uganda, Zambia | tgAAC09 AAV | *gag, PR, RT,* | C | Expanded safety and immunogenicity at three dosage levels and two dosing intervals |
| HVTN 204 | HVTN, NIAID; VRC | September 2005 | USA (7), Jamaica, Brazil (2), South Africa (3), Haiti | VRC-HIVDNA-016 VRC-HIVADV-014 | *gag, pol, nef, env; gag, pol, env* | B, A/B/C | Expanded safety and immunogenicity of multiclade DNA with Ad5 boost (part of Triad study with IAVI V001 and RV 172) |
| HVTN 502/ Merck 023 | HVTN, Merck; Merck | December 2004 | US (12), Canada, Peru (2), Dominican Republic, Haiti, Puerto Rico, Australia, Brazil (2), Jamaica | MRKAd5 HIV-1 gag/pol/ nef | *gag, pol, nef* | B | Proof-of-concept study to assess HIV acquisition in 1,500 at-risk volunteers |
| ANRS VAC 18 | ANRS; Aventis | September 2004 | France (6) | LIPO-5 | 5 lipopeptides containing CTL epitopes (*gag, pol, nef*) | B | Immunogenicity of 3 doses of LIPO-5 versus placebo |
| *Phase I/II (Mid-sized trials in low-risk populations; test vaccine safety, immunogenicity)* | | | | | | | |
| RV 172 | WRAIR, NIAID; VRC | May 2006 | Uganda, Tanzania, Kenya | VRC-HIVDNA-016 VRC-HIVADV-014 | *gag, pol, nef, env; gag, pol, env* | B, A/B/C | Safety and immunogenicity of multiclade DNA with Ad5 boost (part of Triad study with IAVI V001 and HVTN 204) |
| HVTN 050/ Merck 018 | HVTN, NIAID; Merck | September 2004 | Brazil (2), Haiti, Malawi, Peru, Puerto Rico, South Africa (2), Thailand (2), US (12) | MRKAd5 HIV-1 | *gag* | B | Expanded safety and immunogenicity of 3 dose regimen of Ad-5 HIV-1 gag vaccine |
| GTU-MultiHIV | FIT Biotech | February 2004 | Finland | GTU-MultiHIV B clade | *nef, rev, tat, gag, pol, env,* CTL epitopes | B | Immunogenicity of GTU-MultiHIV clade B DNA after intradermal and intramuscular injection |
| N/A | UNSW; AVC | June 2003 | Australia | pHIS-HIV-B rFPV-HIV-B | *gag, RT, rev, tat, vpu, env gag, RT, rev, tat, vpu, env* | B, B | Safety, immunogenicity of DNA Vaccine with fowlpox boost |

*Phase I (small trials in low-risk populations; test vaccine safety, immunogenicity)*

| Trial | Sponsor | Date | Location | Vaccine | Genes/Antigens | Clade | Objective |
|---|---|---|---|---|---|---|---|
| HVTN 065 | HVTN, NIAID: Geovax | March 2006 | US (5), Thailand | DNA pGA2/JS7<br>MVA-HIV 62 | gag, pro, RT, Env, tat, rev, vpu<br>gag, pol, env | B<br>B | Safety, immunogenicity of multigenic DNA in combination with MVA boost |
| HVTN 068 | HVTN, NIAID; VRC | January 2006 | US (6) | VRC-HIVDNA-009<br>VRC-HIVADV-014 | gag, pol, nef, env;<br>gag, pol, env | B, A/B/C | Assessment of Immunogenicity kinetics induced by multiclade DNA prime, Ad5 boost regimen |
| HVTN 064 | HVTN, NIAID; Pharmexa-Epimmune | January 2006 | US (3), Peru (2) | EP-1043 protein<br>EP HIV-1090 DNA | env, gag, pol, vpu<br>T-helper epitopes;<br>env, gag, pol, vpr | B | Safety, immunogenicity of recombinant protein vaccine EP-1043 and EP HIV-1090 DNA given alone or in combination |
| IAVI D001 | IAVI; Therion | December 2005 | India | TBC-M4 | env, gag, tat-rev, nef-RT | C | Safety, immunogenicity of TBC-M4 (modified vaccinia Ankara (MVA) vaccine |
| IAVI V001 | IAVI, NIAID; VRC | November 2005 | Rwanda, Kenya | VRC-HIVDNA-016<br>VRC-HIVADV-014 | gag, pol, nef, env;<br>gag, pol, env | B,<br>A, B, C | Safety, immunogenicity of multiclade Ad5 alone and multiclade DNA with Ad5 boost |
| RV 158 | WRAIR; NIH | November 2005 | US, Thailand | MVA-CMDR | gp160, gag, pol | A, E | Safety, immunogenicity of WRAIR/NIH live recombinant MVA-CMDR administered by intramuscular vs intradermal routes |
| HVTN 063 | HVTN, NIAID; Wyeth | September 2005 | US (7), Brazil (2) | Prime: GENEVAX Gag-2692 +/- IL-15 DNA; Boost: HIV CTL MEP or GENEVAX Gag-2692 + IL-12 DNA | env, gag, nef CTL epitopes from env, gag or nef | B | Safety, immunogenicity of gag DNA vaccine +/- IL-15 DNA, boosted with CTL multiepitope peptide vaccine or HIV-1 gag DNA + IL-12 DNA |
| HVTN 060 | HVTN, NIAID; Wyeth | August 2005 | US (3), Thailand | Prime: GENEVAX Gag-2692 +/- IL-12 DNA Boost: DNA plasmids or HIV CTL MEP +/- RC-529-SE, GM-CSF | env, gag, nef CTL epitopes from env, gag or nef | B | Safety, immunogenicity of DNA vaccine +/- DNA IL-12, boosted with homologous plasmids or CTL multiepitope peptide vaccine +/- RC-529-SE and GM-CSF |
| RV 156 | WRAIR, NIAID: VRC | November 2004 | Uganda | VRC-HIVDNA-016 | gag, pol, nef, env | B | Safety, immunogenicity of multiclade DNA vaccine alone |
| HIVIS 02 | WRAIR, NIAID, Karolinska Inst. | 2005 | Stockholm | DNA +/- GM-CSF MVA-CMDR | n/a | A, B, C<br>A, B, C | Safety, immunogenicity of adjuvanted multiclade DNA via biojector with MVA boost |
| HVTN 054 | HVTN, NIAID; VRC | April 2005 | US (4) | VRC-HIVADV014 | gag, pol, env | B<br>A, B, C | Dose escalation safety and immunogenicity of multiclade Ad5 vaccine in participants with low pre-existing titers of Ad5 neutralizing antibodies |
| N/A | Guangxi CDC | March 2005 | China | DNA plasmids | n/a | B, C | Safety and immunogenicity of a multiclade DNA plasmid vaccine |
| N/A | St. Jude, NIAID | February 2005 | US | EnvDNA | Env | A, B, C, D, E | Safety and tolerability of a multi-envelope DNA plasmid vaccine |

Table 11.2 Continued

| Trial no. | Sponsor/ manufacturer | Start date | Sites (no.) | Vaccine(s) | Antigen | Clade | Comment |
|---|---|---|---|---|---|---|---|
| IAVI C002 | IAVI; ADARC | January 2005 | US (2) | ADMVA | env/gag-pol, nef-tat | C | Safety, immunogenicity of an MVA vector vaccine |
| VRC 009 | NIAID, VRC | January 2005 | US | VRC-HIVADV014 | gag, pol, env | B A, B, C | Rollover safety, immunogenicity study of VRC 004 multiclade DNA recipients to receive Ad5 boost |
| HVTN 059 | HVTN, NIAID; AlphaVax | October 2004 | US (5), South Africa, Botswana | AVX101 (VEE) | gag | C | Safety, immunogenicity of an alphavirus replicon |
| HVTN 055 | HVTN, NIAID; Therion | July 2004 | US (6) | TBC-M358 (MVA) TBC-M335 (MVA) TBC-F357 (FPV) TBC-F349 (FPV) | env, gag tat, rev, nef, RT env, gag tat, rev, RT | B | Safety, immunogenicity of MVA-HIV and rFPV-HIV alone or in combination. |
| N/A | WRAIR, NIAID; Avant | May 2004 | US | LFn-p24 | LFn gag p24 protein | B | Safety, immunogenicity of anthrax-derived polypeptide vaccine |
| HVTN 056 | HVTN, NIAID; Wyeth | April 2004 | US (7) | HIV CTL MEP +/- RC-529-SE, GM-CSF | CTL epitopes from env, gag or nef | B | Safety of and immune response to a new HIV vaccine: HIV CTL MEP |
| VRC 008 | NIAID; VRC | April 2004 | US | VRC-HIVDNA-016 VRC-HIVADV-014 | gag, pol, nef, env; gag, pol, env | B A, B, C | Safety and immunogenicity of multiclade DNA with Ad5 boost |
| HVTN 049 | HVTN, NIAID; Chiron | December 2003 | US (8) | Gag and Env DNA/PLG Oligomeric gp140/MF59 | gag, env DNA/ PLG; Oligomeric gp140 | B B | Safety, Immunogenicity of DNA/PLG and env DNA/PLG prime, oligomeric gp140/MF59 boost |
| HVTN 044 | HVTN, NIAID; VRC | December 2003 | US (3) | VRC-HIVDNA-009-00-VP | gag, pol, nef env | B A,B,C | Safety, immunogenicity of a multiclade DNA Vaccine with IL-2/Ig DNA adjuvant |
| IAVI A001 | IAVI; Targeted Genetics | December 2003 | Belgium (2), Germany (2), India | tgAAC09 AAV | gag, protease, RT | C | Dose escalation, safety and immunogenicity of adeno-associated HIV vaccine |
| N/A | Merck; Aventis | September 2003 | US (17) | Prime: MRKAd5 HIV-1 Boost: ALVAC vCP205 | gag env, gag, pol | B | Safety, immunogenicity of Merck Ad5 gag boosted with ALVAC vCP205 canarypox vaccine |

ADARC, Aaron Diamond AIDS Research Center; AFRIMS, Armed Forces Research Institute of Medical Sciences, Bangkok, Thailand, is a joint US–Royal Thai Army Command; AlphaVax, AlphaVax Human Vaccines Inc.; ANRS, Agence Nationale de Recherche sur le SIDA; AVANT, AVANT Immunotherapeutics, Inc.; AVC, Australian Vaccine Consortium; Aventis: Aventis Pasteur; CA,: Canada; Chiron, Chiron Corporation; CTL, cytotoxic T-lymphocyte; Pharmexa-Epimmune, Pharmexa-Epimmune, Inc.; Geovax: Geovax, Inc., GSK: GlaxoSmithKline; HVTN,: HIV Vaccine Trials Network; IAVI, International AIDS Vaccine Initiative; Merck: Merck & Co., Inc.; MoH, Ministry of Health (Thailand); NIAID, US National Institute Allergy and Infectious Diseases; SAAVI, South African AIDS Vaccine Initiative; St Jude's: St Jude's Children's Hospital; Targeted Genetics: Targeted Genetics Corporation; Therion, Therion Biologics Corporation; UNSW, University of New South Wales; VaxGen, VaxGen, Inc.; VEE: Venezuelan equine encephalitis; VRC, Vaccine Research Center, NIH; WRAIR,: Walter Reed Army Institute of Research; Wyeth, Wyeth Vaccines, Inc.

to some potential redundancy in the pipeline, especially with DNA and poxvirus-vectored candidate vaccines and, at the same time, to a scarcity of envelope-based candidate vaccines.

With only two efficacy trials ongoing and data not expected from those trials until 2008–2009, the HIV vaccine design field will be limited in the near future to testing hypotheses in animal models and phase I/II clinical trials. If any of the currently available CTL-based candidates is successful in suppressing viral load to a level comparable to that observed in SHIV challenged macaques, the decade of 2010–2020 will be focused on an iterative process aimed at improving the efficacy of these candidates, and ideally to licensing and determining through phase IV effectiveness trials the potential for one or more of these vaccines to provide a significant public health benefit. In contrast, should the data from the first series of CTL-based vaccines be similar to the lack of efficacy observed in the VaxGen gp120 trials and to the lack of efficacy observed when monkeys immunized with CTL-based vaccines were challenged with SIV Mac 239 (Koff et al., 2006), then the field will be searching for new vaccine design strategies and paradigms.

Given the extent of the HIV pandemic, global stakeholders must assume both scenarios are possible and plan accordingly, thus making prioritization of finite resources that much more challenging. Thus, two fundamental breakthroughs will be required in the next few years to accelerate HIV vaccine development: (1) demonstration of vaccine efficacy in human clinical trials, and (2) development of candidates capable of eliciting broadly neutralizing antibodies. Both issues are currently being actively pursued.

## References

Amara, R.R., Villinger, F., Altman, J.D., Lydy, S.L., O'Neil, S.P., Staprans, S.I., Montefiori, D.C., Xu, Y., Herndon, J.G., Wyatt, L.S., Candido, M.A., Kozyr, N.L., Earl, P.L., Smith, J.M., Ma, H.L., Grimm, B.D., Hulsey, M.L., Miller, J., McClure, H.M., McNicholl, J.M., Moss, B., and Robinson H.L. (2001). Control of mucosal challenge and prevention of AIDS by a multiprotein DNA/MVA vaccine. Science 292, 69–74.

Beddows, S., Schulke, N., Kirschner, M., Barnes, K., Franti, M., Michael, E., Ketas, T., Sanders, R.W., Maddon, P.J., Olson, W.C., and Moore, J.P. (2005). Evaluating the immunogenicity of a disulfide-stabilized, cleaved, trimeric form of the envelope glycoprotein complex of human immunodeficiency virus type 1. J. Virol. 79, 8812–8827.

Berman, P.W., Gregory, T.J., Riddle, L., Nakamura, G.R., Champe, M.A., Porter, J.P., Wurm, F.M., Hershberg, R.D., Cobb, E.K., and Eichberg, J.W. (1990). Protection of chimpanzees from infection by HIV-1 after vaccination with recombinant glycoprotein gp120 but not gp160. Nature 345, 622–625.

Cao, H., Kaleebu, P., Hom, D., Flores, J., Agrawal, D., Jones, N., Serwanga, J., Okello, M., Walker, C., Sheppard, H., El-Habib, R., Klein, M., Mbidde, E., Mugyenyi, P., Walker, B., Ellner, J., Mugerwa, R. and the HIV Network for Prevention Trials (2003). Immunogenicity of a recombinant human immunodeficiency virus (HIV)-canarypox vaccine in HIV-seronegative Ugandan volunteers, results of the HIV Network for Prevention Trials 007 Vaccine study. J. Infect. Dis. 187, 887–895.

Casimiro, D.R., Tang, A., Chen, L., Fu, T.M., Evans, R.K., Davies, M.E., Freed, D.C., Hurni, W., Aste-Amezaga, J.M., Guan, L., Long, R., Huang, L., Harris, V., Nawrocki, D.K., Mach, H., Troutman, R.D., Isopi, L.A., Murthy, K.K., Rice, K., Wilson, K.A., Volkin, D.B.,

Emini, E.A., and Shiver, J.W.(2003). Vaccine-induced immunity in baboons by using DNA and replication-incompetent adenovirus type 5 vectors expressing human immunodeficiency virus type 1 gag gene. J. Virol. 77, 7663–7668.

Check, E. (2003). AIDS vaccines, back to "plan A." Nature 423, 912–914.

Emini, E.A., Schleif, W.A., Nunberg, J.H., Conley, A.J., Eda, Y., Tokiyoshi, S., Putney, S.D., Matsushita, S., Cobb, K.E., and Jett, C.M. (1992). Prevention of HIV-1 infection in chimpanzees by gp120 V3 domain-specific monoclonal antibody. Nature 355, 728–730.

Esparza, J., and Bhamarapravati, N. (2000). Accelerating the development and future availability of HIV vaccines, why, where, when and how? Lancet 355, 2061–2066.

Esparza, J., and Osmanov, S. (2003). HIV vaccines, a global perspective. Curr. Mol. Med. 3, 183–193.

Esparza, J., Russell, N., and Gayle, H (2006). The challenge of developing and HIV vaccine. In HIV Vaccine Research and Development in Thailand. Pitisuttithum, P., Francis, D.P., Esparza, J., and Thongcharoen, P., ed. (Bangkok, Thailand, Faculty of Tropical Medicine, Mahidol University), pp. 3–26.

Flynn, N.M., Forthal, D.N., Harro, C.D., Judson, F.N., Mayer, K.H., and Para, M.F. (2005). Placebo-controlled phase 3 trial of a recombinant glycoprotein 120 vaccine to prevent HIV-1 infection. J. Infect. Dis. 191, 654–665.

Francis, D.P., Heyward, W.L., Popovic, V., Orozco-Cronin, P., Orelind, K., Gee, C., Hirsch, A., Ippolito, T., Luck, A., Longhi, M., Gulati, V., Winslow, N., Gurwith, M., Sinangil, F., and Berman, P.W. (2003). Candidate HIV/AIDS vaccines, lessons learned from the world's first phase III efficacy trials. AIDS 17, 147–156.

Gilbert, P., and Esparza, J. (2002). HIV-1 vaccine testing, trial design, and ethics. In AIDS in Africa. Essex, M., Mboup, S., Kanki, P.J., Marlink, R.G., and Tlou, S.D., ed. (New York, US, Kluwer Academic/Plenum Publishers), pp. 612–630.

Gilbert, P.B., Peterson, M.L., Follmann, D., Hudgens, M.G., Francis, D.P., Gurwith, M., Heyward, W.L., Jobes, D.V., Popovic, V., Self, S.G., Sinangil, F., Burke, D., Berman, P.W. (2005). Correlation between immunologic responses to a recombinant glycoprotein 120 vaccine and incidence of HIV-1 infection in a phase 3 HIV-1 preventive vaccine trial. J. Infect. Dis. 191, 666–677.

Girard, M.P., Osmanov, S.K., and Kieny, M.P. (2006). A review of vaccine research and development, The human immunodeficiency virus (HIV). Vaccine 24, 4062–4081.

Goepfert, P.A., Horton, H., McElrath, M.J., Gurunathan, S., Ferrari, G., Tomaras, G.D., Montefiori, D.C., Allen, M., Chiu, Y.L., Spearman, P., Fuchs, J.D., Koblin, B.A., Blattner, W.A., Frey, S.E., Keefer, M.C., Baden, L.R., and Corey, L. (2005). Recombinant canarypox vaccine expressing human immunodeficiency virus type 1 protein given at a high dose in seronegative human participants. J. Infect. Dis. 192, 1249–1259.

Graham, B.S. (2002). Clinical trials of HIV vaccines. Annu. Rev. Med. 53, 207–221.

Gupta, K., Hudgens, M., Corey, L., McElrath, M.J., Weinhold, K., Montefiori, D.C., Gorse, G.J., Frey, S.E., Keefer, M.C., Evans, T.G., Dolin, R., Schwartz, D.H., Harro, C., Graham, B., Spearman, P.W., Mulligan, M., Goepfert, P. and the AIDS Vaccine Evaluation Group. (2002). Safety and immunogenicity of a high-titered canarypox vaccine in combination with rgp120 in a diverse population of HIV-1 uninfected adults, AIDS Vaccine Evaluation Group Protocol 022A. J. Acquir. Immune. Defic. Syndr. 29, 254–261.

Hanke, T., McMichael, A.J., Mwau, M., Wee, E.G., Ceberej, I., Patel, S., Sutton, J., Tomlinson, M., and Samuel, R.V. (2002). Development of a DNA-MVA/HIVA vaccine for Kenya. Vaccine 20, 1995–1998.

Johnston, M.I., and Flores, J. (2001). Progress in HIV vaccine development. Curr. Opin. Pharmacol. 1, 504–510.

Klausner, R.D., Nabel, G.J., Gayle, H., Berkley, S., Haynes, B.F., Baltimore, D., Collins, C., Douglas, R.G., Esparza, J., Francis, D.P., Ganguly, N.K., Gerberding, J.L., Johnston, M.I., Kazatchkine, M.D., McMichael, A.J., Makgoba, M.W., Pantaleo, G., Piot, P., Shao, Y., Tramont, E., Varmus, H., and Wasserheit, J.N. (2003). The need for a global HIV vaccine enterprise. Science 300, 2036–2039.

Koff, W.C., Johnson, P.R., Watkins, D.I., Burton, D.R., Lifson, J.D., Hasenkrug, K.J., McDermott, A.B., Schultz, A., Zamb, T.J., Boyle, R., and Desrosiers, R.C. (2006). HIV vaccine design, insights from live attenuated SIV vaccines. Nature Immunol. 7, 19–23.

Kent, S.J., Zhao, A., Best, S.J., Chandler, J.D., Boyle, D.B., and Ramshaw, I.A. (1998). Enhanced T-cell immunogenicity and protective efficacy of a human immunodeficiency virus type 1 vaccine regimen consisting of consecutive priming with DNA and boosting with recombinant fowlpox virus. J. Virol. 72, 10180–10188.

Livingston, B., Crimi, C., Newman, M., Higashimoto, Y., Appella, E., Sidney, J., and Sette, A. (2002). A rational strategy to design multi-epitope immunogens based on multiple Th lymphocyte epitopes. J. Immunol. 168, 5499–5506.

Mascola, J.R., Snyder, S.W., Weislow, O.S., Belay, S.M., Belshe, R.B., Schwartz, D.H., Clements, M.L., Dolin, R., Graham, B.S., Gorse, G.J., Keefer, M.C., McElrath, M.J., Walker, M.C., Wagner, K.F., McNeil, J.G., McCutchan, F.E., Burke, D.S. (1996). Immunization with envelope subunit vaccine products elicits neutralizing antibodies against laboratory-adapted but not primary isolates of human immunodeficiency virus type 1. The National Institute of Allergy and Infectious Diseases AIDS Vaccine Evaluation Group 1996. J. Infect. Dis. 173, 340–348.

Mascola, J.R. (2003). Defining the protective antibody response for HIV-1. Curr. Mol. Med. 3, 209–216.

Moodie, Z., Rossini, A.J., Hudgens, M.G., Gilbert, P.B., Self, S.G., Russell, N.D. (2006). Statistical evaluation of HIV vaccines in early clinical trials. Contemporary Clinical Trials 27, 147–60.

Mulligan, M.J., Russell, N.D., Celum, C., Allen, M., Kahn, J., Rubin, A., Noonan, E., Montefiori, D., Ferrari, G., Weinhold, K., Smith, J.M., Amara, R., and Robinson, H.L. for the NIH/NIAID/DAIDS HIV Vaccine Trials Network (2006). Excellent safety and tolerability of the human immunodeficiency virus type 1 pGA2/JS2 plasmid DNA priming vector vaccine in HIV-1 uninfected Adults. Aids Res. Hum. Retroviruses 22, 678–683.

Nabel, G., Makgoba, W., and Esparza, J. (2002). HIV-1 diversity and vaccine development. Science 296, 2335.

Nanda, A., Lynch, D.M., Goudsmit, J., Lemckert, A.A., Ewald, B.A., Sumida, S.M., Truitt, D.M., Abbink, P., Kishko, M.G., Gorgone, D.A., Lifton, M.A., Shen, L., Carville, A., Mansfield, K.G., Havenga, M.J., and Barouch, D.H. (2005). Immunogenicity of recombinant fiber-chimeric adenovirus serotype 35 vector-based vaccines in mice and rhesus monkeys. J. Virol. 79, 14161–14168.

Pitisuttithum, P., Nitayaphan, S., Thongcharoen, P., Khamboonruang, C., Kim, J., de Souza, M., Chuenchitra, T., Garner, R.P., Thapinta, D., Polonis, V., Ratto-Kim, S., Chanbancherd, P., Chiu, J., Birx, D.L., Duliege, A.M., McNeil, J.G., Brown, A.E. and the Thai AIDS Vaccine Evaluation Group (2003). Safety and immunogenicity of combinations of recombinant subtype E and B human immunodeficiency virus type 1 envelope glycoprotein 120 vaccines in healthy Thai adults. J. Infect. Dis. 188, 219–227.

Putkonen, P., Thorstensson, R., Ghavamzadeh, L., Albert, J., Hild, K., Biberfeld, G., and Norrby, E. (1991). Prevention of HIV-2 and SIVsm infection by passive immunization in cynomolgus monkeys. Nature 352, 436–438.

Ratto-Kim, S., Loomis-Price, L.D., Aronson, N., Grimes, J., Hill, C., Williams, C., El Habib, R., Birx, D.L., and Kim, J.H. (2003). Comparison between env-specific T-cell epitopic responses in HIV-1-uninfected adult immunized with combination of ALVAC-HIV (vCP205) plus or minus rgp160MN/LAI-2 and HIV-1-infceted adults. J. Acquir. Immune. Defic. Syndr. 32, 9–17.

Roberts, D.M., Nanda, A., Havenga, M.J., Abbink, P., Lynch, D.M., Ewald, B.A., Liu, J., Thorner, A.R., Swanson, P.E., Gorgone, D.A., Lifton, M.A., Lemckert, A.A., Holterman, L., Chen, B., Dilraj, A., Carville, A., Mansfield, K.G., Goudsmit, J., Barouch, D.H. (2006). Hexon-chimaeric adenovirus serotype 5 vectors circumvent pre-existing anti-vector immunity. Nature 441, 239–243.

Shiver, J.W., Fu, T.M., Chen, L., Casimiro, D.R., Davies, M.E., Evans, R.K., Zhang, Z.Q., Simon, A.J., Trigona, W.L., Dubey, S.A., Huang, L., Harris, V.A., Long, R.S., Liang, X., Handt, L., Schleif, W.A., Zhu, L., Freed, D.C., Persaud, N.V., Guan, L., Punt, K.S., Tang, A., Chen, M., Wilson, K.A., Collins, K.B., Heidecker, G.J., Fernandez, V.R., Perry, H.C., Joyce, J.G., Grimm, K.M., Cook, J.C., Keller, P.M., Kresock, D.S., Mach, H., Troutman, R.D., Isopi, L.A., Williams, D.M., Xu, Z., Bohannon, K.E., Volkin, D.B., Montefiori, D.C., Miura, A., Krivulka, G.R., Lifton, M.A., Kuroda, M.J., Schmitz, J.E., Letvin, N.L., Caulfield, M.J., Bett, A.J., Youil, R., Kaslow, D.C., and Emini, E.A. (2002). Replication-incompetent adenoviral vaccine vector elicits effective anti-immunodeficiency-virus immunity. Nature 415, 331–335.

Srivastava, I. K., Stamatatos, L., Kan, E., Vajdy, M., Lian, Y., Hilt, S., Martin, L., Vita, C., Zhu, P., Roux, K.H., Vojtech, L., C.M.D, Donnelly, J., Ulmer, J.B., and Barnett, S.W. (2003). Purification, characterization, and immunogenicity of a soluble trimeric envelope protein containing a partial deletion of the V2 loop derived from SF162, an R5-tropic human immunodeficiency virus type 1 isolate. J. Virol. 77, 11244–11259.

Voss, G., Manson, K., Montefiori, D., Watkins, D.I., Heeney, J., Wyand, M., Cohen, J., and Bruck, C. (2003). Prevention of disease induced by a partially heterologous AIDS virus in rhesus monkeys by using an adjuvanted multicomponent vaccine. J. Virol. 77, 1049–1058.

# Clinical Site Development and Preparation for AIDS Vaccine Efficacy Trials in Developing Countries

## 12

Patricia E. Fast, Jean-Louis Excler, Mitchell Warren, and Nzeera Ketter

## Abstract

High-quality clinical trials can be conducted in resource-poor settings. The world's second AIDS vaccine efficacy trial was conducted successfully in Thailand, and phase I AIDS vaccine trials have been carried out in several non-industrialized countries. However, preparation for clinical trials in resource-poor settings requires investment in infrastructure, equipment, training and health care. Regulatory pathways should be clear before a trial is proposed for approval. Most of all, such trials require a committed team of individuals including effective local scientists and staff and, particularly in the initial phases, experienced clinical trials professionals. It is also critical to create an enabling environment, including political support, partnerships with community organizations such as NGOs and CBOs, and outreach to the community at large through strategic use of the media.

## Introduction

AIDS vaccines are needed globally, but nowhere more than in Africa, Asia, the Caribbean and Latin America (Esparza, 2005). Vaccines intended for these regions must be tested for safety and efficacy in the populations for whom they are intended. Clinical trials are now being conducted in eastern and southern African countries, Thailand, India, China, Haiti, Brazil and Peru, and some vaccine candidates now incorporate genes from HIV-1 subtypes C and A and AE, predominant in Africa and Asia (Rodriguez-Chavez et al., 2006) (Table 12.1). Wide participation in clinical trials will pave the way for rapid acceptance and deployment when a safe and effective vaccine is identified.

Worldwide capacity for testing preventive interventions is far from sufficient. To expand this capacity, those who remain at risk for HIV-1 infection despite behavioral interventions must be identified, and the natural history of HIV infection described in light of rapidly changing access to treatment. State-of-the-art laboratories and clinical trial operations in resource-poor settings can match those in developed countries, given appropriate investment and training (Excler, 2006).

Preparation for efficacy trials involves not only science and logistics, but also garnering societal support at several levels. A consensus must be reached among politicians, public health officials, physicians and others to whom people turn for medical advice, civic and religious leaders, the press, community members at large, and most important those who will participate in the trial. Where a strong tradition of clinical research and clearly delineated legal and regulatory procedures are lacking, additional support is required to conduct trials with the utmost ethical and scientific rigor and efficiency.

## Epidemiology studies, site, and community preparation

Vaccine trials should be conducted in the context of an overall prevention program and include risk reduction counseling throughout the trial to ensure that there is no presumption that the study vaccine is protective. Excellent guidelines have been developed in several countries and quality assurance programs are now available to ensure consistent and high quality VCT (Taegtmeyer, 2003). Innovative counseling methods may be required in communities with low literacy and little exposure to research. As demonstrated in both Rwanda and Zambia, HIV transmission to the negative partner in discordant couples is largely from their HIV-infected partner. Joint HIV testing and counseling has decreased stigma, reduced transmission of HIV, and other sexually transmitted diseases and reduced unwanted pregnancies, with an improvement in condom use (Allen et al., 2003; Mehendale et al., 2006). Additional interventions, such as vaccines, are required to improve protection.

The first step in preparing for AIDS vaccine efficacy trials is to conduct a thorough assessment of strengths, assets and needs for infrastructure and training, and to determine whether a population at sufficiently high risk of HIV infection is accessible and willing to participate (see www.iavi.org for a site assessment tool). An action plan will involve not only preparation but ongoing re-assessment of capabilities including the evaluation of services throughout the conduct of epidemiological and/or small-scale clinical studies (feasibility studies). Feasibility studies are being initiated in several countries to prepare sites for future preventive AIDS vaccine efficacy trials. These may not be cohort or incidence studies in the true

**Table 12.1** HIV preventive vaccine trials conducted in Africa, Asia, Caribbean and Latin America* (as of May 2006)

| Region | Country | Vaccine | US government | IAVI | Industry or other | Match circulating subtypes | Test of concept or efficacy trial? |
|---|---|---|---|---|---|---|---|
| Africa | Uganda | Canarypox | X | | | Yes | |
| | | DNA/MVA | | X | | Yes | |
| | | Adenovirus-associated virus capsid | | X | | Yes | |
| | Kenya | DNA/MVA | | X | | Yes | |
| | | DNA/rAd5 | X | X | | Yes | |
| | Rwanda | DNA/rAd5 | X | X | | Yes | |
| | Botswana | DNA (multi-epitope) | X | | | Yes | |
| | | Alphavirus replicon | X | | | Yes | |
| | South Africa | VEE replicon particles | X | | | Yes | |
| | | DNA/MVA | | X | | No | |
| | | Adenovirus 5 | X | | | No | |
| | | Adenovirus 5 | X | | X | No | |
| | | Adenovirus-associated virus capsid | | X | | Yes | |
| | | DNA plus adenovirus 5 | X | | | Yes | |
| | | Alphavirus replicon | X | | | Yes | |
| | Zambia | Adenovirus-associated virus capsid | | X | | Yes | |
| | Malawi | Adenovirus 5 | X | | X | No | |
| Asia | China | Peptides | | | X | Yes | |
| | | DNA | | | X | Yes | |
| | Thailand | Peptides | X | | X | Yes | |
| | | gp120 | X | | X | Yes | Yes |
| | | ALVAC Canarypox +/- gp120 | X | | | Yes | Yes |
| | | DNA with or without IL-12 boost with homologous plasmids or multiepitope vaccine plus GM-CSF | X | | | *** | |
| | | Adenovirus 5 | X | | X | No | |

| Region | Country | Vaccine | | | |
|---|---|---|---|---|---|
| Caribbean | Haiti | ALVAC canarypox +/– gp120 | X | | Yes |
| | | DNA plus adenovirus 5 | X | | Yes |
| | Puerto Rico | Adenovirus 5 | X | X | Yes |
| | | gp120 | | X | *** |
| | | Adenovirus 5 | X | X | *** |
| | Cuba | Adenovirus 5 | | X | *** |
| | Dominican Republic | Adenovirus 5 | X | X | *** |
| | Trinidad and Tobago | DNA plus adenovirus 5 | X | | *** |
| | Jamaica | DNA plus adenovirus 5 | X | | *** |
| | | Adenovirus 5 | X | X | *** |
| Latin America | Brazil | Adenovirus 5 | X | X | *** |
| | | DNA plus adenovirus 5 | X | | *** |
| | | DNA (multi-epitope) with or without IL-15 boost | X | | *** |
| | | MVA/fowlpox | X | | *** |
| | Peru | Canarypox +/– gp120 | X | | *** |
| | | Adenovirus 5 | X | X | *** |
| | | Recombinant protein EP-1043 | X | | *** |

*Preventive trials enroll HIV-uninfected volunteers.

**Trials in Europe, United States, Canada, and Australia are not included.

***Subtype B predominates in Latin America and the Caribbean, therefore vaccines based on US/European strains are "matched."

*Resources:*

An up-to-date list of AIDS vaccine trials is available at www.iavi.org. IAVI has placed the following resources on its website (www.iavi.org).

- a site readiness assessment tool;
- a laboratory readiness assessment tool;
- a community readiness assessment tool.

Additional information is available at the following web sites: www.hvtn.org; www.kavi.org; www.saavi.org; www.aidsvaccineclearinghouse.org.

sense but are designed to prepare the site personnel to recruit, counsel, test for HIV, and retain participants over a minimum of 2 years. The studies will simulate some of the procedures in a trial.

HIV prevalence will estimate the number of HIV-unin-fected individuals; incidence can be documented by sequential testing using serology. Direct viral detection may identify acute infections prior to antibody production in populations with high incidence (Li *et al.*, 2006; Pilcher *et al.*, 2005). The willingness of potential volunteers to participate in a vaccine trial may be evaluated once information on research, clinical trials and AIDS vaccine trials has been shared and understood, by the individual and others in the family and community. Participation in epidemiological studies and AIDS vaccine trials should avoid stigmatizing individuals or communities.

If HIV incidence is not known, it must be estimated in a population similar or identical to the anticipated trial participants (Ghys *et al.*, 2006). The power to detect a significant result in an efficacy trial depends on the sample size, the incidence rate of HIV infection, and the follow-up over time. Selection of communities or individuals at higher risk can significantly decrease the size of the trial, which in turn results in a shorter time of enrollment, completion and analysis. The willingness of the community to participate in the trial and the expected follow-up rates must also be considered. Incidence may or may not decline prior to or during the trial due to increased AIDS awareness and enhanced prevention (Choopanya *et al.*, 2003).

Efficacy trials can enrich for at-risk populations by focusing recruitment efforts to ensure higher incidence. Higher incidence can be found, despite counseling, in HIV-discordant couples in Zambia and Uganda, with an incidence of > 5/100 person-years (Allen *et al.*, 2003; Nyblade *et al.*, 2001), while sex workers in the N9 microbicide efficacy studies in the Cameroon had incidence rates of 1.5–5/100 per year (Roddy *et al.*, 2002). High incidences are generally observed in injecting drug users, for example in China varying from 3% to 8% (Ruan *et al.*, 2005). Substantial declines in injection risk behavior have been observed after risk reduction counseling during cohort studies with intravenous drug users (IDUs). This information is important in the evaluation of possible adverse behavioral effects of participation in future preventive AIDS vaccine trials (Choopanya *et al.*, 2003). Other studies have shown that those attending clinics for sexually transmitted diseases have a high HIV incidence, but follow-up may be difficult. In some countries, adolescents are at high risk of HIV infection (Singh *et al.*, 2006), whereas in others the incidence in this age group appears to be decreasing (Kirungi *et al.*, 2006). Enrollment of adolescents in prevention trials will encounter challenges in obtaining consent and delivering effective risk reduction counseling, recruitment and retention, but is especially important as this group could be a primary audience for eventual vaccine access and use (Jaspan *et al.*, 2005).

Infants of HIV-infected mothers continue to be at risk during breastfeeding. Although several trials using antiretrovirals in the mother, formula feeding and early weaning are under way; an efficacious neonatal vaccine could augment the progress already made with drugs during the period of breast feeding. The availability of a vaccine with adequate safety data and a rapid immune response (during a short period of anti-retroviral treatment) would permit consideration of this group for vaccine trials (Luzuriaga, 2006; Safrit, 2003).

During the feasibility studies, participants who become HIV infected during the follow-up period despite risk reduction counseling can be followed to document key disease modification outcome measures such as viral load set point, CD4 and symptoms or clinical endpoints. This will help to ensure that the data will be properly collected in a clinical trial, and that there is adequate information on the natural history of HIV in specific populations with other underlying acute and chronic conditions such as tuberculosis, malaria and sexually transmitted diseases. Appropriate care referral networks need to be put in place for the diagnosis, care and treatment of HIV and opportunistic infections. The feasibility study provides an opportunity to ensure that trial inclusion and exclusion criteria are clinically relevant and that adverse events can be properly interpreted using clinical safety laboratory data.

*Scientific and laboratory preparation*

Efficacy trials require laboratory infrastructure that meets international best practices (Table 12.2). Laboratory capacity will need to be augmented for evaluation of vaccine safety by routine laboratory tests; definitive diagnosis of illnesses that affect trial eligibility or occur during trials (adverse events); measurement of vaccine-induced immune responses; diagnosis of HIV infection in vaccine trial participants and evaluation of HIV infection (CD4 and virus load). All of these laboratory functions must be quality-assured. Some may be centralized to assure efficiency and quality control, but ideally they will be regional or local and provide an opportunity to improve diagnostic services for the general community. Field laboratories are usually integrated into local health facilities of the medical referral system for trial participants. They will benefit from early quality control procedures, good clinical laboratory practices training prior to, and during the trial, will maintain high-quality standards and reliability of trial result. Definition of consensus equipment, validation of techniques and development of standard operating procedures along with quality control of all assays and laboratories are critical steps to ensure reliability of results, especially in multi-center trials (Cox, 2002; Maecker *et al.*, 2005).

Routine safety assessments of biochemistry and hematology parameters require high through-put assays, the newly developed Good Clinical Laboratory Practices and an international quality assurance program. Likewise, definitive diagnostic facilities for common illnesses must be available. Expert microscopy for parasitic diseases, microbiology for sexually transmitted diseases and newer detection assays for tuberculosis and hepatitis, for example, will clarify the nature of adverse events during the trials.

Assessments of immunogenicity require sophisticated immunology assays such as ELISPOT assays, flow cytometry, and antibodies that bind or neutralize HIV. Sample processing for storage and shipment of serum, plasma and especially mononuclear cells, should be undertaken immediately at the field site, to avoid loss of immunological responses (Gilmour *et al.*, unpublished data, 2006). Using frozen PBMC requires validated freezing and thawing procedures, and validated shipment conditions if testing is to be performed centrally. Several groups are working together to standardize these assays by exchanging panels of samples and to standardize and optimize these methods.

Diagnostic testing for HIV infection may be more complex in vaccinated individuals. Most HIV screening tests are antibody based. Vaccines that induce primarily cell-mediated immunity may not alter these tests, but vaccines that induce antibody may cause certain screening tests to become positive, depending on the titer of antibody and the specific antigens included in the test kits. Confirmatory Western blot may reveal "vaccine antibody bands" that may be difficult to interpret. Antibody testing results that could un-blind the treatment assignment must not be accessible to the study team; however, a definitive diagnosis of HIV infection must be made in a timely fashion and shared with the team and the participant. Diagnosis of HIV infection in vaccine trial participants will be a challenge if standard diagnostic tests are false positive; for some vaccine candidates, a new assay may provide specific diagnosis of HIV infection in the face of vaccine-induced antibodies (Khurana *et al.*, 2006), while for others direct virus detection by a sensitive nucleic acid-based assay may be required to detect or exclude HIV infection. Diagnostic laboratory services in the vicinity of trial sites must be informed about the difference between vaccine-induced antibodies and those induced by HIV infection, and counsel their clients accordingly if they are vaccine trial participants.

Whether or not certain AIDS vaccines affect the risk of HIV infection, they may modify the subsequent natural history of disease by decreasing HIV replication. Such effects might be of real benefit, both by delaying onset of AIDS and by reducing HIV transmission from the infected person to his or her contacts. To define trial endpoints, feasibility studies will better define the natural history of HIV infection in relevant populations, specifically quantitation of virus in plasma (virus load), decline of CD4 cells, the different HIV-1 subtypes circulating in the population and cofactors of HIV infection and disease progression. The assays should be able to detect virus nucleic acid and quantify it, regardless of HIV-1 subtype. Viral sequencing capacity will also be required, to characterize HIV isolates from the community including volunteers in vaccine trials (Kijak *et al.*, 2004).

## Recruitment

Initial information about a trial may be disseminated by written materials, advertisements, or presentations to large groups. A minority of those initially contacted will opt to learn more, in one-on-one discussion, and only a proportion of those will consent to screening after a detailed explanation of risks, benefits and trial requirements. Some will fail to demonstrate adequate understanding of the material presented (often volunteers must pass a formal assessment of understanding in order to join the trial). Physical examination or laboratory tests at baseline may reveal a condition, such as chronic illness or pregnancy, which precludes trial participation. Hence, the initial pool of potential recruits must be large for efficacy trials (Fig 12.1), as well as for for phase I trials (Fig 12.2). Determination of laboratory reference ranges appropriate for the population may avoid unnecessary exclusion of volunteers.

## Logistics

Logistics is a key element of any successful efficacy trial. Definition of consensus equipment, validation of techniques and development of standard operating procedures along with quality control of all assays and laboratories are critical steps to ensure reliability of results, especially in multi-center trials. None of the components can be considered minor. These include organization of the clinical, laboratory and storage facilities at the central and field level, sample management, shipment procedures, power supply and back up, good quality water for laboratories, reagents, importation of investiga-

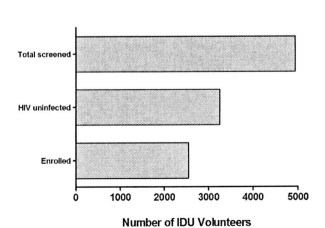

**Figure 12.1** Number of volunteers at different stages of recruitment for AIDSVAX Efficacy trial, Bangkok, Thailand.

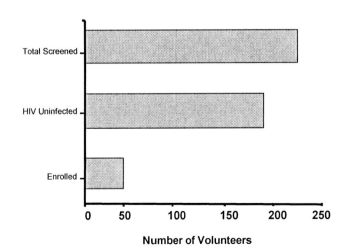

**Figure 12.2** Number of volunteers at different stages of recruitment for IAVI/UVRI phase I trial in Uganda Africa.

**Table 12.2** Laboratory diagnostic and logistical capabilities required for HIV vaccine trials*

*Sample preparation and storage*

Processing of blood samples

Storage of plasma, serum

Isolation of peripheral blood mononuclear cells

Cell freezing and thawing

Shipping procedures

*Basic health indicators*

Physical examination

    Weight and height

    Vital signs

    Examination: skin, respiratory, cardiovascular, nervous system, abdomen, genitourinary

Hematology—full blood count, differential and platelet count

Live function tests: aspartate aminotransferase (AST), alanine aminotransferase (ALT), total and direct bilirubin; optional, GGT or alkaline phosphatase (AP) to confirm cholestasis

Immunology: CD4 and CD8 T cells (percentage and absolute count); optional: gamma globulins

Urinalysis: Dipstick: protein, blood, glucose; optional: ketones, esterase (leukocytes), nitrites to detect urinary tract infection

*Disease diagnostics** (for sub-Saharan Africa)*

Sexually transmitted infections

Malaria

Tuberculosis

Parasitic diseases

Hepatitis

*HIV detection and monitoring*

Rapid or conventional ELISA test for HIV infection

Western blot confirmatory test

CD4 count

Qualitative nucleic acid detection methods for HIV testing***

HIV viral load

HIV subtyping and sequencing capacity

*Evaluation of HIV-specific vaccine responses*

Binding antibodies

Neutralizing antibodies

ELISPOT and/or flow cytometry

Optional: Functional T cell assays (cytolytic, proliferative)

*Logistical requirements*

Core, standardized equipment and reagents

Storage facilities at field and central labs

Sample management procedures

Sample shipment procedures

Power supply and backup

Adequate water quality and reliability

Procedures for importation of vaccines and laboratory reagents, including customs release

Maintenance of cold chain for products, specimens and reagents

Computers, data management and security

Data transfer procedures

Internet access

Established monitoring procedures

Telephone communications

Transportation within trial site region

*For more complete information, see www.iavi.org for:

- a site readiness assessment tool;
- a laboratory readiness assessment tool;
- a community readiness assessment tool.

Additional information is available at the following web sites: www.hvtn.org; www.kavi.org; www.saavi.org.
**This list will vary from region to region, depending on what diseases are prevalent. As an example, the list shown is tailored to sub-Sahara Africa.
***If vaccine induces antibodies, serological assays may not be useful. Ideally conducted at an independent laboratory, to preserve blinding of volunteers' vaccination status.

tional products and customs release, maintenance of the cold chain including local access to dry ice and liquid nitrogen, data management, integrity of the database, data transfer, internet access and computer systems, monitoring tools, communications, and transportation. Most will have been implemented during feasibility studies and the phase I/II trials. A detailed flow chart of events with dry-run exercises is a critical step prior to any trial initiation, and an organizational chart of activities should be displayed at all steps of implementation. A flow chart of cumulated visits should be regularly updated to visualize the peaks of workload and logistical needs over time. The administering of placebos or vaccines requires near perfect blinding of the two products and when this is not possible the staff involved in administration should not be involved in clinical evaluation.

### Medical and health care infrastructure

The type of information collected for a vaccine trial is likely to require assessment and strengthening of the health care infrastructure. This investment will ensure that relevant medical information is collected and that volunteers and community members benefit from the trials.

In developing countries, access to basic medical care is limited, and acute or chronic health conditions may be identified at screening. A suitable medical referral network is needed to ensure the best available care. During a clinical trial, common conditions may occur such as malaria, tuberculosis, diarrhea and sexually transmitted diseases, many of which are treated presumptively, based on clinical algorithms. In Kericho, Kenya, for example, the US Military HIV Research Program has constructed a clinic with up to date laboratory facilities that is available to serve the general community as well as eventual trial participants. The definitive diagnosis of these conditions is critical to ensuring that an adverse event with a clearly identifiable cause is not mistakenly assumed to be due to vaccine. Similarly, autopsy services, either physical or verbal, will need to be expanded, to collect information on the cause of death of any trial participant.

People who become infected with HIV, through risky behavior during a trial will require careful follow up, including support and data collection on disease parameters, treatment or prophylaxis for opportunistic infections and eventually treatment for HIV. Improving referral networks for HIV-infected pregnant women is a very important intervention that could improve maternal and child health. Improvement of care for HIV-infected persons will, in turn, encourage participation in VCT and risk reduction counseling.

### Approval process

#### Political and community support

Successful implementation of AIDS vaccine clinical trials, particularly large-scale trials, requires scientists, policy makers, community groups, and the media, to create an "enabling environment" by implementing wide-spread voluntary HIV counseling and testing (VCT), promoting policies and capacity that support rapid regulatory review and building sufficient community health infrastructure. Consistent, comprehensive information exchange tailored to appropriate audiences is critical for this enabling environment (Francis *et al.*, 2003; Mugerwa *et al.*, 2002; Mugyenyi, 2002; Reeder and Taime, 2003).

International, national and local political commitment and consensus can shorten the approval process. In Uganda, growing political commitment for AIDS vaccines as part of the country's comprehensive response to the epidemic led to the implementation of an effective system for regulatory approvals and cut approval time from over two years for the first trial to less than six months for the second trial. Similarly, strong political commitment and support in Rwanda led to the first AIDS vaccine clinical trial protocol being approved in two months (www.iavi.org).

An important method of demonstrating commitment to the communities where trials will be carried out is to ensure that clinical trials provide an immediate public health benefit to the participating communities, through health education, improving counseling or clinical treatment capacity, thus laying the foundation for subsequent delivery of a proven vaccine and leaving participating communities better off, irrespective of whether the candidate vaccine is shown to be efficacious.

#### Partnerships with researchers

Developing the capacity of individual physicians, scientists, laboratorians, nurses, counselors and data managers, and institutional procedures for review and conduct of clinical trials, is not difficult, given the talent available, but requires time for training and development of confidence and leadership. Career development for professionals should go hand in hand with trials, thus developing credible local expertise and advocacy.

Ultimately, the decision to approve and use an AIDS vaccine will belong to each society. Individuals, who might enroll in large-scale trials or use an approved product, and their governments, want to know that local experts have evaluated the product, and that trials have enrolled a population representative of those who will receive the vaccine.

### Regulatory strategy

The goal of AIDS vaccine clinical trials must remain the development of accessible, affordable interventions for populations at greatest risk. The experience of polio vaccine development in the US, where more than 200 clinical trial sites became the first immediate access points for the vaccine once it was licensed, is an important historical lesson of linking clinical trials to the subsequent distribution and use of a product (Burke, 2004). Nevertheless, the process of regulating trials and approving vaccines requires technical expertise in evaluating the preclinical safety and identity testing of the vaccine, the consistency of manufacture and the design of the research studies. This expertise is rare, and it will be a challenge to provide review that is technically adequate and locally relevant, in a timely manner.

Support for trials in resource-poor countries may be sought from national regulatory agencies in other countries, particularly if clinical trials are also conducted in the United States or Europe. Advice may be sought from the UNAIDS Vaccine Advisory Committee. Trials sponsored by HVTN in the Caribbean and Latin America and by IAVI in Kenya have been carried out under supervision of the US and UK regulatory authorities, respectively, because they were multicenter protocols that included UK or US sites. Proposed mechanisms for obtaining formal advice from experts at US and European regulatory agencies will be of benefit. The regulatory agencies of the United States, Europe and Japan, have cooperated in the International Conference on Harmonization (ICH), and Europe has created a new agency, EMEA (the European Agency for the Evaluation of Medicinal Products) to simplify international clinical research and multinational registration of new products. ICH good clinical practices and good laboratory practices can be applied anywhere in the world.

However, in countries without a strong tradition of pharmaceutical manufacturing and clinical research, expertise is limited in ethics, statistics, and evaluating manufacturing and preclinical data. In most resource-limited countries, regulatory agencies are accustomed to evaluating products that are licensed elsewhere, but less familiar with evaluating novel investigational agents.

WHO is currently evaluating and strengthening national regulatory agencies, and mechanisms for formal consultation with US or European regulatory agencies are planned. Formation of regional agencies to evaluate new products may be essential so that AIDS vaccines designed for those regions can be rapidly approved.

Many AIDS vaccines are DNA plasmids or recombinant viral or bacterial vectors. These vaccines may require three approvals, those required for drugs, for genetically modified plants (even if the vaccines cannot replicate), and for gene therapy agents (even though a vaccine is not designed to alter the human genome). Simplifying these regulations would accelerate AIDS vaccine research. The Ministry of Health normally approves investigational protocols. In some cases Parliament or the office of the head of state has also approved the research. A national AIDS vaccine plan can be invaluable in guiding this process.

## National vaccine plans

A strong system of guidelines and oversight mechanisms has evolved for clinical research. These safeguards require qualified and trusted experts to evaluate manufacturing and preclinical data, study design and procedures. With the help of UNAIDS/WHO and now their African AIDS Vaccine Program (AAVP), many countries are developing National AIDS Vaccine Plans that identify the committees or governmental bodies who must give approval (and in what order), the role of international advisors, and the process for community consultation.

## Ethical approval

Institutional ethics committees (ECs) or institutional review boards (IRBs) at each participating clinical site must approve the study protocol, informed consent document and the process of obtaining informed consent, and the materials used for patient recruitment. Laboratories and data centers also require EC or IRB review. The committees ensure that study procedures are followed, that data are collected and maintained in a secure and confidential manner, and that the laboratory studies are appropriate. Many IRBs or ECs in Africa and Asia have met the standards of the US Office of Human Research Protection in order to approve research supported by grants from the US Government. However, additional support for administrative functions and technical training is important so that these agencies can function efficiently. A balance of careful deliberation and efficient review is warranted, given the widespread impact of the HIV epidemic.

## Building consensus

### Community input and access: role of NGOs and CBOs

Recruitment of volunteers at risk for HIV infection, who are often from stigmatized groups, can be facilitated by acknowledged organizations linked to such groups. Non-governmental organizations (NGOs) and community-based organizations (CBOs) and community advisory boards (CABs) along with community and religious leaders can facilitate communication between government, researchers and communities. To gain their support, and seek their advice, trial sponsors and researchers should set up an informational program on the vaccine and clinical trial design and procedures (Francis et al., 2003; Mugerwa et al., 2002; Mugyenyi, 2002; Reeder and Taime, 2003).

NGO and CBO participation can be effective at three levels. At the strategic level through their networks, community leaders can act as advocates, playing a pivotal role in communication in regional languages, building and sustaining community interest as well as partnership and ownership of the trial, dispelling myths on vaccines and trials, and managing expectations. The process level consists in facilitating community participation, ensuring bilateral flow of communication, and exerting pressure on local politicians, and international stakeholders. Such organizations may ultimately participate in technical activities through prevention education, media work, translations, and providing community perspectives (Kelly, 2006).

Community advisory boards can play a particularly important role in guiding and formalizing the relationship between community and investigators. CABs may review informed consent and study design, advise investigators regarding the participants' perspectives, provide an additional safeguard (in addition to institutional Ethics Committee) for participants' rights, and support volunteer recruitment by disseminating information about the trial (www.iavi.org). As one CAB member eloquently stated: "The CAB is the eyes of the community watching the researchers, and the ears of the researchers to hear what the community is saying about their work" (personal communication, 2005, Zambia-Emory HIV Research Program).

## AIDS awareness, stigmatization, and gender

To enroll sufficient volunteers for a large-scale trial, many thousands of people must have a basic understanding of HIV/AIDS and be motivated to seek out VCT. The community around trial sites should have access to VCT, to minimize stigma and provide a large pool of potential volunteers who already know their status. This will greatly facilitate recruitment of HIV-uninfected individuals for the trial. If numerous HIV-infected people unwittingly present themselves as trial volunteers, it will be difficult to avoid inadvertent identification of those ineligible to join as HIV-infected. Stigmatization and fear of HIV are major barriers to VCT, even where high quality services exist and treatment for HIV infected people is a reality. Encouragement of testing will facilitate risk reduction counseling and medical referrals for those who need them (Liechty, 2005; Mills et al., 2004).

In addition to the general stigma related to HIV/AIDS, there is the added burden of gender inequities exacerbated by the epidemic that further marginalizes women. Investigators in East Africa have found that many women who participate in the screening protocol do not enroll in the vaccine trial. Women's participation can be hindered by: (a) lack of autonomy to make independent decisions about HIV testing or trial enrolment; (b) responsibilities of childcare, care of the elderly and housework may limit their ability to commit time to education sessions or clinic visits; (c) where a woman's fertility is valued, requirements to avoid pregnancy during the trial may discourage participation. Availability of child care and meals at the trial site, and convenient times and locations may be helpful. Engaging couples in the counseling process may select a group of women who can discuss HIV risk factors openly with their partners, thus facilitating participation (Kapoor, 2003).

Community groups, women's organizations, the media and government programs working in the area of HIV/AIDS, reproductive health and general development can be strong allies in helping to mobilize volunteers. These partners can help to assess and shape current attitudes and awareness about AIDS vaccines, help people understand the role vaccines might play in controlling the epidemic and address apprehensions and fears (Green, 2006). They can also help to address some of the stigma and gender-specific issues that may be obstacles to enrolling at-risk populations, including women. The AIDS Support Organization in Uganda and the Kenyan AIDS NGO Consortium are examples of strategic partnerships where AIDS vaccines have been integrated into these NGOs' comprehensive outreach programs. These partnerships improve the current efforts and support future trials.

The print and broadcast press can disseminate accurate information about HIV/AIDS, clinical research and AIDS vaccines and help with specific recruitment activities, provided members of the media are well briefed. The alternative can be the inadvertent spread of misconceptions, and mistrust. Through outreach to key journalists, initially negative press in Uganda and Kenya became generally supportive of the trials.

## Conclusions

1   Additional clinical trial capacity is required in the regions hardest hit by the AIDS epidemic.
2   Targeted prevention and treatment programs have decreased the incidence of HIV infection in most high risk groups over the past 5 years. It is therefore highly likely that AIDS vaccine efficacy trials will need to be multicentric and multicountry in order to enroll sufficient numbers of participants
3   High-quality clinical trials can be conducted in resource-limited settings, given sufficient investment and training and, as appropriate, administrative and technical support for ethical committees and national regulatory authorities.
4   Trial preparedness activities should provide a long-term, sustainable infrastructure and build capacity for research, care and treatment. Trials can focus resources now available to improve awareness, access to diagnosis and treatment of HIV.
5   Engagement of community and political leaders and media to create an enabling environment of trust and open discussion is essential to support large-scale clinical trials of AIDS vaccines.

## Acknowledgments
Christina Schiller and Melissa Simek provided valuable editorial assistance.

## References
Allen, S., Meinzen-Derr, J., Kautzman, M., Zulu, I., Trask, S., Fideli, U., Musonda, R., Kasolo, F., Gao, F., and Haworth, A. (2003). Sexual behavior of HIV discordant couples after HIV counseling and testing. AIDS 17, 733–740.

Burke, D.S. (2004). Lessons learned from the 1954 field trial of poliomyelitis vaccine. Clin. Trials 1, 3–5.

Choopanya, K., Des Jarlais, D.C., Vanichseni, S., Mock, P.A., Kitayaporn, D., Sangkhum, U., Prasithiphol, B., Hiranrus, K., van Griensven, F., Tappero, J.W., and Mastro, T.D. (2003). HIV risk reduction in a cohort of injecting drug users in Bangkok, Thailand. J. Acquir. Immune Defic. Syndr. 33, 88–95.

Cox, J.H., deSouza, M., Ratto-Kim, S., Ferrari, G., Weinhold, K., and Birx, D.L. (2002). Accomplishing cellular immune assays for evaluation of vaccine efficacy in developing countries. In Manual Clinical Laboratory Immunology (Washington, DC, ASM Publications), pp. 301–315.

Esparza, J. (2005). The global HIV vaccine enterprise. Int. Microbiol. 8, 93–101.

Excler, J.L. (2006). AIDS vaccine efficacy trials: expand capacity and prioritize. Throughout Africa, Asia and Latin America state-of-the-art clinics and laboratories...exist where, 4 years ago, there were none. Expert Rev. Vaccines 5, 167–170.

Francis, D.P., Heyward, W. L., Popovic, V., Orozco-Cronin, P., Orelind, K., Gee, C., Hirsch, A., Ippolito, T., Luck, A., Longhi, M., et al. (2003). Candidate HIV/AIDS vaccines: lessons learned from the World's first phase III efficacy trials. AIDS 17, 147–156.

Ghys, P.D., Kufa, E., and George, M.V. (2006). Measuring trends in prevalence and incidence of HIV infection in countries with generalised epidemics. Sex. Transm. Infect. 82, Suppl. 1, i52–56.

Green, E.C., Halperin, D.T., Nantulya, V., and Hogle, J.A. (2006). Uganda's HIV prevention success: the role of sexual behavior change and the National response. AIDS Behav. 10, 335–346.

Jaspan, H.B., Gray, G.E., Robinson, A.K., Coovadia, H.M., and Bekker, L.G. (2005). Scientific justification for the participation of children and adolescents in HIV-1 vaccine trials in South Africa. S. Afr. Med. J. 95, 685–687.

Kapoor, S. (2003). Gender issues in AIDS vaccine trials in India: analyses and recommendations. www.iavi.org

Khurana, S., Needham, J., Mathieson, B., Rodriguez-Chavez, I.R., Catanzaro, A.T., Bailer, R.T., Kim, J., Polonis, V., Cooper, D.A., Guerin, J., et al. (2006). Human immunodeficiency virus (HIV) vaccine trials: a novel assay for differential diagnosis of HIV infections in the face of vaccine-generated antibodies. J. Virol. 80, 2092–2099.

Kijak, G.H., Sanders-Buell, E., Wolfe, N.D., Mpoudi-Ngole, E., Kim, B., Brown, B., Robb, M.L., Birx, D.L., Burke, D.S., Carr, J.K., and McCutchan, F.E. (2004). Development and application of a high-throughput HIV type 1 genotyping assay to identify CRF02_AG in West/West Central Africa. AIDS Res Hum. Retroviruses 20, 521–530.

Kirungi, W.L., Musinguzi, J., Madraa, E., Mulumba, N., Callejja, T., Ghys, P., and Bessinger, R. (2006). Trends in antenatal HIV prevalence in urban Uganda associated with uptake of preventive sexual behaviour. Sex. Transm. Infect. 82 Suppl. 1, i36–41.

Li, B., Decker, J.M., Johnson, R.W., Bibollet-Ruche, F., Wei, X., Mulenga, J., Allen, S., Hunter, E., Hahn, B.H., and Shaw, G.M., et al. (2006). Evidence for potent autologous neutralizing antibody titers and compact envelopes in early infection with subtype C human immunodeficiency virus type 1. J. Virol. 80, 5211–5218.

Liechty, C.A. (2005). The evolving role of HIV counseling and testing in resource-limited settings: HIV prevention and linkage to expanding HIV care access. Curr. Infect. Dis. Rep. 7, 154–158.

Luzuriaga, K., Newell, M.L., Dabis, F., Excler, J.L., and Sullivan, J.L. (2006). Vaccines to prevent transmission of HIV-1 via breastmilk: scientific and logistical priorities. Lancet 368, 511–521.

Maecker, H.T., Rinfret, A., D'Souza, P., Darden, J., Roig, E., Landry, C., Hayes, P., Birungi, J., Anzala, O., Garcia, M., et al. (2005). Standardization of cytokine flow cytometry assays. BMC Immunol 6, 13.

Mehendale, S.M., Ghate, M.V., Kishore Kumar, B., Sahay, S., Gamble, T.R., Godbole, S.V., Thakar, M.R., Kulkarni, S.S., Gupta, A., Gangakhedkar, R.R., et al. (2006). Low HIV-1 incidence among married serodiscordant couples in Pune, India. J. Acquir. Immune Defic. Syndr. 41, 371–373.

Mills, E., Cooper, C., Guyatt, G., Gilchrist, A., Rachlis, B., Sulway, C., and Wilson, K. (2004). Barriers to participating in an HIV vaccine trial: a systematic review. AIDS 18, 2235–2242.

Mugerwa, R.D., Kaleebu, P., Mugyenyi, P., Katongole-Mbidde, E., Hom, D.L., Byaruhanga, R., Salata, R.A., and Ellner, J.J. (2002). First trial of the HIV-1 vaccine in Africa: Ugandan experience. BMJ 324, 226–229.

Mugyenyi, P.N. (2002). HIV vaccines: the Uganda experience. Vaccine 20, 1905–1908.

Nyblade, L.C., Menken, J., Wawer, M.J., Sewankambo, N.K., Serwadda, D., Makumbi, F., Lutalo, T., and Gray, R.H. (2001). Population-based HIV testing and counseling in rural Uganda: participation and risk characteristics. J. Acquir. Immune Defic. Syndr. 28, 463–470.

Pilcher, C.D., Fiscus, S.A., Nguyen, T.Q., Foust, E., Wolf, L., Williams, D., Ashby, R., O'Dowd, J.O., McPherson, J.T., Stalzer, B., et al. (2005). Detection of acute infections during HIV testing in North Carolina. N. Engl. J. Med. 352, 1873–1883.

Reeder, J.C., and Taime, J. (2003). Engaging the community in research: lessons learned from the malaria vaccine trial. Trends Parasitol. 19, 281–282.

Roddy, R.E., Zekeng, L., Ryan, K.A., Tamoufe, U., and Tweedy, K.G. (2002). Effect of nonoxynol-9 gel on urogenital gonorrhea and chlamydial infection: a randomized controlled trial. JAMA 287, 1117–1122.

Rodriguez-Chavez, I.R., Allen, M., Hill, E.L., Sheets, R.L., Pensiero, M., Bradac, J.A., and D'Souza, M.P. (2006). Current advances and challenges in HIV-1 vaccines. Curr HIV/AIDS Rep 3, 39–47.

Ruan, Y., Qin, G., Liu, S., Qian, H., Zhang, L., Zhou, F., He, Y., Chen, K., Yin, L., Chen, X., et al. (2005). HIV incidence and factors contributed to retention in a 12-month follow-up study of injection drug users in Sichuan Province, China. J. Acquir. Immune Defic. Syndr. 39, 459–463.

Safrit, J.T. (2003). HIV vaccines in infants and children: past trials, present plans and future perspectives. Curr. Mol. Med. 3, 303–312.

Singh, J.A., Abdool Karim, S.S., Karim, Q.A., Mlisana, K., Williamson, C., Gray, C., Govender, M., and Gray, A. (2006). Enrolling adolescents in research on HIV and other sensitive issues: lessons from South Africa. PLoS Med. 3, e180.

Taegtmeyer, M., Doyle, V. (2003). Liverpool VCT and Care Kenya, Quality Assurance Manual for Voluntary Counselling and Testing Service Providers).

# Issues in the Design of HIV Vaccine Efficacy Trials

Steven G. Self

13

## Abstract

This chapter discusses several issues in the design of HIV vaccine efficacy trials. It first describes how primary objectives are formulated for phase IIB and phase III studies and how they are used to determine the numbers of volunteers needed for these designs. The discussion then turns to primary efficacy endpoints, and to why and how they differ from those typically used in efficacy trials for other vaccines. Two possible designs for "nested" studies to examine immunologic correlates of protection against HIV/AIDS are described, along with some potential pitfalls in interpreting them. The chapter concludes with some guidelines for planning analyses of subgroups within trial cohorts and for determining the proportion of volunteers to allocate to vaccine versus placebo groups.

## Introduction

Although we are in the third decade of the HIV pandemic, the era of HIV vaccine efficacy trials is still in its infancy. Results from the first two efficacy trials were reported in 2003 (Chapters 14 and 15), a third efficacy trial began in late 2003, a fourth efficacy trial began in late 2004 and a fifth efficacy trial is scheduled to begin in late 2006. The first two efficacy trials used a Phase III design while all subsequent efficacy trials have used a Phase IIB design. From now on the pace is likely to accelerate, given the many candidates moving through phase I/II evaluation.

An effective HIV vaccine will probably be developed iteratively via successive efficacy trials of candidates that represent modest improvements over preceding ones (Klausner et al., 2003). Mathematical modeling (Anderson et al., 1995, 1996; and Chapter 19) suggests that even moderately efficacious HIV vaccines can have significant public health value. Thus, while trials of other types of vaccines are usually designed to assess very high levels of efficacy, HIV vaccine efficacy trials must detect lower levels of protection and modest increments relative to earlier candidates. In this landscape, careful study design and scrupulous trial operations are essential.

Several issues make the design of HIV efficacy trials particularly challenging. First, trials must assess multiple types of vaccine effects that demonstrate the ability to block infection and/or to delay disease progression. Second, since correlates of protection are unknown, efficacy trials will most likely incorporate secondary objectives aimed at identifying possible correlates. Third, the global nature of the epidemic and the genetic diversity of HIV mean that trials must assess heterogeneity in study populations and in infecting virus strains, both of which may affect efficacy. The final trial design will reflect a balance among these and many other considerations, such as characteristics of the vaccine, scientific priorities and programmatic requirements of the sponsor, and resources and infrastructure available for conducting the trial.

## The big picture: primary trial objectives

Vaccine efficacy trials are primarily concerned with directly measuring safety and protection and with assessing whether they suffice for licensure. Tests of concept, analysis of potential correlates of protection and study of whether viral variation affects vaccine efficacy may be important, but are secondary with respect to the principal statistical design considerations.

In this discussion we define a generic vaccine efficacy parameter, VE, as the percent reduction in the rate of occurrence of a primary trial endpoint (e.g., HIV infection or HIV-related morbidity/mortality).

Phase III designs are anchored by two parameters chosen by the trial planners. The first, $VE_0$, is the minimum level of true efficacy that would warrant licensure or public health utilization. The value selected for $VE_0$ is somewhat subjective, but it is not arbitrary. The choice may be guided by mathematical modeling of vaccine impact and should be vetted with relevant communities, investigators and regulators. Generally, the value for $VE_0$ will be greater than 0%, reflecting the differences between a vaccine's efficacy as measured in a controlled clinical trial and its likely effectiveness in a "real world" public health setting (which will be somewhat less than VE). The second anchor point value, $VE_A$, is the minimum level of efficacy the trial should reliably detect.

A third design parameter is the desired level of statistical certainty for the trial outcome; in statistical terms, this means testing the primary null hypothesis that $VE = VE_0$. (i.e., vaccine efficacy equals or exceeds the chosen minimum). Although somewhat arbitrary, the standard value for this parameter is 0.025 for the one-sided nature of the hypothesis being tested. Alternatively, statistical certainty can be expressed as confidence intervals for VE. For example, a significant 1-sided test conducted at the 0.025 level is equivalent to the lower bound of a 95% confidence interval for VE exceeding $VE_0$, which means 97.5% confidence that VE exceeds $VE_0$. If the lower boundary of a more (less) stringent confidence interval for VE exceeds $VE_0$, then this constitutes stronger (weaker) evidence that true efficacy exceeds $VE_0$.

Trials can be designed to deliver different statistical standards of evidence for efficacy. The phrase "robust and compelling" is often used to describe a standard that suffices for licensure, and is commonly met by performing two independent phase III trials which each detect efficacy above $VE_0$ with 97.5% confidence. "Robustness" is reflected in the duplication of a positive result, while the "compelling" aspect is reflected in the combined confidence (99.94%) associated with two positive trials (i.e. $0.999375 = 1-0.025^2$). If it is not feasible to conduct two replicate phase III trials, then other aspects of trial design must be used to meet this standard. For example, robustness can be partly addressed within a single trial by enrolling a relatively heterogeneous study population, which in the case of HIV vaccines could mean cohorts with multiple routes of transmission or multiple viral subtypes. Alternatively, doubling the number of volunteers could deliver strength of evidence comparable to that in replicate phase III trials. Although subject to negotiation with regulators, a practical approach might involve a single trial approximately 50% larger than a standard phase III design. Such a trial would be roughly equivalent to requiring confidence levels of 99.6% (rather than 97.5%) for evidence of efficacy exceeding $VE_0$.

Just as trial designs can be calibrated to provide stronger evidence (e.g., for regulatory purposes), they can also be adjusted if less stringency is required—for instance, when investigators seek some evidence of efficacy as justification for continuing development of a candidate but are reluctant to initiate a phase III trial.

There are several possible reasons for this reluctance. There may be doubts about the likelihood of efficacy, uncertainty about study design parameters (such as selection of endpoints) or other aspects of trial operations. The enormous cost of conducting phase III studies is especially daunting in the face of such questions. However, these doubts must be weighed against the need for direct information about efficacy lest vaccine evaluation remain stalled in phase II.

Since any direct proof of efficacy is likely to have considerable impact on the AIDS vaccine field, even if the evidence is of only moderate statistical strength, the notion of conducting intermediate-sized (phase IIB) efficacy trials has gained support (Rida et al., 1997). The concept of a phase IIB trials has been applied in other settings such as microbicides for HIV prevention (Fleming and Richardson, 2004) and HPV vaccine evaluation (Harper et al., 2005; Koutsky et al., 2002). However the first, and so far only, IIB trial of an HIV vaccine

(Merck's adenovirus-based candidate) began in late 2004 and the second such trial is planned to begin in Fall 2006. Phase IIB trials should be large enough to produce some direct information on efficacy endpoints, but also require fewer volunteers (and perhaps a shorter duration) than phase III studies. The key to these scaled-down designs is clarity over what decisions will be made based on the trial's results, and over the type and strength of evidence required for these decisions. The design must also be conceptually consistent with the aforementioned notion of anchor points for phase III trials.

To illustrate how these factors affect the design of a phase IIB study, consider the example of a trial designed to decide whether to:

a    initiate a phase III trial;

b    initiate discussions with regulators regarding licensure; or

c    discard the vaccine from further consideration.

The first design decision is the type of evidence that would be accepted as sufficient to warrant further study of the candidate (option a). Such evidence can be formalized in terms of two parameters: a minimal level of efficacy (VE) and the strength of evidence (confidence level). For example, VE exceeding 0% with a high level of confidence (97.5%) might be considered sufficient "proof of concept" that the candidate induces at least some protection. Alternatively, one might set the threshold at VE exceeding 15% with a moderate level of confidence (20%).

Once the basis for deciding to pursue or discard a candidate is defined, the second anchor point ($VE_A$) is used to determine the number of volunteers needed. To remain consistent with the concepts underlying phase III design, phase IIB studies must be sized to ensure a correspondingly low probability of discarding a vaccine with true VE at or above the value of $VE_A$. Since the minimum threshold for efficacy is typically set lower for phase IIB studies than for phase III, the former require fewer volunteers. Once the volunteer number is determined, the levels of efficacy required for other decisions can be calculated. For example, evidence that VE exceeds $VE_0$ with 97.5% confidence might be grounds to proceed with a phase III study as a second "replicate" trial, while the same evidence with 99.6% confidence might lead to discussions with regulators about licensure.

To get a sense of how these concepts translate into trial designs, consider a comparison of phase III and IIB designs with HIV infection as the primary endpoint. A phase III trial with the primary objective of distinguishing $VE_0 = 30\%$ from $VE_A = 60\%$ at a 97.5 confidence level and the conditions described in Table 13.1 would require 5,300 volunteers. In contrast, a corresponding IIB trial to determine whether VE exceeds 15% at a 20% confidence level would require 2,160 volunteers to ensure (with a confidence level of 97.5) that a vaccine with 60% efficacy would not be discarded. With this phase IIB design, the probability of discarding a vaccine with

**Table 13.1** Phase III versus IIB designs

| Parameter | Phase III | Phase IIB |
|---|---|---|
| $VE_0$ confidence level | 30%, 97.5 | 15%, 20 |
| $VE_A$ confidence level | 60%, 97.5 | 60%, 97.5 |
| No. of volunteers | 5,300 | 2,160 |

This example assumes a 3-year study in a cohort with 2% annual seroincidence and loss to follow-up of 10%, 5% and 5% in years 1, 2 and 3, respectively.

true VE = 0% is 0.95, and the probabilities of demonstrating VE above 30% at confidence levels of 97.5% and 99.6% when true vaccine efficacy is 60% are approximately 0.53 and 0.24, respectively. If true efficacy is 80% then these probabilities are 0.98 and 0.87.

## Defining efficacy: primary trial endpoints
Although primary endpoints in efficacy trials must capture aspects of both safety and efficacy, we focus here only on efficacy and refer readers to a review (Hudgens et al., 2004) for details on safety endpoints and for a comprehensive discussion of endpoints in vaccine trials. Issues about selection of efficacy endpoints in the specific context of HIV vaccine trials have also been discussed and recommendations given (Gilbert et al., 2003).

### Morbidity and mortality
The direct benefit of a prophylactic vaccine is typically defined as the reduction in pathogen-specific occurrence of clinically significant morbidity and mortality. Thus, the most natural primary endpoint for vaccine efficacy is morbidity or death.

The advantage of using endpoints based on morbidity and mortality is that they directly reflect the clinically relevant outcome of vaccination, independent of the vaccine's mechanism of action. Unfortunately, for HIV vaccines there is a compelling disadvantage: the very long latency period of AIDS means that it would take many years to assess efficacy by morbidity/mortality endpoints. HIV vaccine trial designers therefore look for endpoints that can be measured within a shorter time span.

### Infection
The most straightforward such endpoint is one based on infection (prevention of either initial infection or establishment of chronic infection); the ability to accurately assess these outcomes is therefore a key aspect of trial design. Since HIV vaccines that induce humoral responses have so far induced only a narrow range of HIV-specific antibodies, standard serologic assays for detecting HIV infection (e.g., ELISA, Western blot) can distinguish uninfected vaccinees from infected individuals by their HIV serology profiles. However, future candidates may induce a broader range of antibodies that cannot be reliably distinguished from infection by standard serology. In this case, an alternative will be to detect infection by measuring HIV-specific RNA using ultrasensitive PCR-based assays.

### Post-infection endpoints
Nearly all vaccine candidates now in clinical trials target cell-mediated immunity (CMI), and it is generally believed that they are most likely to act post-infection by delaying disease progression. Incorporating post-infection endpoints into efficacy trials of these candidates is therefore essential for measuring their efficacy.

There is an emerging consensus among trial sponsors, investigators and communities that anti-retroviral (ARV) treatment should be provided to all study participants who become infected through unsafe behavior during efficacy trials, including those conducted in developing countries where ARV treatment is not commonplace. Since clinical symptoms of HIV/AIDS are usually minimal in the first few years after ARV treatment is started, the most feasible post-infection endpoints for efficacy studies are surrogate markers that can be assessed *before* initiation of treatment—especially viral load, as measured by levels of HIV RNA, and CD4 T-cell counts. At the same time, the dangers of using invalidated surrogate endpoints have been well documented (Fleming et al., 1996), while comprehensive analyses aimed at validating HIV RNA levels and CD4 cell counts as surrogate endpoints in the context of ARV treatment have so far not provided a full, empirically based justification for their use (Hughes et al., 1998; Hughes, 2000).

Since a complete validation of surrogate endpoints for HIV vaccine trials may never be available, recent work has focused on defining the most useful combination of post-infection endpoints, including biomarker-based surrogates and/or clinical outcomes (Gilbert et al., 2003, and Chapter 4). This work uses existing data from natural history studies and treatment trials to model the relationship between biomarkers and clinical outcomes while introducing appropriate degrees of caution. Interpretation of analyses across this range of endpoints would consider both the strength of the evidence and its consistency in demonstrating a clinically significant effect on each endpoint. Particular care is needed to interpret results of these analyses as they are based on comparisons of groups defined post-randomization and therefore are subject to potential selection biases. For a detailed description of this problem and analytic methods for its assessment, see Sheppard et al. (2006) and references therein.

Because of the high standard of care for HIV-infected people in developed countries, clinical endpoints will likely be observed only after treatment initiation and long-term follow-up. In these settings, current designs are likely to provide substantial information only on biomarker-based surrogate endpoints and possibly composites of both biomarker and clinical endpoints.

However, in developing countries, the rates of HIV-related clinical events very early in the course of infection may be much higher (Morgan et al., 1998, 2002). If so, the impact of an HIV vaccine on important clinical outcomes may be reliably documented during trials in these settings, even when

ARVs are provided to participants who need them using standard guidelines for initiating treatment (which usually means several years after initial infection, based on various clinical factors). Unfortunately, there is relatively little data available from developing countries on the range of clinical outcomes within the first few years of HIV infection. Filling this information gap will be critical in establishing post-infection endpoints for HIV vaccine efficacy.

## HIV diversity and trial endpoints

Care should be taken in defining endpoints when there is genetic heterogeneity of the pathogen, as with HIV. If a vaccine formulation might protect against some but not all pathogen subtypes, then a natural choice for primary endpoint would be the morbidity/mortality events attributable specifically to the targeted subtype. However, such an endpoint could not assess the possible occurrence of vaccine-induced *enhancement* of morbidity by non-targeted subtypes. Even if there is no enhancement, the overall direct clinical benefit of vaccination is arguably best measured using endpoints attributable to any subtype circulating in the population, since high levels of protection against an uncommon subtype would have only limited public health utility. Thus, the primary endpoint in HIV vaccine efficacy trials would ideally not be restricted to particular subtypes. Nonetheless, data showing protection against subtypes matching the vaccine formulation would represent an important "proof of concept" and could point the way to improved vaccine formulations. Thus, both subtype specificity as well as breadth of protection against all subtypes circulating in a population are important elements to be captured by endpoints in HIV vaccine trials.

## Population heterogeneity and subgroup analyses

There is a natural interest in examining vaccine effects that may be specific to various subgroups within trial populations—for example, among racial subgroups, or in male versus female participants. However, subgroup analyses are notoriously unreliable and are therefore typically conducted as tertiary analyses to generate hypotheses for testing in future studies. Nonetheless, there may be questions regarding subgroup-specific vaccine effects that have important programmatic or regulatory impact and should be formally addressed in the study protocol. Trial planners should also specify what type and strength of evidence for subgroup-specific efficacy will lead to particular decisions, such as initiation of a follow-up subgroup-specific efficacy trial, or subgroup-specific indications for vaccine use.

These criteria can be adjusted based on overall trial results. For instance, investigators might require stronger evidence to establish efficacy in a subgroup when the overall trial results are negative than to confirm consistency with an overall positive result. Confidence levels must also be adjusted for the number of subgroups analyzed, and computation of the statistical power for these adjusted analyses should be documented in the study protocol. These calculations will probably influence design considerations regarding the minimum numbers of volunteers for each subgroup. If there are too few participants in the subgroups of interest, confidence levels fall so low that the analysis cannot provide statistically sound conclusions, as happened in the first VaxGen phase III trial (Chapter 14).

## Design of nested studies to address secondary trial objectives

Once an HIV vaccine trial demonstrates at least a low level of efficacy, investigators will most likely attempt to identify specific immune correlates of protection. This is usually done by comparing immune response profiles of vaccinees that become infected during the trial with those who remain uninfected.

Prospectively performing a full range of immunologic assays on all vaccinees in the study would be very costly and perhaps not feasible operationally. If the assays can be done retrospectively using stored (frozen) samples, then either of two more cost-efficient designs can be used: a matched, nested case–control design (Breslow *et al.*, 1980; Schlesselman, 1982) or the closely related case–cohort design (Prentice, 1986).

In case–control studies, samples are thawed and assays performed for all vaccinees who became infected and for a subset of uninfected vaccinees. The latter group is chosen by randomly sampling K uninfected vaccinees for each infected vaccinee (the index case) at the time point when the infection of the index case was ascertained. Logistic regression models are used to contrast types and levels of immune responses for the index case with those of the matched controls. The relative odds of infection associated with different immune responses, is estimated by combining these contrasts over all case–control sets. This method can estimate the relative odds of infection associated with different levels immune responses measured either at the time of complete immunization or of the last study visit at which the index case was uninfected.

The second type of design is a case–cohort study, which is similar to the case–control described above except that, rather than matching individual uninfected controls to each index case, the comparison group is a random sample drawn from the entire cohort of uninfected vaccinees. Although this design may provide less precise control of confounding factors, it can estimate the absolute infection risk associated with different levels of immune response. This allows direct comparison with infection rates in the placebo group, which is important in interpreting these analyses.

Interpreting analyses of correlates depends not just on gradients in rates of infection across different levels of immune responses but also on the rates among vaccinees without a detectable immune response relative to the placebo group. If the infection rate among these non-responding vaccinees is less than that among placebo recipients, then either there are vaccine-induced protective responses which are not captured in the assays or there are responses that are below the limit of detection but still sufficient to confer some protection. In either case, a significant gradient in infection rate over levels of the assay readout may be established, but would represent only a small fraction of the overall protective effect of the vaccine. In this way, a correlate of protection could be statistically established, but its usefulness in predicting protection based on levels of assay readout would be minimal. Alternatively, there may be a significant gradient over levels of the assay readout but the infection rate among non-responsive vaccinees exceeds that among placebo recipients. This could indicate immune enhancement at very low levels of response but protective effects associated with strong responders. Alternatively, it could mean that the measured immunologic response is a correlate of infection risk but not of protection. In this case, the assay response may merely reflect a general level of immunologic competence, so that weak responders will generally be at higher risk for infection and strong responders at lower risk. Again, such a correlate would not help characterize protective responses to the vaccine. See Gilbert et al. (2006) for a specific example of this problem.

Another important secondary analysis in HIV vaccine efficacy trials is to assess the impact of viral variation on vaccine efficacy. This assessment, called sieve analysis (Gilbert et al., 2001), is most useful when some level of overall efficacy is observed. Sieve analyses compare genotypic or phenotypic characteristics of viruses from vaccinees with those in placebo recipients. The comparisons are performed on scores or "distances" that represent the degree of similarity between each infecting viral strain and the viral sequences used in the vaccine. The underlying assumption is that vaccines should confer stronger protection against viruses which are very similar to the vaccine strain. Formally, these analyses estimate the relative attack rates for viruses classified by their distance to the vaccine immunogen.

## Allocation to vaccine and placebo groups

The VaxGen efficacy trials used different relative allocations of volunteers to vaccine and placebo groups (2:1 in the Thai trial, 1:1 in the North America/Europe trial). There are several reasons to consider unequal allocation to vaccine and placebo. A first consideration is the efficiency of the primary statistical test for efficacy. Although a 1:1 allocation provides the best statistical efficiency of a test for the null hypothesis of zero efficacy, it is not optimal for tests of null hypotheses at vaccine efficacy levels above zero. As shown in Table 13.2, the optimal ratio of volunteers in vaccine to placebo groups rises as efficacy increases (in the simple setting of a binary response.) Thus,

for trials to detect relatively modest levels of efficacy (e.g., one that reduces infection risk by 30%; that is, $VE_S = 30\%$), like those currently considered for the current generation of candidates, there is little to be gained by unequal allocation, and some statistical efficiency could even be lost if a more extreme allocation (e.g., 2:1) is used

A second reason to consider unequal allocation is to increase the statistical power of analyses to assess immune correlates of protection, since power is directly related to the number of infected vaccinees. Taking the number of infected vaccinees as the effective sample size in these analyses and noting that precision increases with the square root of sample size, we can compute a rough guideline for improving precision by unequal allocation to vaccine and placebo groups. For a fixed total trial size, a 2:1 allocation would mean 33% more infected vaccinees relative to a 1:1 allocation and an increase of approximately 15% in precision. A third consideration is the power of sieve analyses, which are most efficient when there are equal numbers of infected vaccinees and infected placebo recipients. Under a null hypothesis of $VE_S = 30\%$, this suggests an optimal allocation of 10:7 (vaccine: placebo).

## References

Anderson, R.M., Swinton, J., and Garnett, G.P. (1995). Potential impact of low-efficacy HIV-1 vaccines in populations with high rates of infection. Proc. Roy.l Soc. Lond. B *261*, 147–161.

Anderson, R.M., and Garnett, G.P. (1996). Low efficacy HIV vaccines, Potential for community-based intervention programmes. Lancet *348*, 1010–1013.

Breslow, N.E., and Day, N.E. (1980). Statistical Methods in Cancer Research. Vol. 1. The Analysis of Case–Control Studies. International Agency for Research on Cancer, Lyon.

Fleming, T.R., and DeMets, D.L. (1996). Surrogate endpoints in clinical trials, Are we being misled? Ann. Intern. Med. *125*, 605–613.

Fleming, T.R., and Richardson, B.A. (2004). Some design issues in trials of microbicides for the prevention of HIV infection. J. Infect. Dis. *190*, 666–674.

Gilbert, P.B., Self, S.G., Rao, M., Naficy, A., and Clemens, J. (2001). Sieve analysis, Methods for assessing how vaccine efficacy depends on genotypic and phenotypic pathogen variation from vaccine trial data. J. Clin. Epidemiol. *54*, 68–85.

Gilbert, P.B., DeGruttola, V., Hudgens, M.G., Self, S.G., Hammer, S.M., and Corey, L. (2003). What constitutes efficacy for a HIV vaccine that ameliorates viremia, Issues involving surrogate endpoints in Phase 3 trials. J. Infect. Dis. *188*, 179–193.

Gilbert, P., Peterson, M., Follmann, D., Francis, D., Gurwith, M., Heyward, W., Hudgens, M., Jobes, D., Popovic, V., Self, S., Sinangil, F., Burke, D., Berman, P. (2005). Immunologic responses to rgp120 vaccine correlate with the incidence of HIV-1 infection in a Phase 3 preventive HIV-1 vaccine trial. J. Infect. Dis. *191*, 666–677.

Harper, D.M., Franco, E.L., Wheeler, C., Ferris, D.G., Jenkins, D., Schuind, A., Zahaf, T., Innis, G., Naud, P., DeCarvalho, N.S., Roteli-Martins, C.M., Teixeira, J., Blatter, M.M., Korn, A.R., Quint, W., Dubin, G., the GlaxoSmithKline HPV Vaccine Study Group. (2005). Efficacy of a bivalent L1 virus-like particle vaccine in prevention of infection with human papillomavirus types 16 and 18 in young women: a randomized, controlled trial. Obst. Gynecol. Surv. *60*, 303–305.

Hudgens, M.G., Gilbert, P.B., and Self, S.G. (2004). Endpoints in vaccine trials. Stat. Methods Med. Res. *13(2)*, 89–114.

Hughes, M., Daniels, M., Fischl, M., Kim, S., and Schooley, R. (1998). CD4 counts as a surrogate endpoint in HIV clinical trials, A meta-analysis of studies of the ACTG. AIDS *12*, 1823–1832.

**Table 13.2** Vaccine efficacy, statistical efficiency and relative sizes of vaccine and placebo groups

| $VE_S^*$ | Optimal ratio in vaccine: placebo groups | Efficiency gain |
|---|---|---|
| 30% | 6:5 | <1% |
| 50% | 3:2 | 4% |
| 75% | 2:1 | 11% |
| 90% | 3:1 | 25% |

*VE is the percent reduction in risk of infection due to vaccine; "s" refers to susceptibility.

Hughes, M. (Corresponding author for The HIV Surrogate Marker Collaborative Group) (2000). HIV RNA level and CD4 counts as prognostic markers and surrogate endpoints, A meta-analysis. AIDS Res. Hum. Retrovirus *16*, 1123–1133.

Klausner, R.D., Fauci, A.S., Corey, L., Nabel, G.J., Gayle, H., Berkley, S., Haynes, B.F., Baltimore, D., Collins, C., Douglas, R.G., Esparza, J., *et al.* (2003). The need for a global HIV vaccine enterprise. Science *300*, 2036–2039.

Koutsky, L.A., Ault, K.A., Wheeler, C.M., Brown, D.R., Barr, El, Alvarez, F.B., Chiacchierini, L.M., and Jansen, K.U. (2002). A controlled trial of a human papillomavirus Type 16 vaccine. N. Engl. J. Med. *347*, 1645–1651.

Morgan, D., Mahe, C., Mayanja, B., and Whitworth, J.A.G. (2002). Progression to symptomatic disease in people infected with HIV-1 in rural Uganda, Prospective cohort study. BMJ *324*,193–197.

Morgan, D., Ross A., Mayanja B., Malamba S., and Whitworth J. (1998). Early manifestations (pre-AIDS) of HIV-1 infection in Uganda. AIDS *12*, 591–596.

Prentice, R.L. (1986). A case–cohort design for epidemiologic cohort studies and disease prevention trials. Biometrika *73*, 1–11.

Rida, W.N., Fast, P., Hoff, R., and Fleming, T.R. (1997). Intermediate-sized trials for the evaluation of HIV vaccine candidates, A workshop summary. J. Acquir. Immune Defic. Syndr. Hum. Retrovirol. *16*, 195–205.

Schlesselman, J.J. (1982). Case–Control Studies, Design, Conduct, Analysis. Oxford University Press, Inc., New York.

Shepherd, B., Gilbert, P., Jemiai, Y., and Rotnitzky, A. (2006). Sensitivity analyses comparing outcomes only existing in a subset selected post-randomization, conditional on covariates, with application to HIV vaccine trials. Biometrics (in press).

# Lessons from the AIDSVAX B/B′ Vaccine Efficacy Trial

## 14

Jonathan D. Fuchs and Susan P. Buchbinder

## Abstract

We have much to learn from the North American phase III trial of VaxGen's AIDSVAX B/B′ vaccine, even though the vaccine proved to have no overall efficacy in preventing HIV-1 infection. The trial was statistically well powered to provide clear answers on its primary and secondary endpoints, and met its goals in recruiting and retaining volunteers over the 3-year study. Unfortunately, premature release of data suggesting vaccine efficacy in certain racial subgroups of the study population (based on statistically unadjusted analyses) caused considerable confusion in the field and the general public. It also highlighted the importance for future trials of selecting the most important subgroup analyses in advance and ensuring that the study has adequate statistical power to resolve them clearly. And it spotlighted the need to enroll volunteers reflecting the diversity of at-risk populations, and to utilize broad biostatistical expertise before releasing results to the media.

Other lessons pertain to working with study participants. Future trials would benefit from having experienced, high-capacity sites and centralized assistance in developing strategies for recruitment and retention. Although risk behavior and HIV seroincidence remained high throughout this trial despite ongoing risk-reduction counseling, future efficacy studies in more prevention-naïve populations may see substantial declines in these parameters, and should be powered accordingly. Trials must continue to provide the best prevention strategies available and to develop methods for limiting potential behavioral "disinhibition" among volunteers. Finally, this trial serves as a reminder of the extreme care that must be taken in working with media to ensure that accurate, clear information is disseminated throughout the study and to prepare communities for the long road to an HIV vaccine.

## Introduction

The world's first HIV vaccine efficacy trial, the VAX004 study conducted in North America and the Netherlands, was completed in late 2002 and results were released in February 2003. While the scientific community was able to agree that the AIDSVAX B/B′ gp120 subunit vaccine had no overall efficacy in preventing HIV infection in the study population [5,108 men who have sex with men (MSM) and 309 high-risk heterosexual women], there was considerable disagreement about the correct interpretation of data analyses based on racial subgroups. This chapter describes the overall study design and objectives, summarizes the controversial subgroup analyses and outlines some important lessons to be learned from this trial in planning future efficacy studies. The lessons learned are many, and include not only issues of study design and analysis, but also operational issues pertaining to recruitment and retention of volunteers, behavioral and social ramifications of trial participation and strategies for communicating results.

## Study overview

The primary objective of the VAX004 trial was to determine whether the AIDSVAX B/B′ subunit vaccine, which contains genetically engineered gp120 from two HIV-1 clade B strains (MN, a laboratory-grown strain, and the GNE8 primary isolate), protects against sexually acquired HIV-1 infection. The trial's secondary objectives were to assess the impact of vaccination on volunteers who became infected (as measured by post-infection HIV-1 viral load and CD4$^+$ count) and to confirm safety of the product. The study also had exploratory research objectives, including comparison of viral sequences in infected vaccine versus placebo recipients (i.e., "sieve analysis"), evaluation of possible immune correlates of protection, and behavioral effects of trial participation. In addition, the US Centers for Disease Control and Prevention (CDC) funded six US trial sites to conduct ancillary virologic, immunologic and behavioral studies, called the VISION study.

To meet the core study objectives, VaxGen contracted with 61 sites in the United States, Puerto Rico, Canada, and the Netherlands to enroll a cohort of 5,417 volunteers, mostly MSM, at risk of sexually transmitted HIV-1 infection. Participants who met basic behavioral and medical eligibility criteria were randomized to receive vaccine or placebo in a 2:1 ratio. Participants received injections at 0, 1, 6, 12, 18, 24 and

30 months of study duration, and were seen for a final visit at 36 months. At each visit, HIV pre-test counseling was performed and blood drawn to assess HIV infection status and immunologic response.

## Efficacy results

Results from this trial were initially reported in a number of ways, including Webcast presentations to study site investigators, journalists and interested members of the public in February 2003, and presentations at key scientific meetings (Berman, 2003; Gilbert *et al.*, 2003; Popovic *et al.*, 2003). Efficacy results were published in 2005 in two companion articles (Gilbert *et al.*, 2005b; The rgp120 HIV Vaccine Study Group, 2005).

The AIDSVAX B/B′ vaccine appeared to be safe, with no significant difference in the incidence of serious or non-serious adverse events reported by vaccine and placebo recipients. HIV seroincidence in the trial was 2.6/100 person-years (py) through the 36-month follow-up period; (2.7/100 py in men and 0.8/100 py in women). Infection rates were not different in vaccine and placebo groups, indicating that the vaccine had no efficacy against HIV-1 infection in the cohort as a whole (Table 14.1). The data also showed no overall effect on post-infection (secondary) endpoints, including plasma viral load, CD4$^+$ T-cell count and time interval from infection to initiation of antiretroviral therapy (Gilbert *et al.*, 2005a).

## Subgroup analyses

The issue that raised confusion within and outside the scientific community was VaxGen's suggestion of significant vaccine efficacy in the subgroup of black study participants, and the company's unusual combination of Black, Asian and other racial/ethnic subgroups into one group. Although VaxGen initially stated that these findings achieved statistical significance, subsequent reports indicated that their analyses did not adjust for multiple comparisons, and that when appropriate adjustments were made, these associations between race/ethnicity and vaccine efficacy did not achieve or even approach statistical significance (Graham and Mascola, 2005).

Questions remained about whether the data nevertheless indicate a "real" difference in HIV susceptibility between vaccine and placebo recipients in these racial/ethnic subgroups (even if this difference did not achieve statistical significance, due to the small numbers of volunteers in these subgroups) or rather, represent random variation without any true biological meaning (a spurious result, also more likely to occur with small sample size). Supplemental analyses have ruled out various measurable reasons for a spurious association, including maldistribution in the process of randomizing volunteers to vaccine versus placebo groups, or differential loss to follow-up. Analyses have also explored possible mechanisms by which race could influence vaccine efficacy. Unfortunately, these analyses did not uncover any underlying biological explanation that would support a true difference in infection rates between black vaccine and placebo recipients attributable to vaccine (Gilbert *et al.*, 2005b). For example, while the point estimates for vaccine efficacy were somewhat greater among volunteers reporting higher risk behavior compared to those reporting less risky behavior, black participants reported less risk-taking than white participants, so this finding cannot support claims of increased vaccine efficacy in blacks. VaxGen raised another possibility shortly after the initial results were released when they reported that black vaccine recipients had higher titers of antibodies to gp120 than white vaccinees, and speculated that these higher levels might lead to increased protection in blacks (Berman, 2003). However, non-white volunteers had only minor increases in antibody titers (i.e., on average, one-quarter log$_{10}$), and the relationship between antibody values and vaccine efficacy were not different between *all* racial/ethnic subgroups (Follman, 2004; Gilbert *et al.*, 2003).

Thus, we are left not knowing definitively whether this statistically non-significant suggestion of vaccine efficacy in black participants is real or spurious, although the bulk of scientific opinion is that there is insufficient evidence to support these claims. The US National Institutes of Health (NIH) has convened a series of meetings with scientists and community representatives to review all of the subgroup analyses and discuss whether additional steps to resolve this issue are merited. Regardless of the outcome, there is much to be learned from the handling of the subgroup analysis and the conduct of the study overall, both to avoid similar confusion and concern in future trials and to build on the strengths of this trial.

**Table 14.1** Infections in the VAX004 trial and vaccine efficacy by racial/ethnic group

| Group | No. infected | % infected, vaccinees | % infected, placebo | Vaccine efficacy (%) | Adjusted *P*-value |
|---|---|---|---|---|---|
| Overall | 368 | 6.8 | 7.0 | 6 | >0.5 |
| White/non-Hispanic | 309 | 7.0 | 6.6 | -6 | >0.5 |
| All non-white | 59 | 5.0 | 9.4 | 47 | 0.13 |
| Hispanic | 23 | 5.9 | 7.0 | 15 | >0.5 |
| Black/non-Hispanic | 15 | 2.6 | 7.8 | 67 | 0.24 |
| Asian/Pacific Islander | 6 | 5.4 | 14.3 | 66 | >0.5 |
| Other | 15 | 9.2 | 17.8 | 50 | >0.5 |

## Lessons learned

### Trial design

*The VAX004 trial was successful in providing a definitive answer to the primary research objectives*
VaxGen is to be commended for conducting a well-designed trial adequately powered to meet primary and secondary objectives (vaccine efficacy in preventing HIV-1 infection and post-infection endpoints, respectively). This success was predicated, in part, on having accurate information about HIV seroincidence prior to launching the study (Seage *et al.*, 2001) and on working with some sites experienced in accessing high-risk populations. Currently there are only limited data on HIV seroincidence in many populations being considered for inclusion in future HIV vaccine trials, and only limited experience in recruiting difficult-to-reach populations. Success in future trials will therefore require focused preparatory work in these populations, as well as trial designs based on conservative estimates of HIV seroincidence, to ensure that these studies have sufficient power to evaluate primary and secondary endpoints.

*Trials should be designed with adequate power to answer the highest-priority supplemental research questions*
Regardless of the lack of data supporting racial/ethnic subgroup differences, this trial underscored the notion that differential vaccine efficacy *could* occur within subgroups based on gender, risk group, geographic region (defined by predominant circulating viral subtype) or race/ethnicity, to name a few possibilities. However, the human and monetary cost of powering a study to obtain even moderately precise estimates of vaccine efficacy within many individual subgroups is likely to be prohibitive. From a practical standpoint, early efficacy trials are likely to be able to provide estimates of efficacy for one or two subgroups at most. This limitation must be recognized before initiating trials, and any additional subgroup analyses should be undertaken with caution. Procedures to make statistical adjustments for multiple comparisons should be pre-specified in the analysis plan, and all adjustments made before releasing results to the media.

*For the trial to yield efficacy data which is most applicable to the populations that will ultimately use the vaccine, recruitment strategies should ensure that diverse members of these populations are adequately represented in the study cohort*
This means that special efforts should be undertaken in populations heavily impacted by the HIV epidemic and traditionally under-represented in clinical trials, and that speed and ease of enrollment should not take priority over cohort diversity. Because under-representation of particular groups often stems from community mistrust of medical research in general or HIV vaccine research in particular, investigators will need to build ongoing relationships with community groups, engage community members in Community Advisory Boards,

and spend sufficient time, creativity and resources in developing novel approaches to accessing these populations. Issues of adequate representation are likely to become even more challenging in attempting to test a vaccine for global use, which will necessitate inclusion of many trial sites around the world. Success in this global arena will require investing time and resources on strategies that ensure cohort diversity.

*Teams of biostatisticians, representing different organizations and areas of expertise, should be closely involved in the design and analysis of efficacy studies to ensure the best, most appropriate use of trial data*
VaxGen initially engaged outside statisticians in developing its data analysis plan. After the trial results were announced, they worked with a team of biostatisticians from the NIH and the Seattle-based Statistical Center for HIV and AIDS Research and Prevention (SCHARP) to confirm the overall primary and secondary efficacy results and to perform exploratory analyses, including potential immune correlates of protection, sieve analyses and analysis of behavioral factors associated with HIV infection. VaxGen also collaborated with investigators at the CDC to evaluate changes in risk behavior over time. Having an external team of scientists from multiple organizations analyzing the same dataset has lent credibility to the trial's final results and brought greater depth of expertise in analyzing the full range of data collected during this trial.

### Recruitment and retention

Recruitment efficiency can be enhanced by having an adequate number of trial sites ready before trials begin, by creating and disseminating to the sites a range of recruitment strategies and materials developed with site and community collaboration, and by limiting inclusion of low-capacity sites. The VAX004 trial accrued its 5417 MSM and female volunteers over 17 months, from June 1998 to October 1999. The 61 study sites enrolled anywhere from 8–307 participants each, with approximately two-thirds of sites enrolling fewer than 100 participants. Enrollment was relatively slow at first and only reached optimal levels at about one year; roughly half of the volunteers were enrolled in the last 4 months of the accrual period. Some of the delay was to be expected, as sites needed time to build their lists of interested and eligible participants. However, other factors in the slow start may have been unique to this trial, reflecting the pace at which new sites were brought on, use of sites without prior experience recruiting the target population, minimal centralized assistance or sharing of recruitment materials and techniques, and limited enthusiasm within some communities about the particular vaccine being tested. Future trials involving less well-studied populations than MSM may present additional recruitment hurdles, including community mistrust of HIV vaccine research and difficulty identifying populations with the highest, most sustained HIV seroincidence (McLellan *et al.*, 2003).

Study sites used a wide range of recruitment strategies. These included face-to-face outreach by trained recruiters at venues attracting high-risk MSM and women, referrals from other study participants (a practice known as "snowballing") and targeted advertising in local and national newspapers. In response to the slow initial recruitment, VaxGen conducted a print media campaign entitled "Let's talk about sex," which displayed a toll-free telephone number that referred callers to their nearest US vaccine trial sites. Perceptions of the recruitment process, as reported later by MSM participants in interviews conducted at the six CDC-funded VISION sites, suggest that materials using sexual imagery were effective at reaching the MSM population, but that such images may reinforce negative stereotypes about MSM and contradict safer sex messages (Neidig et al., 2002). This qualitative study also concluded that future recruitment strategies should emphasize the opportunity for personal involvement in the fight against AIDS, a factor motivating over 90% of all participants in the VAX004 trial (Colfax et al., 2005), and that messages should reach out to a more diverse group of participants—which often requires targeted outreach and media strategies, as well as ongoing relationships with communities. A later recruitment campaign organized by VaxGen did focus on altruistic motives, and was widely perceived as more successful.

*Sites need a range of data management tools and long-term strategies to ensure that participants remain in trials for follow-up visits after injection visits are complete*

Retention rates (in excess of 85% over 3 years) were impressive in this large, three-year study of high-risk individuals. Factors that may have contributed to this success include the dedication of study volunteers and staff, streamlined study procedures that minimized participant burden, and provision of services to particularly high-risk individuals, such as referrals to drug treatment programs, child welfare and employment services (Gaitanis et al., 2003). All of these factors can and should be replicated in future trials.

It is possible that the administration of booster doses over a period of 30 months also boosted retention rates. But such a long immunization course is unlikely for future trials, and supplemental retention strategies may therefore be required after the immunization course is complete. In addition, with at least 10% of the volunteers relocating two or three times during the study, the wide geographic distribution of participating trial sites allowed these participants to transfer to a new site, preventing loss to follow-up (Francis et al., 2003). Future studies that attempt to improve recruitment efficiency through use of fewer sites enrolling larger numbers of participants will need to develop alternative strategies for retaining participants who move away from the study site. In one successful example, an NIH-funded study of whether intensive individualized risk-reduction counseling lowers HIV infection rates (the EXPLORE study), six sites enrolled 624–743 participants each. These sites had mechanisms for follow-up of relocating participants, such as long-distance collection of blood samples from volunteers, and they achieved retention rates above 80%

over 48 months. To achieve such impressive retention rates in this very complex and time-consuming behavioral intervention, sites needed to develop and share novel retention strategies and implement data management strategies to track study visit windows.

## Behavioral and social risk

*High-risk volunteers may be relatively resistant to risk reduction messages*

The VAX004 trial enrolled a very high-risk population: at baseline: 58% of the participating MSM had engaged in unprotected anal sex in the 6 months prior to enrollment, and 55% of the women in unprotected vaginal sex (Bartholow et al., 2005). During the trial, all participants received semi-annual risk reduction counseling. Overall HIV seroincidence in the men was 2.7/100 person-years in the MSM, somewhat higher than the seroincidence measured in an 18-month vaccine preparedness study prior to the VAX004 trial that used similar eligibility criteria (Seage et al., 2001).

Concerns have been raised about the potential for behavioral disinhibition among vaccine trial volunteers—that is, the risk of absolute or relative increases in risk behavior, fueled by the belief that trial participation confers some protection against HIV. These misperceptions can be more difficult to correct when frequent news releases tout the success of these experimental products in *in vitro* assays or preclinical studies, as occurred throughout the VAX004 trial. Sites attempted to prevent behavioral disinhibition through extensive informed consent procedures and ongoing risk reduction counseling, which repeatedly reminds participants that the vaccine's efficacy is unknown and that they might be receiving placebo rather than vaccine. Analysis of the VAX004 behavioral data showed that the prevalence of reported unprotected sexual practices decreased between enrollment and the 6-month visit, only to rise slowly thereafter and approach baseline risk levels at 36-months (Bartholow et al., 2005).

To further explore the possibility of behavioral disinhibition among VAX004 volunteers, the CDC funded six VAX004 sites to enroll a control group of study volunteers into the VISION study. These control volunteers met the same eligibility criteria and underwent the same study procedures as the VAX004 participants (informed consent, counseling, etc.), but without receiving injections of either vaccine or placebo. Preliminary data suggest that several risk behaviors (number of sex partners, unprotected anal sex) declined to a greater extent in this control group than in the VAX004 participants (Buchbinder et al., 2003). One of many possible explanations for this finding is that vaccine trial participants may be relatively less susceptible to risk reduction counseling messages over time. Novel behavioral strategies and more frequent reinforcement of key concepts reviewed during the informed consent process may be required to further reduce risk among trial volunteers and to prevent behavioral disinhibition.

*Although HIV-1 seroincidence remained stable throughout the VAX004 trial, future trials may see declining rates of infection if they enroll populations with less prior exposure to risk reduction messages*

While all vaccine trials must deliver state-of-the-art risk reduction counseling and referrals to all study participants, the effectiveness of these interventions—and, in turn, the change in infection rates over the course of a trial—can vary greatly, depending on several factors. This may become especially apparent in future efficacy trials conducted in resource-poor settings, where most populations have had far less exposure to risk reduction counseling compared with VAX004 participants. Future trial designs must take into account the potential impact of risk reduction counseling and community-wide access to antiretroviral therapy in projecting HIV seroincidence rates, and must power trials accordingly.

*Most social harms during trials arose from negative reactions by trial participants' families, friends or co-workers*

In addition to monitoring behavioral risk during this study, trial-related discrimination, or social harm, was assessed regularly. Participants enrolled in earlier phase I/II trials have reported negative reactions from friends and family, often fueled by a misperception that the vaccine itself can cause infection or that the volunteer may be at behavioral risk for acquiring HIV (Allen *et al.*, 2001). Few incidents from these earlier studies were related to problems with health/life insurance or employment arising from vaccine-induced seropositivity, although this concern was voiced by potential volunteers in vaccine preparedness studies. A preliminary analysis from the phase III trial revealed that negative social impacts were reported infrequently. The most commonly cited social harms were attributed to disturbances in personal relationships, while study-related employment and insurance issues were the least common (Fuchs *et al.*, 2004). More complete trial data are currently being analyzed to determine the prevalence of these and other social harms over the course of the study and to ascertain whether specific demographic or risk characteristics are predictive of reporting a social harm.

Study staff can often anticipate potential social harms arising from trial participation and counsel participants about whether and how to disclose their participation to social contacts. Staff may already be doing an excellent job of preventing social harms arising from positive HIV tests due to vaccine-induced antibodies (e.g., difficulties obtaining insurance) by counseling participants on this issue throughout the trial. Such monitoring should be implemented in future trials, since different populations may experience different types or severity of social harms.

## Communication of trial results

*Great caution should be exercised in releasing preliminary or exploratory results to the media*

Different media reports offered conflicting interpretations of the VAX004 trial results in the days and months following VaxGen's initial announcement of the study's findings (Pollack and Altman, 2003; Sternberg, 2003). Leading up to February 24, 2003, VaxGen, the study investigators, CDC and vaccine advocacy groups engaged one another in discussions exploring potential trial outcomes, including the possibility that the vaccine would be only partially efficacious (AIDS Vaccine Advocacy Coalition, 2002; Hu *et al.*, 2003). What could not be predicted was VaxGen's early reports of differential efficacy among specific racial groups. A flurry of commentaries about the significance of these results and how they were initially shared and interpreted inadvertently resulted in a backlash from some African-American groups, which claimed that a potentially efficacious vaccine was being withheld (Collins and Wakefield, 2003). This is particularly unfortunate, given final results of the analyses which found both no significant efficacy in any of the racial or ethnic subgroups, nor any biologic plausibility to explain differences in efficacy estimates between racial groups (Follman *et al.*, 2004). Community advocacy groups became involved in disseminating information about the trial. In particular, the AIDS Vaccine Advocacy Coalition created two publications that were quite helpful in explaining trial results to the layperson and clinician communities (AIDS Vaccine Advocacy Coalition, 2002; AIDS Vaccine Advocacy Coalition, 2003). Several vaccine groups attempted to deal with these concerns through community discussion forums, and NIH sponsored a series of meetings to discuss the preliminary trial results and receive input from various stakeholder groups on actions to be taken.

Efficacy trials of products from publicly held companies will inevitably involve restrictions on the mechanisms and timing of releasing results. However, sufficient investigator input into reviewing and interpreting study results should occur prior to any announcement, and community members should be consulted in planning how results are disseminated. Appropriate statistical adjustments should be made before release of data to the media, and caution exercised in discussing equivocal results.

Trial sponsors must also pay attention to the social and historical context in which vaccine trials are conducted and, ultimately, how the results are both reported and interpreted. Failure to do so may further erode the trust communities of color have in the clinical research enterprise, and may undermine our ability to recruit diverse populations for future studies. Comprehensive community education efforts must be an integral part of HIV vaccine research, and should target both key media outlets and broad community groups, giving them tools with which to interpret trial results and preparing them for the long road to the development of a safe, highly efficacious HIV vaccine.

## Conclusions

Future vaccine trials are likely to be more scientifically, operationally and ethically complex than the VAX004 trial, as they will evaluate vaccines designed to elicit cellular rather than humoral immunity, use a broader array of trial sites with less research experience and infrastructure, ensure access to treatment and care for infected trial participants in resource-poor settings and attempt to coordinate multiple vaccine and non-vaccine prevention trials. These trials will benefit from the many lessons in study design, implementation and communication provided by the world's first HIV vaccine efficacy trial.

## References

AIDS Vaccine Advocacy Coalition. (2002). Anticipating the news on AIDSVAX: Results from the world's first AIDS vaccine efficacy trial: What will they mean? (AIDS Vaccine Advocacy Coalition).

AIDS Vaccine Advocacy Coalition. (2003). Understanding the Results of the AIDSVAX Trial (AIDS Vaccine Advocacy Coalition).

Allen, M., Israel, H., Rybczyk, K., Pugliese, M.A., Loughran, K., Wagner, L., and Erb, S. (2001). Trial-related discrimination in HIV vaccine clinical trials. AIDS Res. Hum. Retroviruses *17*, 667–674.

Bartholow, B., Buchbiner, S., Celum, C., Goli, V., Koblin, B., Para, M., Marmor, M., Novak, R.M., Mayer, K., Creticos, C., Orozco-Cronin, P., Popovic, V., Mastro, T.D. (2005). HIV sexual risk behavior over 36 months of follow-up in the world's first HIV vaccine efficacy trial. J. Acquir. Immune Defic. Syndr. *39*, 90–101.

Berman, P.W. (2003). Preliminary results of the phase III efficacy trial of AIDSVAX B/B. Paper presented at: Keystone Symposia: HIV vaccine development: Immunological and biological challenges (Banff, Alberta, Canada).

Buchbinder, S., Wheeler, S., Vittinghoff, E., McKirnan, D., Celum, C., Mayer, K., Fuchs, J., Para, M., Novak, R., and Bartholow, B. (2003). Declines in risk behavior are smaller in phase III vaccine trial participants than in a non-vaccine trial control group. Paper presented at: AIDS Vaccine (2003) (New York, New York).

Colfax, G., Buchbinder, S., Vamshidar, G., Celum, C., McKirnan, D., Neidig, J., Koblin, B., Gurwith, M., and Bartholow, B. (2005). Motivations for Participating in an HIV Vaccine Efficacy Trial. J. Acquir. Immune Defic. Syndr. *39*, 359–364.

Collins, C., and Wakefield, S. (2003). Extra-science lessons from the AIDSVAX trial. Paper presented at: AIDS Vaccine (2003) (New York, NY).

Follman, D. (2004). An Independent Analysis of the Effect of Race in VAX004. Paper presented at: 11th Conference on Retroviruses and Oppputunistic Infections (San Francisco, San Francisco).

Francis, D.P., Heyward, W.L., Popovic, V., Orozco-Cronin, P., Orelind, K., Gee, C., Hirsch, A., Ippolito, T., Luck, A., Longhi, M., et al. (2003). Candidate HIV/AIDS vaccines: Lessons learned from the world's first phase III efficacy trials. AIDS *17*, 147–156.

Fuchs, J., Durham, M., McLellan-Lemal, E., Vittinghoff, E., Buchbinder, S., and Vax004 Study Team. (2004). Younger HIV vaccine trial participants report negative social impacts. [ThPeC(7444)]. Paper presented at: the XV International AIDS Conference (Bangkok, Thailand).

Gaitanis, M., Alvarez, S., Mayer, K., and Lally, M. (2003). Selective case management use among high-risk women in two studies: a retrospective analysis [498]. Paper presented at: AIDS Vaccine (2003) (New York, NY).

Gilbert, P.B., Ackers, M.L., Berman, P.W., Francis, D.P., Popovic, V., Hu, D.J., Heyward, W.L., Sinangil, F., Shepherd, B.E., and Gurwith, M. (2005a). HIV-1 virologic and immunologic progression and initiation of antiretroviral therapy among HIV-1-infected subjects in a trial of the efficacy of recombinant glycoprotein 120 vaccine. J. Infect. Dis. *192*, 974–983.

Gilbert, P.B., Peterson, M.L., Follmann, D., Hudgens, M.G., Francis, D.P., Gurwith, M., Heyward, W.L., Jobes, D.V., Popovic, V., Self, S.G., et al. (2005b). Correlation between immunologic responses to a recombinant glycoprotein 120 vaccine and incidence of HIV-1 infection in a phase 3 HIV-1 preventive vaccine trial. J. Infect. Dis. *191*, 666–677.

Gilbert, P.B., Popovic, V., Gurwith, M., Heyward, W.L., Francis, D., Sinangil, F., Peterson, M., and Berman, P.W. (2003). Immunologic responses to rgp-120 vaccine and correlation with the risk of HIV infection—Results from the world's first HIV vaccine efficacy trial. Paper presented at: AIDS Vaccine (2003) (New York, NY).

Graham, B.S., and Mascola, J.R. (2005). Lessons from failure—preparing for future HIV-1 vaccine efficacy trials. J. Infect. Dis. *191*, 647–649.

Hu, D.J., Vitek, C.R., Bartholow, B., and Mastro, T.D. (2003). Key issues for a potential human immunodeficiency virus vaccine. Clin. Infect. Dis. *36*, 638–644.

McLellan, E., Ackers, M., Goli, V., Barthelow, B., and Team, V.S. (2003). HIV Vaccine Efficacy Trials: Women at Heterosexual Risk. Paper presented at: AIDS Vaccine (2003) (New York, N.Y.).

Neidig, J., McLellan, E., Pickard, R., Dyslin, K., and VaxGen Study Team. (2002). Best Recruitment Approaches: The Perceptions of Men Enrolled in the First HIV Vaccine Efficacy Trial. Paper presented at: Society for Applied Anthropology Annual Meeting (Atlanta, GA).

Pollack, A., and Altman, L.K. (2003). Large Trial Finds AIDS Vaccine Fails to Stop Infection. In The New York Times (New York), p. 1.

Popovic, V., Gurwith, M., Heyward, W.L., Gilbert, P.B., Berman, P.W., and Francis, D. (2003). Evaluation of vaccine efficacy in populations with high-risk behavior and high HIV incidence—Results from the world's first phase III trial of an HIV vaccine. Paper presented at: AIDS Vaccine (2003) (New York, NY).

Seage, G.R., 3rd, Holte, S.E., Metzger, D., Koblin, B.A., Gross, M., Celum, C., Marmor, M., Woody, G., Mayer, K.H., Stevens, C., et al. (2001). Are US populations appropriate for trials of human immunodeficiency virus vaccine? The HIVNET Vaccine Preparedness Study. Am. J. Epidemiol. *153*, 619–627.

Sternberg, S. (2003). Vaccine for AIDS appears to work; Blacks, Asians receive protection. In USA Today, pp. 1.

The rgp120 HIV Vaccine Study Group (2005). Placebo-controlled phase 3 trial of recombinant glycoprotein 120 vaccine to prevent HIV-1 infection. J.Infect. Dis. *191*.

# The Thai VaxGen Trial: What Have We Learned?     15

Chris Beyrer

## Abstract

One year after VaxGen launched its phase III vaccine trial in 5,000 North Americans and Europeans at risk for sexual transmission of HIV (Chapter 14), a second trial began in 2,500 intravenous drug users in Thailand. In November 2003, analysis of final results from the Thai trial showed clearly that the gp120-based AIDSVAX vaccine had no efficacy in this population, in agreement with results from the first phase III study. Despite these disappointing findings, the trial yielded invaluable information about conducting large-scale studies in IDU populations—something many researchers thought could not be done—and offers compelling insights into the conduct of future efficacy trials in developing countries.

## Introduction

Success in clinical trials can be defined as the extent to which the results of a study give clear answers to the fundamental questions the trial was designed to address. To succeed, a trial must recruit and enroll participants at a reasonable pace, retain them long enough to maintain the study's statistical power, and generate enough critical endpoints so that trial outcomes are clear. By these measures, the now completed phase III HIV vaccine trial of the AIDSVAX B/E gp120 candidate in Thailand was a success, despite the failure of the product to have any impact on HIV infection risk.

For efficacy trials of prevention technologies, including HIV vaccines, these components of success each raise difficult scientific, operational, and human challenges (Excler and Beyrer, 2000). Such trials are enormous collective undertakings, and all of us who care about the AIDS pandemic are in debt to those individuals, organizations, and communities who undertake them. Since development of a safe and effective AIDS vaccine will most likely require many more phase III trials in the future, it is imperative that the field absorbs the lessons of these first efficacy trials.

Landmark clinical trials have had enormous impacts on HIV/AIDS. Recall the world before ACTG 076, the trial which demonstrated that AZT can reduce the rate of mother-to-child transmission of HIV. Prior to that study, health care providers had precious little to offer anxious expectant mothers living with the virus. Less than a decade later, vertical transmission rates in developed countries are well below 3% of infected mothers, and pediatric AIDS has become uncommon. I would argue that the Thailand VaxGen efficacy trial is a landmark study, despite the final outcome. The trial has already answered some of the most persistent questions in HIV research in developing countries, most notably the feasibility of injecting drug users as trial participants. And it is rich in lessons for a field in urgent need of "real world" findings to further refine its science.

The Thailand trial of AIDSVAX® B/E is the first HIV vaccine efficacy trial conducted in a developing country. It is also the first one to focus exclusively on a study population of injection drug users (IDU) (Greenberg, et al., 2005). The primary question was simple: whether or not the vaccine protects against primary HIV infection in uninfected, at-risk Thai IDU. The vaccine was also relatively simple: Bivalent protein subunits of two different recombinant gp120 antigens, one from subtype B (the laboratory-grown MN strain) and the other from subtype E (the A 244 primary isolate), grown in CHO (Chinese hamster ovary) cells and formulated with alum, a common vaccine adjuvant. These particular strains were chosen because B and E represent the most common circulating subtypes in Thailand.

Almost nothing else about the trial was simple. The study screened over 4,900 IDU and enrolled 2,545 seronegative IDU at 17 clinical trial sites in the greater Bangkok metropolitan area (Vanichseni, et al., 2004). Enrollment began early in 1999 (roughly a year after the U.S. AIDSVAX B/B trail opened) and was completed in August 2000. Seroincidence during the trial was 3.1% annually in both the placebo and vaccine arms, which was slightly lower than expected: the study design assumed a 4% annualized seroincidence. Despite declines in many risk behaviors over time (Thailand MOPH-US CDC Collaboration, 2003; Greenberg, et al., 2005), there were, unfortunately for participants, substantial numbers of infections during the trial: 106 volunteers became infected in the vaccine group, and 105 in the placebo arm. The retention rate was outstanding, with less than 3% of the volunteers lost at the sixth immunization (Thailand MOPH-US CDC Collaboration, 2003), and over 90% completing the full 3 years of the study.

## Lessons learned: the lead-in to efficacy trials

It is certainly no coincidence that the first phase III HIV vaccine trial to be conducted in a developing country was done in Thailand. In 1993, the Kingdom became the first country worldwide to include a plan for HIV vaccine research in its national plan to combat AIDS (Excler and Beyrer, 2000). The Thai HIV/AIDS epidemic began relatively late compared to the US or Africa, with the first extensive spread documented only in mid-1988. Yet a social mobilization against AIDS was under way by 1990, and an unprecedented national level prevention program, the now justly famous "100% Condom Campaign," was implemented in 1992 (Ainsworth et al., 2000). HIV infection rates among young adults peaked in 1993 and have been declining for roughly a decade—surely one of the most impressive "turn-around" in the global history of AIDS (Ainsworth et al., 2000).

A striking feature of this response was Thailand's openness to research and to international collaboration. In the HIV vaccine research arena alone, Thai institutions partnered with WHO, UNAIDS, the US CDC and NIH, the Walter Reed Army Institute for Research (WRAIR) and the Armed Forces Research Institute for Medical Sciences (AFRIMS) (collaborations supported by Japan, Australia, the Netherlands) and with the vaccine manufacturers VaxGen, Merck, Chiron, UBI and Aventis Pasteur. Partnerships between U.S. universities and Thai research groups also featured prominently in the Thai vaccine research landscape, and included Johns Hopkins, Harvard, UCLA and many others. The VaxGen trial itself was implemented through an infrastructure and with a cohort developed jointly with the US CDC, the Thai Ministry of Public Health, the Bangkok Metropolitan Authority and Mahidol University, based on several years of collaborative epidemiology and behavioral research (Pitisuttithum, 2005). Prior to the actual trial, studies launched in 1995 with a large "pre-trial" IDU cohort (1,209 participants) helped establish the knowledge base for the trial (Kitayaporn et al., 1998).

This is perhaps the key first lesson learned from the VaxGen trial: Thai scientists and the national government were deeply committed to HIV/AIDS and open to lasting international collaborations. The political will and scientific savvy of the Thais created a highly conducive "enabling environment" that made HIV vaccine research possible (Pitisuttithum, 2005). It need hardly be said, but perhaps must be, that political and collaborative barriers in a range of Asian, African, and Latin American states with serious HIV epidemics have hindered the kind of long-term commitment necessary to implement phase III trials. Should we be surprised that the *next* HIV vaccine efficacy trial to be conducted in a developing country is also taking place in Thailand? This trial, conducted by the Thai Ministry of Public Health and US Military HIV Research Program, is testing the canarypox-based vaccine vCP1521) with an AIDSVAX® gp120 B/E boost and remains under way (Karnasuta et al., 2005).

The enormous genetic diversity of HIV; and its rapid rate of genotypic and phenotypic change, is a major challenge to both treatment and prevention (Chapter 10). For this reason,

a second lesson concerns the continuously changing molecular epidemiology of HIV-1 among Thai drug users and its impact on trial planning. In the early years of the Thai epidemic there was a marked segregation of HIV-1 subtypes and risk groups: IDU were infected predominately with a subtype B virus showing only minor differences to strains found in the Americas and Western Europe (Limpakarnjanarat et al., 1998). In contrast, heterosexual transmission involved mostly subtype E (later reclassified as a recombinant form of two older African parental strains derived from subtypes A and E, and therefore renamed Circulating Recombinant Form 01, or CRF01_A/E. However, "E," although clearly a misnomer, is still commonly used and will be used here for simplicity). This segregation initially led VaxGen investigators to conclude that an IDU trial in Thailand could be done in subtype-"matched" fashion with the same candidate they were planning to test in US gay and bisexual men.

But by 1997, as trial preparations got under way and the large pre-trial cohort of IDU was being enrolled across Bangkok, the molecular picture had shifted dramatically (Limpakarnjanarat et al., 1998; Nguyen et al., 2002). The CDC-Thai team leading the molecular effort found that among newly infected IDU, subtype B had been largely replaced: instead, nearly all new infections were with the E subtype (Nguyen et al., 2002). Segregation by route of transmission had clearly ended, and indeed, subtype E had come to predominate across all risk groups and regions of Thailand. In response VaxGen produced an E subtype antigen, to maintain a closer match between circulating virus and the candidate vaccine, and the trial was launched with a bivalent candidate containing gp120 antigens from both B and E.

The key lesson here is that even well-established, well-characterized HIV epidemics can change quickly, and that HIV genetic variation must therefore be evaluated in real time during the lead-in to trials—regardless of whether the vaccine approach involves matching to circulating subtypes. There is also very real possibility that widespread use of a partially effective vaccine (which might differentially protect against one variant over another) could shift the molecular picture of HIV in populations where trials are taking place, an effect which could really only be recognized if the range of circulating strains is evaluated prior to trial launch. The uncertainty as to whether HIV-1 subtypes and circulating recombinants will turn out to have functional significance for vaccines lends more urgency to the argument that molecular surveillance should be done before, during, and after HIV vaccine trials. If HIV genetic variation can lead to immune evasion, which in turn might impact vaccine failure or success, we certainly need to know what this variation is—and such data will only come from thoroughly analyzed phase III trials, including detailed information on the molecular epidemiology of HIV among infected trial participants and their wider networks.

The Thai VaxGen trial was implemented within just this kind of scientific setting—with the US CDC and its Thai partners providing an extraordinarily detailed scientific base of molecular epidemiology, and several years of intensive research across an array of disciplines (Greenberg, *et al.*, 2005). This approach may well be too demanding and expensive a model to replicate for every phase III HIV vaccine trial and therefore future trials may implement only parts of such thorough research plans. Nevertheless, the shift in the Thai epidemic during product design is a lesson no developer can afford to ignore.

## Lessons learned from the volunteers

"Addictophobia" is a name that can be given to irrational fear of drug users. It is a surprisingly common disorder, one that can affect governments, regulatory agencies, researchers and clinicians. A common symptom is the belief that drug users make poor patients and worse research participants. In the HIV/AIDS world, addictophobia often manifests itself in the thinking that drug users are isolated from their communities, or that an HIV epidemic in IDU in a given country or region will have little impact on the general population and can therefore be ignored.

Africa aside, there are significant IDU components in virtually all HIV epidemics worldwide, including those in North and South America, Western, Central and Eastern Europe (Crofts *et al.*, 1998). Moving east across Eurasia to Russia, Ukraine, Belarus, Central Asia, Iran, China, and Southeast Asia, the majority of reported and/or estimated cases in most Asian states are in IDU (Aceijas *et al.*, 2004). But there are exceptions: for example, Cambodia and Papua New Guinea have serious HIV epidemics with little or no IDU component, and Thailand and Burma have both had widespread epidemics where IDU were significant but minor risk groups (Aceijas, *et al.*, 2004). If it is indeed true that IDU epidemics will be ignored, or that the vaccine field will wait until there is an effective vaccine against sexual transmission before worrying about efficacy against blood-borne transmission, then the world may be watching one of the great natural experiments in HIV infection take place. Although the enormous populations of Asia are predominately exposed to HIV spread through IDU networks, Hong Kong is the only place across the entire region that provides comprehensive HIV prevention programs for drug users (Beyrer, b, 2003).

The Thai trial did not, of course, target IDUs out of any ideological position. The investigators simply went where there was political will and the infrastructure to do trials, infection rates were high in a well-characterized and established cohort, and where they could answer their primary question with the greatest expediency. Overall, the Thai trial was about half the size of the US trial, because IDU seroincidence rates in the Thai lead in cohort were higher, at 5–6% per year, and sustained (Vanichseni *et al.*, 2001). Thailand's second efficacy trial, launched in late 2003, targets reproductive age adult men and women at presumed sexual risk for HIV infection and has 16,000 participants and 4 years of follow up after immunization.

The strong participation of IDU in the Thai trial, and their impressive rates of retention, should help reduce addic-

tophobia, at least in the HIV vaccine research arena. It is an outcome devoutly to be wished. The extent to which IDU trials in other settings will be as feasible as the Bangkok trial is an open question. Nevertheless, the trial sets a useful benchmark for further work with these populations.

## Drug treatment, harm reduction, and ethical considerations

A challenge for all HIV prevention research with endpoints of infection and/or post-infection clinical measures (such as initial viral load or CD4 cell decline) is that researchers are obligated to provide high-quality risk-reduction counseling, HIV prevention measures such as condom promotion and distribution, and frequent HIV testing and counseling. These efforts have generally meant that infection rates in HIV study cohorts decrease over time (especially in studies involving volunteers for whom risk reduction counseling and messages are new; see chapter by Buchbinder and Fuchs), and may eventually reach such low levels that efficacy trials are no longer feasible (Excler and Beyrer, 2000). It is widely accepted internationally that the balance between working with at-risk populations and conducting a successful trial with sufficient incidence must favor maximum protection of individual research participants over the interests of the trial. Tragically for many high-risk individuals, but importantly for researchers, many men and women at risk for HIV have been unwilling or unable to significantly reduce their HIV infection risks, despite the best available counseling and preventive services.

In the VaxGen trial among US, Canadian, and Dutch gay and bisexual men, HIV infection rates remained substantial throughout the course of the trial, with over 5% of all trial participants becoming HIV infected despite continuous risk-reduction counseling (Francis *et al.*, 2003). This meant enough infections for a clear trial outcome, at least in terms of the overall study cohort: infection rates were nearly identical in the vaccine and placebo arms, and there was ample statistical power to show that the vaccine had no impact on preventing HIV infection. The claim of differences in subsets of the trial participants was, in contrast, sharply underpowered to be substantiated.

In both trials, risk reduction counseling was provided to study participants, along with condom promotion and distribution and frequent HIV testing. From the perspective of reducing sexual risks among these participants, the studies appear to have reached a high standard (Choopanya *et al.*, 2003). But the Thai cohort was not a population selected for sexual risks, and the cohort study which preceded the vaccine trial found that injection drug use, needle sharing and incarceration, rather than sexual risks, were most closely associated with HIV seroconversion (Vanichseni *et al.*, 2001).

Based on these findings, a state-of-the-art, evidence-based preventive program for IDUs would target safer injection practices, needle and syringe exchange, and drug treatment at a reasonable international standard, including methadone maintenance therapy in addition to acute detoxification. Consistent with this notion, a large and growing body of literature from Australia, Europe, the US and Hong Kong suggests that HIV spread among IDUs can be dramatically reduced through widespread implementation of comprehensive prevention programs for drug users.

But many of these proven prevention tools were unavailable to the VaxGen researchers and trial participants, due to legal restrictions. For example, Thai policy limits the use of methadone to a 45-day short-course "tapering-off" protocol, which has been repeatedly shown to be ineffective as long-term substitution therapy (Vanichseni et al., 1991). It is also important to remember that trial participants were recruited through public drug treatment centers where methadone taper protocols were in use, and that a return to drug use was common about halfway through the 45 days. Furthermore, needle and syringe exchange (NEP) programs are prohibited by Thai law and policy, although injection equipment can be purchased easily in pharmacies.

Taken together, these limitations meant that the VaxGen investigators had the best available tools to help participants avoid sexual exposure to HIV, but significantly less for reducing parenteral exposure. Nevertheless, HIV risks for *both* sexual and injecting risks did not increase among trial participants who remained under study (van Griensvan et al., 2004), and indeed, IDU use decreased from 93.8% at baseline to 66.5% at 12 months ($P < 0.001$) and needle sharing declined from 33.0% to 17.5% over the same period ($P < 0.001$). Still, these issues remain highly relevant for future trials in IDU populations in other countries, where provision of state-of-the-art prevention services may be drastically restricted by law. For example, Russia is actively engaged in preparing for HIV vaccine trials, and the country has a predominant IDU epidemic. Yet *all* methadone treatment, even taper programs, are illegal in Russia, Malaysia, and across Central Asia (Archibald et al., 2003). Even in the US, federal law bans funding for needle and syringe exchange, which would make it difficult, if not impossible, to incorporate needle/syringe exchanges in a federally funded vaccine trial. The federal ban on needle exchange has continued under the President's Emergency Plan for AIDS Relief (PEPFAR) and in the one PEPFAR target country with a predominant IDU epidemic in 2006, Vietnam.

## Incarceration and HIV risk

A last, crucial lesson from the Thai IDU trial is perhaps the most difficult and contentious one, and is also related to the criminalization of drug users. Possession of illicit drugs is a crime virtually everywhere on earth—and heroin, the drug of choice for injectors across Asia, is an illicit drug throughout the region. Hence IDU in most countries are at extremely high risk for arrest, detention, and incarceration.

While the VaxGen team did not recruit volunteers from Thai prisons, their earlier cohort work had shown unequivocally that arrest of already-enrolled IDU volunteers was common, and that being jailed was a major cause of loss to follow-up (Vanichseni et al., 2001)—and therefore, that that the

ability to follow participants who had been arrested or were in detention was critical to the success of any HIV vaccine trial in Thai IDU. After wide consultation and extensive work with police, prison authorities and local government, the team developed a protocol that allowed for study visits, immunizations, and blood draws among participants who agreed to ongoing follow-up while incarcerated.

As predicted, this emerged as a key element for the study's high retention rate, since incarceration rates during the study were extremely high (roughly 20 per 100 person-years of follow-up in the pre-trial cohort; Choopanya et al., 2002). Had the arrested participants been lost to follow-up, the trial would have collapsed; instead, the high arrest and incarceration rate did not have an adverse impact on the trial (Thailand MOPH-US CDC Collaboration, 2003). Furthermore, having regular visits from study nurses and staff while in detention was highly valued by participants, and seen by them as an important protection and communication channel. Our group used a similar practice for following IDU volunteers in a Chiang Mai cohort, and those who had been arrested overwhelmingly welcomed jail visits from trial staff (Beyrer et al., 2003). Whether and how such visits would work, in other settings such as China or Russia is unknown.

The problem of limited HIV prevention services for IDU in Thailand is, however, even more extreme in the prison system (Beyrer et al., 2003). Condom distribution is not allowed in Thai prisons, where situational homosexual sex and rape are common. Needle and syringe access is also extremely limited. But access to illicit drugs is not, and the prisons are notorious for widespread availability and use of drugs (Beyrer et al., 2003). This is a potent combination that makes time spent in Thai prisons extremely high risk for acquisition of HIV, and most likely accounted for the much of the trial's high seroincidence rate. The Thai-US CDC group has published an analysis of HIV seroincidence in and out of incarceration among Bangkok IDU, with striking results (Choopanya et al., 2002). HIV infection rates outside of prison were modest, but soared to 35 per 100 person-years during incarceration, an astonishingly high rate (Choopanya et al., 2002). And, of course, preventive education is of little benefit if drug users cannot access condoms, clean injection equipment or methadone treatment, but can easily get heroin.

## Conclusions

We have learned a great deal from the Thai VaxGen trial. The results demonstrate that phase III trials in developing country IDUs are feasible, efficient, and can be conducted ethically. The trial grew out of longstanding collaborative relationships and significant investments in feasibility studies, molecular epidemiology, and behavioral research. Risk reduction counseling was effective in reducing seroincidence, but 3.1% per year remains an unacceptably high rate of infection and underscores the urgent need for a vaccine in this highly vulnerable population.

## References

Aceijas, C., Stimson, G.V., Hickman, M., Rhodes, T. and the United Nations Reference Group on HIV/AIDS Prevention and Care among IDU in Developing and Transitional Countries. (2004). Global overview of injecting drug use and HIV infection among injecting drug users. AIDS *18*, 2295–303.

Ainsworth, M., Beyrer, C., and Soucat, A. (2000). Thailand's Response to AIDS, Building on Success, Confronting the Future. Thailand Social Monitor V, The World Bank Thailand Office, Bangkok.

Archibald, C., Bastos, F., Beyrer, C., Crofts, N., Des Jarlais, D., Grund, J.P., Hacker, M., Heimer, R., and Saidel, T. (2003). The nature and extent of HIV/AIDS among injecting drug users. In Evidence For Action, Establishing the Evidence-Base for Effective HIV Prevention among Injecting Drug Users. World Health Organization, Geneva.

Beyrer, C., Juttiwutikarn, J., Teokul, W., Razak, M.H., Suriyanon, V., Srirak, N., Pripaipan, T., Vonchuk, T., *et al.* (2003). Drug use, increasing incarceration rates, and prison associated HIV risks in Thailand. AIDS & Behavior 2, 153–161.

Beyrer C. Human Immunodeficiency Virus infection rates and heroin trafficking, Fearful symmetries. (2003) Bulletin on Narcotics, The science of drug use epidemiology 2, 400–417.

Choopanya, K., Des Jarlais, D.C., Vanichseni, S., Kitayaporn, D., Mock, P.A., Raktham, S., Hireanras, K., Heyward, W.L., Sujarita, S., and Mastro, T.D. (2002). Incarceration and risk for HIV infection among injection drug users in Bangkok. J. Acquir. Immune Defic. Syndr. 29, 86–94.

Choopanya, K., Des Jarlais, D.C., Vanichseni, S., Mock, P.A., Kitayaporn, D., Sangkhum, U., Prasithiphol, B., Hiranrus, K., *et al.* (2003). HIV risk reduction in a cohort of injecting drug users in Bangkok, Thailand. J. Acquir. Immune Defic. Syndr. 33, 88–95.

Crofts, N., Reid, G., and Deany, P. (1998). Injecting drug use and HIV infection in Asia. The Asian Harm Reduction Network. AIDS 12, Suppl. B, S69–78.

Excler, J.L. and Beyrer, C. (2000). HIV vaccine development in developing countries, Are efficacy trials feasible? J. Hum. Virol. 3, 193–214.

Francis, D.P., Heyward, W.L., Popovic, V., Orozco-Cronin, P., Orelind, K., Gee, C., Hirsch, A.., Ippolito, T., Luck, A., *et al.* (2003). Candidate HIV/AIDS vaccines, lessons learned from the World's first phase III efficacy trials. AIDS 17, 147–156.

Greenberg, A.E., Tappero, J., Choopanya, K., van Griensven, F., Martin, M., Vanichsenbi, S., Santibanez, S., Molotilov, V., Hader, S., and Broyles, L.N. (2005). CDC International HIV prevention research activities among injection drug users in Thailand and Russia. J. Urban Health 82 (3 Suppl. 4), iv24–33.

Karnasuta, C., Paris, R.M., Cox, J.H., Nitayaphan, S., Pitisuttithum, P., Thongcharoen, P., Brown, A.E., Gurunathan, S., Tartaglia, J., Heyward, W.L., McNeil, J.G., Birx, D.L., de Souza, M.S.; Thai AIDS Vaccine Evaluation Group, Thailand. (2005). Antibody-dependent cell-mediated cytotoxic responses in participants enrolled in a phase I/II ALVAC-HIV/AIDSVAX B/E prime-boost HIV-1 vaccine trial in Thailand. Vaccine 23, 2522–2529.

Kitayaporn, D., Vanichseni, S., Mastro, T.D., Raktham, S., Vaniyapongs, T., Des Jarlais, D.C., Wasi, C., Young, N.L., Sujarita, S., *et al.* (1998). Infection with HIV-1 subtypes B and E in injecting drug users screened for enrollment into a prospective cohort in Bangkok, Thailand. J. Acquir. Immune Defic. Syndr. *19*, 289–295.

Limpakarnjanarat, K., Ungchusak, K., Mastro, T.D., Young, N.L., Likhityingvara, C., Sangwonloy, O., *et al.* (1998). The epidemiological evolution of HIV-1 subtypes B and E among heterosexuals and injecting drug users in Thailand, 1992–1997. AIDS 12, 1108–1109.

Nguyen, L., Hu, D.J., Choopanya, K., Vanichseni, S., Kitayaporn, D., van Griensven, F., Mock, P.A., Kittikraisak, W., *et al.* (2002). Genetic analysis of incident HIV-1 strains among injection drug users in Bangkok, evidence for multiple transmission clusters during a period of high incidence. J. AIDS. 30, 248–256.

Pitisuttithum, P. (2005). HIV-1 prophylactic vaccine trials in Thailand. Curr. HIV Res. *3(1)*, 17–30.

Thailand MOPH-US CDC Collaboration. (2003). Annual Report for (2002). Thailand MOPH-US CDC Collaboration.

van Griensvan, F., Keawkungwal, J., Tappero, J.W., Sangkum, U., Pitisuttithum, P., Vanichseni, S., Suntharasamai, P., Orelind, K., Gee, C., Choopanya, K.; Bangkok Vaccine Evaluation Group. (2004). Lack of increased HIV risk behavior among injection drug users participating in the AIDSVAX B/E HIV vaccine trial in Bangkok, Thailand. AIDS 18, 295–301.

Vanichseni, S., Wondsuwan, B., Choopanya, K., and Wongpanich, K. (1991). A controlled trial of methadone maintenance in a population of IDU in Bangkok, implications for prevention of HIV. Int. J. Addict. 26, 1313–1320.

Vanichseni, S., Kitayaporn, D., Mastro, T.D., Mock, P.A., Raktham, S., Des Jarlais, D.C., Sujarita, S., Srisuwanvilai, L.O., Young, N.L., *et al.* (2001). Continued high HIV-1 incidence in a vaccine trial preparatory cohort of injection drug users in Bangkok, Thailand. AIDS 15, 397–405.

Vanichseni, S., Tappero, J.W., Pitisuttithum, P., Kitayaporn, D., Mastro, T.D., Vimutisunthorn, E., van Griensvan, F., Heyward, W.L., Francis, D.P., Choopanya, K.; Bangkok Vaccine Evaluation Group. (2004). Recruitment, screening and characteristics of injection drug users participating in the AIDSVAX B/E HIV vaccine trial, Bangkok, Thailand. AIDS 18, 311–316.

# Part V

# From Testing to Deployment

# Regulatory Issues for AIDS Vaccine Development

## 16

Jim Ackland

## Abstract

The development and licensure of a successful HIV vaccine involves meeting various regulatory requirements that were put in place to protect individuals from unsafe or ineffective pharmaceutical products. Regulatory agencies such as the US Food and Drug Administration (FDA), the European Medicines Evaluation Agency (EMEA) and the South African Medicines Control Council must approve vaccine products before they are tested in clinical trials or licensed for general use. Approval is based on a scientific assessment of risks and benefits, and involves a review of manufacturing, preclinical and clinical information. In this article I discuss possible ways to expedite regulatory approval at all stages of development and to involve regulatory agencies in the development process—important steps in reducing the time it will take until an effective HIV vaccine can become widely available.

## Introduction

Regulatory agencies and health departments around the world have a responsibility to protect the public from unreasonable risk and to promote the development of medicines that improve health. Thus they are involved in the approval of clinical trials, the assessment of new products prior to licensure, and post-licensure review of the products' performance and quality.

However, their level of involvement varies among countries, based on the availability of expertise and resources. In the US, the FDA encourages meetings with a vaccine's developers/sponsors at three specific points during the development process: before the first clinical trial and submission of the clinical trial application (Investigational New Drug (IND); after the phase II clinical trial; and before the marketing (licensure) application. In addition, a comprehensive summary of all relevant information on manufacturing, preclinical and clinical experience must be submitted before starting every clinical trial, and assessed by the FDA. In some countries the level of involvement by regulators is far less—limited, for example, to review of a free sale certificate, a Certificate of Pharmaceutical Product or an assurance that the product has been approved by a recognized foreign government agency.

## Typical issues during vaccine development

Traditionally, vaccines were developed and manufactured within large pharmaceutical companies; however, recent years have seen increasing involvement from non-traditional players. In the case of HIV vaccines, an unprecedented number of approaches are being pursued at universities, research institutions and start-up biotech companies, which usually have limited experience or expertise in product development and regulatory processes. Yet a well-thought-out regulatory strategy that meets the requirements of agencies from all countries involved with the vaccine's development is essential for preventing lengthy delays, which can arise if regulators determine that any data are inadequate, and therefore that certain studies must therefore be repeated.

Table 16.1 lists circumstances that could cause a vaccine development program to be stopped until additional work is completed. Both the length of the list and the varied scenarios it includes illustrate how crucial it is to get expert advice on regulatory requirements starting very early in the development process.

Alongside these types of problems, which can arise with any vaccine, AIDS vaccines raise some additional regulatory issues. One is that an AIDS vaccine may be developed in Europe or the US but intended for use elsewhere (most likely Africa, Asia or another less developed region). Although vaccines must always meet fundamental requirements for safety, their risk–benefit considerations—a key issue from the regulatory perspective—vary with a country's infection rate and other local factors. For example, vaccines against epidemic diseases are often used in the general population, a practice which could bring tremendous benefits for communities in slowing or stopping the AIDS epidemic. Yet some vaccinated individuals may have little or no risk of exposure to HIV and therefore would derive little personal benefit from immunization. This is why the risk profile of candidate HIV vaccines must be carefully evaluated from both the individual and the public health perspectives. Large regional differences in infection rates and in the particular HIV subtypes which predominate locally suggest that vaccines developed and manufactured in the U.S. or

**Table 16.1** Examples of potential regulatory problems

| | |
|---|---|
| Manufacture | Exposure of the cell line or product components to adventitious agents such as transmissible encephalitis (TSE) or other viruses |
| | Inadequate documentation relating to cell line, virus seed history or vector construction |
| | Residual high levels of toxic raw materials |
| | Poor-quality chemical raw materials with inadequate specifications |
| | Animal-derived raw materials without adequate certification regarding TSE |
| | Stoppers made from unacceptable rubber formulation, or inadequately prepared vials and stoppers |
| | Processes, equipment, services or facilities that have not been validated |
| | Unacceptable chromatography resins or filters which leach out toxic chemicals |
| | Inadequate separation of products or processes within manufacturing facility, leading to unacceptable risk of contaminating the vaccine |
| | Unstable intermediate or final product, requiring that product is reformulated |
| | Assays that are not proven to demonstrate product stability, not validated and/or unreliable |
| | Inadequate product or process characterization |
| | High levels of process contaminants, such as endotoxin |
| | Poor manufacturing consistency |
| | Inadequately defined manufacturing process or analytical procedures |
| | Lack of compliance with GMP |
| Preclinical | Poorly designed or controlled toxicology studies, leading to results which cannot be interpreted without additional studies, do not meet regulatory requirements and/or do not support the proposed clinical studies |
| | Inadequate documentation of preclinical studies, with inadequate quality oversight and failure to meet GLP requirements |
| Clinical | Poorly designed clinical studies which have inadequate control groups or produce data that cannot be interpreted |
| | Studies which lack sufficient statistical power |
| | Inappropriate endpoints |
| | Inadequate identification and investigation of adverse events |
| | Lack of compliance with GCP |
| | Inadequate blinding, leading to bias in data analysis or interpretation |
| | Poor product accountability |
| | Poor documentation, which decreases regulators' confidence in the results |

Europe may not be approved for use in their home country. Another complicating factor for regulators is the many different types of HIV vaccines being developed, and which are often combined with one another—resulting in complicated dosing regimens and even non-traditional delivery devices.

Addressing these issues in a timely way for each vaccine entering clinical development presents challenges for both vaccine developers and regulatory agencies, as described below.

## Working with regulatory agencies on HIV vaccine development

Today the development of new vaccines is a complex and lengthy process involving many stages, which are described in other chapters of this volume. Each stage may take significant time and resources to complete, although some can be done in parallel. Depending on the data obtained at each stage, it may be necessary to repeat certain steps to improve a vaccine's performance. This results in multiple (iterative) cycles of development, requiring more time and funds.

Regulatory approval of a product for both clinical trials and licensure involves scientific review of the available data on preclinical studies, manufacture and clinical evidence of safety and efficacy, followed by a decision based on this evidence in the context of a risk/benefit assessment. Thus there are many opportunities for developers to involve regulatory agencies in

discussing the requirements for a new vaccine. Such interactions are important in the development process: they allow regulatory agency staff to become familiar with the product, which can lead to faster regulatory decisions later on, and they can help the developers of novel products by providing validation of and feedback on the development strategy.

Interaction with regulatory agencies generally takes the form of developers providing scientific information and justification of their strategy to the regulators, who then provide guidance or make an informed decision. For meetings of developers and regulators to have a productive outcome, it is essential that developers show a sound scientific approach and a good understanding of the regulatory guidelines. They should also appreciate that staff at regulatory agencies deal with many different types of products and cannot be experts on all types of novel products. Organizations with insufficient regulatory expertise may hire an experienced outside consultant to advise them on regulatory expectations and development strategy, and to assist in interactions with the regulators.

## Meetings with regulators

As mentioned above, the US FDA encourages meetings with sponsors of investigational products on three specific occasions during the development of a pharmaceutical product. These statutory meetings and the issues they generally cover are:

‣ Pre-IND meeting:
  – validation of initial clinical strategy and proposal;
  – feedback on adequacy of preclinical safety; and
  – comment on product manufacture and control.
‣ Post-phase II clinical study meeting:
  – discussion of phase I/II results; and
  – validation of design for planned efficacy studies.
‣ Pre-marketing application meeting:
  – review of clinical information and labeling;
  – any remaining manufacturing issues; and
  – format of applications.

The FDA may also grant additional meetings with developers to deal with specific issues. Its website provides specific guidelines on the conduct of these meetings (FDA, 2000). These guidelines provide details on how to request meetings with the agency and on the sponsors' and developer's expectations of the FDA.

The situation outside the U.S. is somewhat different, and is country specific. Within Europe, each member state has a regulatory agency that may meet with developers. Some countries, such as Sweden and the UK, have specific guidelines that spell out the procedures, while others have a less formal process. However, regulators in most countries usually welcome the opportunity to discuss new product development issues with developers.

In Europe the EMEA, reviews all marketing applications for biotechnology products and has a formal process for providing scientific opinion to developers of new products. Recently the EMEA has established a program for providing scientific advice on Emerging Therapies and Technologies. This program will provide informal opinion on new therapies in development.

However, the key principle for vaccine developers when they meet with regulators remains the same regardless of whether the country has a formal process or a more ad hoc one: The better prepared they are, and the better they prepare the information that forms the basis of discussion, the better the outcome (Tables 16.2 and 16.3).

## Common topics of discussion with regulatory agencies

### Manufacturing

HIV vaccines are likely to be complex biological products produced by biological processes, which makes them difficult to fully characterize—and presents challenges to both regulators and developers.

For this reason, vaccine developers typically seek advice early on potentially difficult manufacturing issues, such as the use of novel cell lines for producing viral vectors; the safety of specific HIV gene sequences or their protein products; characterization of the product; in-process controls; validation requirements for assays, equipment, processes and facilities; and final product specifications.

**Table 16.2** Basic principles for successful meetings with regulatory agencies

*Prepare well*

Know the product and the issues it raises

Review the relevant guidelines

Prepare a comprehensive but succinct information package

Carefully consider the questions that may be asked and

Rehearse and anticipate potential responses

*Conduct of the meeting*

Bring the right company personnel and technical experts

Be prepared to disclose information on the product and to ask the difficult questions

Use clear scientific evidence to defend positions and respond to questions and

Before the meeting ends, summarize any important agreements reached

*Meeting minutes*

Take your own notes

Share these notes with the regulatory agency and

*Respond to and resolve any discrepancies with the agency's minutes*

### Preclinical studies

Although vaccines are generally made from naturally occurring substances (e.g., proteins or nucleic acids), they are powerful immune stimulants and therefore might potentially cause unexpected reactions in some vaccinated people. To determine if a product may be harmful, preclinical toxicological studies are required. While clearly necessary, such studies are complex, expensive and difficult to perform, especially since they must be carried out under the stringent conditions of good laboratory practice (GLP).

Preclinical studies for new pharmaceutical chemical products traditionally involved involve a fairly standard set of assessments. Usually this means the use of two animal species (one rodent and one non-rodent) in single-dose acute and repeat-dose chronic dosing studies, along with genotoxicity, reproductive toxicity and long-term carcinogenicity studies. Exceptions have been made for vaccines that contain only very small quantities of naturally occurring products, in which case requirements may be limited to studying repeat dosing in one species and monitoring for local and systemic effects. Prior to granting marketing approval of vaccines that will be used in women of childbearing age; regulators may also require an assessment of reproductive toxicity. However, the various national agencies still have different requirements for preclinical vaccine safety, despite gradual harmonization of guidelines through the International Congress of Harmonization (ICH).

### Clinical trial designs

Early in clinical development, small phase I studies explore vaccine safety and immunogenicity, including the best dose

**Table 16.3** Expectations of regulatory agencies and of companies developing vaccines

| Stage of development | Developers' needs from regulatory agency | Regulatory agency expectations of developer |
|---|---|---|
| Research/pre-clinical development | Advice on design of preclinical studies. | Sound science, knowledge of regulatory guidelines |
| Clinical development phase 1 | Advice on phase I clinical trial design | Assure that subjects are not exposed to unnecessary risk—safety |
| Clinical development phase 2/3 | Advice on design of pivotal clinical trials | Assure that subjects are not exposed to unnecessary risk—safety |
| Approval to use/market | Rapid review of available data on quality, safety and efficacy | Evidence of acceptable risk/benefit and durable protection<br>Evidence of manufacturing consistency and control<br>Information about impact on other vaccine schedules |
| Post approval | Rapid approval of manufacturing changes | Ongoing consistency, with clinical evidence of safety and efficacy<br>Pharmacovigilance<br>Post-approval manufacturing changes<br>Ongoing assessment of GMP compliance |

and immunization schedule for inducing immune responses. Later-stage (phase II and III studies) expand these safety studies and also explore the vaccine's clinical utility, either in trials designed to give preliminary evidence of efficacy (proof of concept) or in larger studies that measure efficacy more precisely (Chapter 13).

One of the key difficulties at the later stages is how to best measure vaccine efficacy within a reasonable time period—in particular, how to choose appropriate endpoints for these trials, since the onset of disease (a typical vaccine trial endpoint) takes many years in the case of AIDS; some vaccines may not protect against infection, another typical endpoint; and there is no clear immune correlate of protection against HIV/AIDS. This situation is not unique: for example, the pertussis vaccines currently in widespread use are highly effective, although the immune responses they are known to elicit do not correlate with protection. The lack of an immune correlate complicates not only testing efficacy, but also the assessment of optimal vaccine dose and schedule. Depending on what populations the vaccine is intended for, additional clinical studies may also be needed to assess possible interactions with other routine vaccines.

## Regulatory guidelines

Regulatory agencies around the world publish technical guidelines to assist developers and manufacturers. These guidelines are generally not legally binding, and alternative approaches may be acceptable to regulators providing these alternatives are scientifically well-justified. Guidelines cover general aspects of development and manufacturing, including good manufacturing practices (GMPs), good laboratory practice (GLP) and good clinical practices (GCPs), as well as specific aspects of product development such as points specific for particular technologies (e.g., DNA vaccines), clinical evaluation of new vaccines, gene transfer medicinal products, and pharmacology/toxicology studies of vaccine candidates.

However, guidelines do not provide a rigid prescription for developing a product; rather, they are living documents that

spell out the agencies' expectations, and need to be interpreted/adapted for each particular product. These expectations tend to evolve as technologies and scientific understanding improves. Unfortunately, guidance documents do not always keep pace and may quickly become outdated, while new practices become unwritten requirements. It is therefore important for developers to have a good understanding not only of current written requirements, but also of unwritten ones.

Licensure is more complicated when it comes to registering a new product in different countries, which involves meeting both the technical and the submission requirements of each national regulatory agency. Fortunately there is a growing trend among regulatory agencies towards harmonization of these requirements—a step which would reduce the need to duplicate testing carried out during R&D, facilitate more economical use of human, animal and material resources and reducing unnecessary delays. This harmonization process is being managed by the International Conference on Harmonisations of Technical Requirements for Registration of Pharmaceuticals for Human Use (ICH). The group's "Technical Requirements for Registration of Pharmaceuticals for Human Use" is a unique project that brings together the regulatory authorities of Europe, Japan and the US with experts from the pharmaceutical industry in the three world regions. The ICH makes recommendations on ways to achieve greater harmonization in the interpretation and application of technical guidelines and in requirements for product registration. (http://www.ich.org/)

Guidelines can be accessed online through the following websites:

| US | http://www.fda.gov/cber/guidelines.htm |
|---|---|
| European | http://www.emea.eu.int/ |
| International | http://www.ich.org |

Yet despite tremendous progress in harmonization, there are still region-specific requirements, especially in relation to the clinical data.

## Regulatory strategy for licensing vaccines in developing countries

Traditionally the development of novel pharmaceutical products has been directed towards initial market entry in the US, Japan and major European countries—a strategy driven by the companies' need to recoup the huge costs associated with developing a single pharmaceutical product, estimated to average US$800 million (Center for the Study of Drug Development report, November 2001). In addition, many regulatory agencies in developing countries rely on approval by the FDA or other recognized regulatory agencies before they accept novel products (often because they lack the resources or expertise to review some or all of the data). These strategies, combined with the high prices of most new pharmaceutical products, usually result in very slow introduction of new products into developing countries. They would be particularly counter-productive once an effective HIV vaccine is developed, since the vaccine is most critically needed in those countries now generally excluded from the first wave of new product introduction. In other words, a new paradigm for rapid dissemination is needed for a new and effective vaccine to have the most impact.

For countries that rely on World Health Organization (WHO), EMEA or the FDA for assistance in the approval process, various new mechanisms are being considered. One is for the EMEA to review marketing applications and provide opinion on the merits of a pharmaceutical product (including HIV vaccines) even when it is intended for use outside the European Union. (Article 58 of Regulation (EC) No 726/2004 1) This opinion would be based on a review of the available information on the new vaccine, and could be made available to target countries either directly or through WHO. Another potential strategy is for developers to seek initial approval as a travel vaccine or a vaccine for use in high risk individuals in the US or Europe. This approval could then be used as the basis for approval in other countries. A third option would be to seek approval in a country which has some resources and regulatory competence, although it may not be recognized as widely as the US or Europe. Countries such as India, China, Australia, Canada, Brazil and South Africa have regulatory processes that may be suitable for use in particular regions. The location of manufacturing facilities may also influence the choice of countries for initial approval.

Approval of a new product requires that the following basic requirements are satisfied:

* evidence of an acceptable clinical risk–benefit in the target population;

* trials conducted to ICH GCP with appropriate ethical and regulatory approval;
* consistent manufacture under GMP; and
* regulatory approval to market or use in target countries.

There must also be ongoing regulatory oversight to monitor continued compliance with GMP and to assess any safety issues that may arise during large-scale use of the product.

## Risk–benefit considerations in the target populations

Clinical trials are conducted to determine both the benefits and risks of a product. All pharmaceutical products have potential risks associated with their use, and even the safest products have a capacity to cause an unwanted outcome. When a product effectively treats a serious disease, physicians, patients and regulatory agencies are usually willing to accept some degree of risk. For example, terminal cancer is often treated with highly toxic pharmaceutical products that commonly have very serious side effects.

In contrast, since vaccines are intended for healthy people, regulators require that the risk of a serious reaction to immunization is extremely low, and that data to support this conclusion are gathered throughout clinical development, including in large safety trials. A rough guide to determining the presence of a adverse event (AE) (see Table 16.4) is the rule of three: when there are zero adverse and undesirable events out of $n$ operations (vaccinations), a 95% upper confidence limit for the true probability that an adverse event will occur is $3/n$ (for $n > 30$) (Hanley and Lippman-Hand, 1983). On the other hand, if an event occurs at a rate of 1 in 100, the clinical database should include at least 300 individuals to give 95% confidence that the adverse event will be seen. If the event occurs at 1 in 1000 (0.1%), then 3,000 individuals are needed, while a rate of 1 in 10,000 requires 30,000 people.

Another factor influencing the decision on the necessary size of the safety database (i.e., number of individuals) is the anticipated benefit of the vaccines to the individual and to the population. For example, the benefit may be quite small to populations with a low incidence of disease, and of exposure to disease. To illustrate, in a population with a 0.1% incidence (i.e., only 1 person in 1000 would be infected yearly), only one out of every 1000 people vaccinated actually need protection, while the other 999 do not (although of course it is impossible to know in advance who will be exposed).

In considering risk versus benefit, it is also important to note that vaccines which are only partially effective at prevent-

**Table 16.4** Determining adverse events

| Indicator | Estimated rate of AE | | | |
| --- | --- | --- | --- | --- |
| | 0.001% | 0.01% | 0.1% | 0.1% |
| Size of clinical database to detect an AE (no. of individuals monitored) | 300,000 | 30,000 | 3,000 | 300 |
| No. of AEs per 1,000,000 people vaccinated | 10 | 100 | 1,000 | 10,000 |

**Table 16.5** Vaccine efficacy and its effect on reducing disease burden

| Indicator of vaccine effectiveness | Rate of infection | | |
|---|---|---|---|
| | 0.1% | 1% | 5% |
| Number of new HIV infections per 1 million people | 1,000 | 10,000 | 50,000 |
| Number of HIV infections prevented per 1 million people with a vaccine of 50% protective efficacy | 500 | 5,000 | 25,000 |

ing infections may still be highly effective at preventing or slowing an epidemic. For example, Table 16.5 shows that a vaccine which is only 50% effective will still prevent 500 new infections per 1,000,000 vaccinated people where the incidence is 0.1% (see also Chapter 19 by Anderson and Plotkin).

A vaccine's risk–benefit ratio depends on the underlying pathogen's rate of infection, the vaccine's protective efficacy and the rate of serious AEs associated with vaccine use. The cost of generating a large safety database can be prohibitively expensive. In addition, generating a large clinical safety database is time-consuming and may add years to the clinical development program. For HIV vaccines in a region with high incidence, rates, consideration should be given to introducing even a vaccine with a limited clinical safety database (for example 3,000) under a system of controlled release, with active monitoring for serious AEs as a mechanism to generate more safety data.

## Conclusions

Reducing the time until an effective HIV vaccine is widely available will bring tremendous benefits to whole populations and to millions of individuals. Having vaccine developers work closely with regulatory agencies should shorten timelines through the creative design of clinical trials and a shared understanding of a new vaccine's risk–benefit ratio. Approval of a novel vaccine for use in the countries in most need will require a paradigm shift in the regulatory approval process, for example by having different regulatory agencies work together to provide a rapid review and assessment of the new product.

## References

FDA. Guidance for Industry Formal Meetings with Sponsors and Applicants for PDUFA Products, February. (2000). http://www.fda.gov/cber/gdlns/mtpdufa.pdf.

Hanley, J.A., and Lippman-Hand, A. (1983). If nothing goes wrong, is everything alright? JAMA 259, 1743–1745.

November 30, 2001 Tufts Center for the Study of Drug Development Pegs Cost of a New Prescription Medicine at $802 Million. http://csdd.tufts.edu/NewsEvents/RecentNews.asp?newsid=6 Press release.

# Vaccine Scale-up and Manufacturing

17

Donald F. Gerson, Bhawani Mukherjee, and Rattan Banerjee

Abstract

Vaccine licensing and manufacturing are interdependent. The vaccine product and license depend on the process, equipment and facility. Vaccines typically are complex mixtures of epitopes, antigens, impurities, and adducts, making the reproducibility of the vaccine substance dependent on the manufacturing process. Regulators worldwide are aware of these issues, and operate on the precept that the process defines the vaccine. Creating a new robust, reproducible vaccine manufacturing process is key to successful long-term vaccine supply. Process development, equipment selection, and facility design define the final vaccine manufacturing process, and must embody the science behind the vaccine. The long lead-times in manufacturing process design, facility implementation, and start-up necessitate parallel investment in vaccine discovery and industrialization, simultaneously increasing financial risk and ensuring expedient delivery of the vaccine product to the population upon licensure. Success in new vaccine development can only be defined by the sustained long-term provision of consistent vaccine to billions of people.

## Introduction

There are two major parallel pathways in vaccine development. Product development is the pathway from discovery research to clinical evaluation of putative protective antigens. Process development is pharmaceutics, process evaluation, production optimization, stabilization, assay validation, packaging and other practical activities required to turn an antigen into a vaccine.

There are three major stages in the development of a vaccine: research leading to antigen discovery, development leading to a small-scale manufacturing process for clinical materials, and manufacturing leading to large-scale mass production of the vaccine for worldwide use.

During process development, exploratory research determines scaleable methods that will produce the same antigen made during discovery research. The techniques and methodologies are used for the production of phase I, II and III clinical materials, and ultimately define the manufacturing process.

The establishment of manufacturing involves the simultaneous development of cGMP facilities and equipment, process engineering for scale-up, refinement of QC methods, validation and proof the mass produced vaccine is bioequivalent (Gerson, 1998).

Optimality criteria for the manufacturing process are based on the technology and the expected economics of the product. Manufacturing economics are very different for a high-priced vaccine for the developed world and for a low-priced vaccine for the developing world. With a high-profit vaccine, reduced process development reduces initial investment, speeds product introduction and gives fast financial return, covering high capital and operational costs. With a low-priced vaccine, enhanced process development increases initial investment, reduces operational costs later on, and allows a low sales price. The total cost to society is least in the long run if operational costs are minimized. Balances between investments in development, capital cost and operating cost are made in all cases, but decisions depend on the price and volume expectations for the product. Most probably, an AIDS vaccine for the developing world will always be produced in large volumes and purchased at low cost with, essentially, donated funds.

Low-cost manufacturing for the developing world raises concern for the balance of quality and need. Just because the need is great or urgent, just because the price is low, just because the location is the developing world, there is no reason to assume, encourage or allow low quality manufacturing. Well designed processes and facilities can produce very large quantities of low cost, high quality vaccines. The requirements for quality, purity, good manufacturing practices, and regulatory compliance no longer differ around the world. Manufacturing facility design and construction is converging on a worldwide standard of acceptability, and long-term planning for AIDS vaccine manufacturing must take this into account.

## Process development

Once a vaccine candidate is selected by preclinical testing and phase I/II clinicals, process development should begin. The current regulations are that clinical materials must closely represent the intended final product and be made in cGMP compliance.

HIV vaccine development projects have not given clear-cut results, making decisions on process development and manufacturing preparedness problematical. VaxGen had the courage to proceed with process development and facility planning and construction on the basis of positive immunogenicity results. Unfortunately there was no protection: had there been protection, VaxGen would have been ready to begin manufacturing upon licensure. Should process development and manufacturing preparedness be delayed until proof of efficacy, there will be about a 5-year gap before product is available for distribution.

## Progression from laboratory method to large-scale manufacturing

Fig. 17.1 shows diagrammatically the progression from laboratory method to large-scale manufacturing.

Following antigen discovery, systematic, iterative process development studies transform the discovery process into a practical, highly reproducible, robust, cost-effective large-scale manufacturing process that will make hundreds of millions of doses of vaccine.

Manufacturing clinical grade vaccines using a well-defined process in an appropriate facility, under increasingly stringent good manufacturing practices (cGMP), is the basis for the success of phase III clinical trials. Licensure depends on successful proof of efficacy and documented proof of the optimization and reproducibility of the manufacturing process, and the compliance of the manufacturing facility.

The transition from laboratory method to industrial process adds many layers of scientific, technical, regulatory and organizational knowledge and implementation to the vaccine production method. Knowledgeable and wise application of the multiple fields of endeavor involved in vaccine industrialization usually yields a successful product. However, numerous failures at this transition attest to the difficulties.

Process development occurs in incremental steps from discovery through clinical trials, and continues as process im-

provement after licensed manufacturing begins. This progression from discovery laboratory through process development laboratories to large-scale manufacturing facilities and product launch is shown diagrammatically in Fig. 17.2.

Emphasis on process development is a major success factor in being first to market and profitable with new vaccines and biopharmaceuticals. Inadequate process development is associated with late-stage product development failure, or for high production costs for successful products (Pisano, 1997).

Inadequate attention to process development details may result in failure or abandonment of a good product due to unforeseen manufacturing difficulties or unnecessary high cost, with tragic consequences. Cost estimates made before process development can lead to the abandonment of a perfectly good product on the basis of incorrectly perceived high production costs. Costs can almost always be brought into line with expectations if the process is subjected to an appropriate level and duration of process development by those skilled in this aspect of new vaccine development. Manufacturing process development involves an iterative optimization of each sequential process step to define methodologies appropriate to the scale of production. A properly implemented manufacturing process development program contributes significantly to product success by providing engineering data, prospective process validation at a manufacturing scale, and accurate cost information for sound economic decisions.

At the present time, global capabilities are less than adequate for process development, clinical materials manufacturing and eventual large-scale manufacture of a successful HIV vaccine. With the vaccine production technologies available today, it is possible to design and construct flexible, generic production facilities that could make any of the HIV (or TB or malaria) vaccine products currently envisioned. Once the precise product has been decided upon, procedures to implement the required process in such a generic plant could be developed.

Pre- construction of facilities for clinical materials manufacturing, and most importantly for large-scale manufacturing could be done by a contract manufacturing organization,

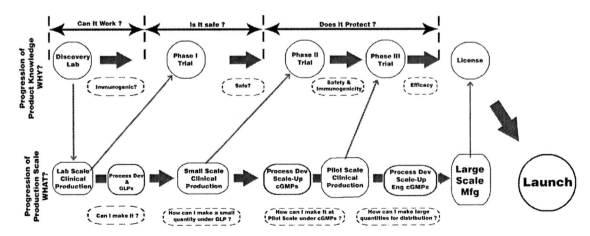

**Figure 17.1** The progression of product and process development from laboratory method and phase I trials, to large-scale manufacturing process and phase III trials, leading to licensed product launch.

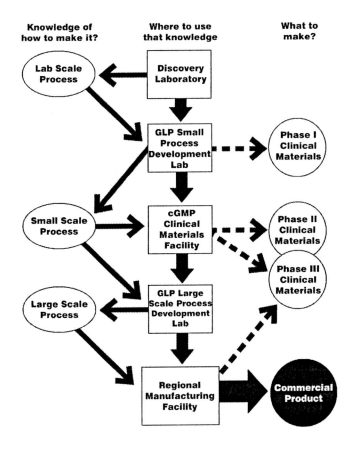

**Figure 17.2** Interplay between product and process knowledge development, appropriate facilities and the production of clinical materials in the development of a commercial vaccine product.

would result in beneficial use. A contract manufacturing organization independent from a vaccine development company, devoted to the eventual large-scale manufacturing of an AIDS vaccine, would greatly accelerate the introduction of all successful vaccines to the developing world.

## Large-scale manufacturing technologies

### Current status of AIDS vaccine manufacturing processes

Most current AIDS vaccine manufacturing processes are in early stages of process development, and considerable efforts will be required for effective scale-up.

The processes to be used for AIDS vaccines under development to date involve three major categories of production technology: microbial fermentation, cell culture or egg-based production. In each production technology, a given host organism may carry one of many possible HIV-specific gene constructs. This is an advantageous situation: unlike traditional vaccine manufacturing in which vaccines were made from the respective pathogens, each having unique and unusual physiologies and requiring highly specific, specialized processing approaches, the processes for AIDS vaccines fall into only 3 distinctly different categories. In addition, each methodology is of average nature within its type. This situation greatly reduces the risk involved in early decisions to proceed with manufacturing facility design and construction. A plant designed to meet the average needs and to have greater operational latitude could be accommodated to whichever product is successful.

### Large-scale manufacture of HIV vaccines

The generalized processing steps involved in the manufacture of an AIDS vaccine are as follows (Fig. 17.3):

The conceptual manufacturing steps are as follows:

CMO, on either a profitable or not-for-profit basis, and used by the first successful vaccine to be licensed. In this way, the risk of capital expenditure would be separated from any one individual product, greatly increasing the probability that it

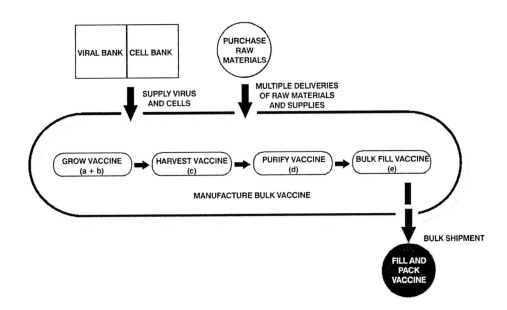

**Figure 17.3** The generalized processing steps involved in the manufacture of an AIDS vaccine: Seed Banks, Growth, Harvest, Purification, Bulk formulation, and filling and packaging.

a   Master and working seed banks: To ensure that the starting materials are identical for each batch, all biological processes begin with a vial from a certified seed bank system for microbial or animal cells, or virus.

b   Growth: Fermentation in a series of increasingly large bioreactors develops the desired quantities of cells to produce the product. In viral processes, the cells are usually grown to maximum density, then infected with the virus and maintained to maximize virus production.

c   Harvest: The active vaccine intermediate is separated from the growth media using cross-flow or dead-end filtration, or centrifugation.

d   Purification: The active vaccine intermediate is purified by filtration and chromatography.

e   Bulk filling: Purified vaccine intermediate is formulated to final bulk, or API, specifications and filled into appropriate sterile bulk containers.

f   Final product filling and packaging: Final formulated vaccine is filled into syringes, vials or other final delivery containers, lyophilized if necessary, labeled, packaged and prepared for shipment to the final destination.

Three bulk vaccine intermediate manufacturing technologies encompass all vaccine candidates under consideration at this time: microbial, cell and egg. While traditional vaccines have utilized multiple doses of the same antigen, it appears at this time that an AIDS vaccine immunization series may involve multiple doses of different antigens and that the antigens may be produced by different production technologies. It is foreseen that manufacturing technologies for chick embryo cells will become the same as the manufacturing technology for other animal cells, and that primary cells will be replaced by avian or other cell lines, further reducing the complexity of planning.

In the following section, each process technology is described in greater detail.

## Cell culture-based viral vector vaccine manufacturing (Fig. 17.4)

Animal cells can be replicated in a bioreactor with appropriate media and controlled operating conditions.

All nutrients and supplements required for cell growth are mixed with highly purified, pharmaceutical grade water in Media Preparation Tanks before being sterilized and transferred to the bioreactors. The production of purified water and other process utilities is a major part of any manufacturing facility. Cell inoculum from the cell bank is placed into the first seed fermentor to initiate the process.

Growth of animal cells in bioreactors is a difficult and exacting process, requiring equipment with precise operational variable control and absolute sterility. Equipment failure due to inadequate design is the most common cause of manufacturing failures or interruptions. Once the number of cells has increased by 5–10 times, the cells are transferred to the next stage leading to the production bioreactor, where the cells increase another 5- to 10-fold. Usually, there is a series of fermentors, each 5–10 times larger than the previous leading to the penultimate production volume. A 10-fold multiple balances the economics of production with the technical difficulties of scale-up; other multiplication factors have been used industrially but if smaller, add capital cost, or if larger, add scale-up risk, without significant benefit. By the time the cell growth step ends, the total number of cells has increased thousands of times.

At the final growth step, the cells in the production bioreactor are infected with genetically modified virus containing genes for the desired HIV antigen, and the virus is allowed to multiply.

At the end of the virus growth cycle, the contents of the production bioreactor are centrifuged or filtered to separate the cells from the supernatant. Depending on the process, either the cells or the supernatant will contain the virus. The product is held in a harvest hold tank for further processing

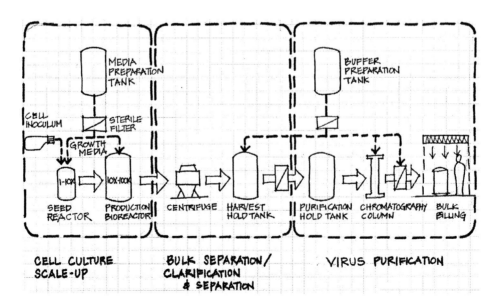

**Figure 17.4** Cell culture-based viral vector vaccine manufacturing.

and cross-flow filtration to separate the virus from most cellular contaminants.

Virus purification proceeds by isolating the virus from most of the remaining contaminants by chromatographic separation or cross-flow filtration. Typically, large quantities of buffer are required at this step, and one of the objectives of process development is to reduce processing requirements to achieve the desired level of purity at minimum total cost.

Following virus purification, the active vaccine Intermediate is formulated to its final composition and prepared for bulk filling into sterile transfer vessels. Bulk vaccine intermediate is then stored prior to final filling and packaging.

Equipment turn-around requires automated cleaning cycles and batch-to-batch maintenance.

## Microbial-based manufacturing (Fig. 17.5)

Microbial production is very similar to, but slightly less stringent than, cell culture. The seed fermentor containing sterile media is inoculated with recombinant microbial cells containing appropriate HIV constructs and is controlled to promote optimal microbial cell growth. An important difference between animal cell cultivation and microbial cell growth is that microbial cells usually require an order-of-magnitude more agitation and aeration, significantly changing the nature of the fermentation and utility supply equipment. The cells multiply in a series of 10-fold steps leading to the production bioreactor.

At the end of cultivation, the biomass is centrifuged to separate the product from media and other contaminants. If the vaccine is the cells, they are recovered, washed and sent to bulk filling. In another possible process, the cells are processed in a homogenizer to release the target plasmids or protein. Lysed cell paste from the homogenizer is then resuspended with a suitable buffer solution in the lysate hold tank. Residual cell debris is then removed from the lysate by cross-flow filtration. The product, rDNA or protein vaccine intermediate is stored in the clarified broth tank before being purified on a

chromatography column. Purified product is then formulated, filled into transfer vessels and stored prior to final filling and packaging.

## Egg-based viral vector vaccine manufacturing (Fig. 17.6)

In this process, chicken embryo fibroblast (CEF) cells are utilized as host cells to grow MVA, or another virus that has been genetically modified to include genes for HIV antigens. MVA has been adapted to grow exclusively on chicken embryo cells and will not grow on human cells, making it a suitable live viral vaccine vector for use in populations with unsuspecting HIV-positive individuals.

A major issue with virus production from eggs is sterility control. Eggs come from a non-sterile environment and are difficult to open without occasional contamination. MVA is a very large virus, and cannot be terminally filter sterilized, so the only protection from contamination is aseptic technique and the quality of the facility and environment. All MVA processes require aseptic operations in clean rooms: processes that are facilities, personnel and training intensive, hard to maintain and expensive to operate.

This situation illustrates a classical quandary in production: while eggs appear to be inexpensive and offer the promise of low operating costs, the required large and high-quality facilities, the high operational expenses, the impossibility of economies of scale, and the relatively high frequency and cost of batch failures combine to make it questionable whether the apparent savings can be realized. Fermentor and cell-culture based operations may appear to be more complex and expensive at the lab level, but at full-scale they result in lower fixed and variable facilities costs, true economies of scale and much lower batch failure rates, resulting in low unit manufacturing costs.

This process begins with fertilized specific pathogen-free eggs (SPF eggs) produced in a highly specialized chicken population and facility. The size of an SPF chicken and egg

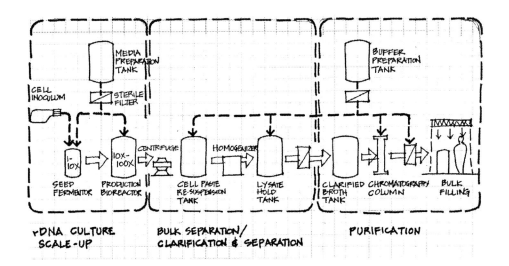

**Figure 17.5** Microbial-based vaccine manufacturing.

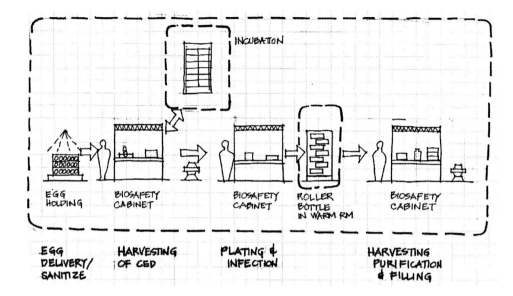

**Figure 17.6** Egg-based viral vector vaccine manufacturing.

production facility appropriate to the quantities of HIV vaccine required has yet to be estimated, however, approximately 20 million eggs/year could be required for a full scale facility. SPF eggs are shipped to the manufacturing facility, checked for viability and sanitized.

Chicken embryos are harvested from surface sanitized chicken eggs. The embryos are incubated with trypsin to separate the CED cells, which are recovered from the filtrate by centrifugation. All these operations are manual and are conducted in a biosafety hood in a class B environment.

The recovered CED cells are infected with virus seed in roller bottles, and incubated in a warm room. The cells do not grow in this system, but the virus multiplies. At the end of the incubation period the cells and virus are harvested and centrifuged to begin the purification process. The recovered cells are broken to release the target virus particles, then clarified and purified by centrifugation. Bulk formulated vaccine is prepared and filled into transfer vessels under aseptic conditions. All these operations are carried out under aseptic conditions in a class B environment.

## Filling and packaging

Filling and packaging is always a costly, space- and labor-consuming activity. Fig. 17.7 compares the benefits and detriments of multi-dose and single-dose presentations of the vaccines. In terms of facility planning, this is an extremely important consideration: filling and packaging space is clean room space and is very expensive to build and operate. For many traditional vaccines for the developing world, multi-dose presentations have been optimal: cost per dose is minimized for manufacturing, shipping and storage. However, multi-dose vials require many syringes and must be entered many times. If a needle is used twice, the entire contents of the vial could be contaminated and disease could be spread between vaccinees. Given the known danger of HIV transmission by multiple uses of the same needle, greater social safety will be achieved by a single dose pre-filled syringe presentation. Use of a pre-filled plastic disposable syringe device such as the BD Uniject™ injection device (BD and Uniject are trademarks of Becton Dickinson and Company) will be highly desirable. This device has the additional advantage that it is designed to prevent secondary use, reducing the dangers associated with the unauthorized recycling and re-use often associated with traditional syringe devices (Gerson, 2005).

## Manufacturing facility

Combining the characteristics described above with reasonable estimates of process yields and the manufacturing space

| Dosage Presentation | Features |
|---|---|
| Single Dose | • More expensive<br>• Increased Safety |
| Multi-Dose | • Less Expensive<br>• Decreased Safety |

**Figure 17.7** Risk and cost table for single dose and multi-dose final product presentations of an AIDS vaccine.

requirements for different basic types of manufacturing activities, it is possible to derive a basic estimate of the facilities requirements for an AIDS vaccine manufacturing facility. The usual estimate of the capacity of a vaccine facility assumes the need to immunize approximately 5% of the population each year, this is 50 million immunization schedules per billion persons. Early in the lifecycle of a new vaccine, this is low, as the population is unimmunized, and considerably more catch-up doses are required to immunize a wider age range than would be needed in a steady-state situation. Once only those entering the target age-class require immunization, capacity may appear to be high, providing the opportunity to export vaccine to other areas or to make other vaccines. Later in the product and plant life cycle, the population will have increased, reducing the excess capacity.

Any manufacturing facility for the developing world must meet the same quality standards as a vaccine facility in the developed world. To meet standard vaccine facility design criteria at minimum cost and with maximum flexibility, a facility should be composed of production, quality, service and administrative modules along a central spine, facilitating construction, process flow, personnel flow and potential expansion (Fig. 17.8). The overall size of an HIV vaccine facility, with a capacity of 50 million immunizations per year, and thus servicing a billion people, is approximately 425,000 sq ft (42,500 m²). The expected number of employees, based on staffing standards in the USA, is approximately 500. The capital cost would be expected to be approximately US$350 million, if constructed in the USA (Mukherjee and Gerson, 2004).

The impact of different locations on the cost is subject to analysis based on factors for construction, equipment, utilities and operational costs for pharmaceutical facilities around the world. Preliminary estimates indicate that costs are less sensitive to location than may have been imagined. This is primarily due to the lack of tax considerations, the insensitivity of equipment costs to location, and the need for well-educated workers. Clearly, this topic requires full economic location analysis at the appropriate time.

## Summary and conclusions

Vaccine development involves multiple parallel pathways. Product development, from laboratory to clinical proof of efficacy is one pathway, and process development from laboratory method to pilot plant studies to manufacturing facility design and start-up is another. Regulatory development leading from IND or equivalent to licensure, and economic and social development leading to a social desire and a financial ability to purchase and administer the vaccine are also parallel elements of vaccine development. The only useful measure of vaccine development success is delivery to and protection of millions or billions of people. All these, and many other parallel efforts comprise the multi-dimensional scientific, manufacturing, and social effort required to effectively develop a vaccine product that will benefit mankind.

## Acknowledgments

The authors would like to thank Luke Gong, Nancy Borda-Diaz, and Mark Chmielewski for their skill and patience in making the figures.

## References

Gerson, D.F., *et al.* (1998). Transfer of processes from development to manufacturing. Drug Information J. *32*, 19–26.

Gerson, D.F. (2005). Safety Guides New Syringe Designs. Pharma Manufacturing, April 2005, 255.

Mukherjee, B. and Gerson, D.F. (2004). Manufacturing Vaccines for the Developing World. BioPharm Int. *17(10)*, 24–30.

Pisano, G.P. (1997). The Development Factory. Harvard Business School Press, Boston, MA.

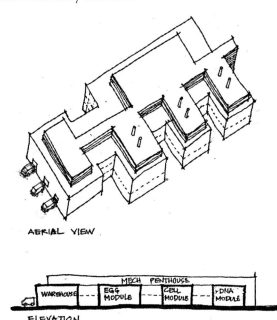

**Figure 17.8** Design for an economical AIDS vaccine production facility, composed of production, quality, service and administrative modules along a central spine with linear product, process, and personnel flows.

# Global Access to Vaccines: Deployment, Use, and Acceptance 18

Jon Kim Andrus and Ciro A. de Quadros

## Abstract

Rapid introduction of a safe and effective HIV vaccine will be critical for curbing the global HIV epidemic and the massive number of deaths from AIDS. The slow "trickle-down" process by which new vaccines from developed countries have historically been introduced into developing nations must be circumvented once an effective HIV vaccine is licensed. This article examines some of the obstacles that impede widespread access to vaccines, and then draws upon the lessons learned to formulate a set of recommendations for achieving rapid global access to a future AIDS vaccine.

## Introduction

It typically takes two decades or more for new vaccines to be introduced into developing countries. A variety of factors are responsible for this long delay, including:

+ insufficient political commitment;
+ growing number of new vaccines;
+ cost of new vaccines;
+ insufficient vaccine supply;
+ insufficient capacity of public laboratories to augment vaccine production by private industry; and
+ country-to-country disparities in coverage.

Political commitment is crucial for the timely introduction of new vaccines and for implementing strategies meant to ensure the best use of vaccines (Andrus, 2004). Although obtaining this commitment for public health interventions may be difficult, highly visible disease control initiatives like smallpox and polio eradication have often helped stimulate this commitment quickly. Most Ministers of Health would like to be perceived as the force behind reaching and protecting every child in their constituency against feared infectious diseases. Historically, this has certainly been the case in the Americas.

In 1990, the recommendations from the World Health Organization (WHO) for vaccines to be included in the im-munization schedules of developing countries included only six antigens: BCG, polio, diphtheria, pertussis, tetanus, and measles. This situation existed even though many developed countries had already introduced (in addition to those listed) vaccines for hepatitis B, *Haemophilus influenzae* type b (Hib), pneumococcus and influenza. Since then the only addition to the WHO recommendations for developing countries is hepatitis B vaccine, even though many developed countries have rapidly added other new vaccines (such as varicella and hepatitis A) and made improvements in old ones (e.g., acellular pertussis vaccine).

The experience of the Americas, Europe, and many parts of Asia demonstrates how disease eradication strategies pioneered in the Americas can exert a "pull" to add other new vaccines into routine immunization programs. These strategies also involve addressing issues of inequity, because municipalities with poor coverage are usually those with underserved, impoverished and minority populations. One common strategy is to couple eradication programs for a specific disease with expanding routine coverage. For example, sustaining high-level routine immunization rates has been a critical strategy of measles elimination; municipalities are identified as high-risk for measles outbreaks when coverage drops below 95% (Centers for Disease Control, 2003). Targeted efforts to improve measles immunization rates in these areas also incorporate other antigens, such as DPT and polio vaccines, so that coverage for three doses of all these vaccines is increased to very high levels.

This relationship between accelerated disease eradication strategies and routine immunization may partly explain why the introduction of Hib and HepB vaccines occurred so rapidly in the Americas. A pentavalent vaccine with components for diphtheria, whole cell pertussis (wP), tetanus, Hib and HepB was initially made available to countries of Latin America in 1994, when Uruguay introduced this vaccine into its national immunization schedule. While this vaccine was being introduced, countries of the Americas were also immersed in a measles eradication initiative, with the goal of eliminating indigenous transmission throughout the region by 2000 (PAHO, 2003). Critical to the success of this campaign was ensuring high measles immunization coverage in all municipalities. The result was that by 2001, 95% of the children born in Latin America were living in countries that routinely included the pentavalent vaccine in childhood immunizations, and coverage for three doses of pentavalent vaccine rapidly increased to over 85% throughout the region.

Rapid introduction of a new vaccine also requires effective community activism. In the case of HIV therapeutics, the explosive increase of HIV/AIDS cases early in the US epidemic stimulated activism that played a crucial role in accelerating drug development and then in expanding access to antiviral drugs. Similarly, worldwide activism for rapid introduction of HIV vaccines, particularly in less developed countries, would focus critically needed attention on addressing inequities in global access to health technologies.

But as demand for the newer vaccines increases, so does the challenge of supplying enough vaccine to meet these demands. Success will require that international agencies, governments, public health authorities, academic research institutions and vaccine manufacturers form effective partnerships and be committed to serving *all* populations—rich or poor—with new technologies (Andrus, 2005). It also means that data must be gathered on target populations, particularly those at high risk, so that manufacturers can accurately forecast future demand for the product. These data are typically generated through the existing epidemiological surveillance infrastructure of the national health systems and by medical research institutions.

However, maintaining adequate supply of a new vaccine also requires alternative strategies to address and counterbalance the recent radical changes in global vaccine supply. The experience in the US, which reflects a global trend, is worth highlighting: Approximately 30 years ago, more than 25 manufacturers were involved in vaccine production in the US. Today, only three remain. This trend puts great stress on the capacity of immunization programs to deliver vaccines on time. For example, the resulting paucity of supply sources resulted in the influenza vaccine shortage in the US in 2004. (For a more complete discussion of manufacturing issues, see Chapter 17.)

## The role of public sector vaccine manufacturers

Developing country purchases now account for more than 50% of the global vaccine market. Governments of developing countries are therefore highly concerned about the precarious state of vaccine supply. One approach to help ensure adequate supply, especially for underserved populations, is to increase support of government-owned manufacturers. India and Indonesia have each demonstrated that this is possible. Other countries, including Brazil, China, Vietnam and Mexico, have a longstanding tradition of producing and supplying their populations with essential vaccines.

However, public vaccine laboratories in developing countries work against enormous odds to meet the demands of providing potent and safe, cost-effective vaccines to their underserved populations. One reason is that shrinking financial support severely hampers their capacity to keep up with the development of new technologies. Another is that these laboratories do not possess the technical capacity to investigate and develop new vaccine technologies, such as recombinant and genetic technologies (Homma *et al.*, 1998).

In general, the only clients of public laboratories are the governments that support them. The adverse consequences of this limited arrangement include insufficient political support, diminishing resources and insufficient attention to sorely needed aspects of modernization. In contrast, private companies have been able to completely revamp and modernize their production facilities to use state of-the-art-technologies. Compared with the public laboratories, the production capacity of private manufacturers typically results in larger quantities of high-quality products. It is clear that countries with public laboratories must find ways to radically re-organize and revitalize their networks if they are to survive and to play an important role in ensuring the availability of new vaccines.

Several Latin American countries have initiated activities to address the constraints of public bureaucracies and inflation. For example, in 1989 the Instituto Butantan, a public vaccine production laboratory in Sao Paulo, Brazil, created the Butantan Foundation as a private entity charged with securing the financial sustainability of the Institute. The public sector Instituto Butantan is now benefiting from the association with its private sister foundation by the recent construction of new DPT and hepatitis B vaccine facilities; the financial support to make this happen largely resulted from the efforts of the private foundation. In addition, the Institute has embarked on a program targeting the development of new vaccines.

Cuba has taken the approach of increasing direct public support for manufacturing. Over the past 10 years it has significantly accelerated the construction of new vaccine production facilities costing more than US$200 million. Cuba now has the capacity to make polysaccharide vaccine (e.g., against pneumococcus) as well as recombinant vaccines against bacterial and viral infections, such as hepatitis B.

Mexico is the one country in Latin America that produces all antigens listed in its vaccination schedule: polio, measles, DwPT, diphtheria-tetanus, tetanus toxoid and BCG. Approximately 10 years ago the Gerencia General de Biologicos y Reactivos (GGBR) began implementing a plan to modernize the production facilities. This facility was transformed into the Biologicos y Reactivos Mexicanos (BIRMEX), and since 1997 has produced DwPT. To achieve financial stability, the facility was recently converted to a mixed entity that is 51% public and 49% private.

Looking ahead to the challenges in ensuring adequate supplies of HIV vaccines, policy makers will need to consider not only the issues discussed above but also additional factors which distinguish HIV vaccines from routine childhood vaccines. A key difference is that HIV vaccines (at least the initial products) will likely have lower efficacies than the childhood vaccines. The act of getting vaccinated against HIV may therefore create a false perception in some individuals that they are completely protected, leading to continued (or increased) risk behavior—despite preventive counseling (which will need to accompany immunization) on the continued need to avoid risky behaviors. Vaccine failure in this setting could lead to a public backlash against HIV vaccines. Ultimately, manufacturers would be strapped with the difficulties of trying to re-adjust supply and demand estimates; if demand decreases, prices would invariably escalate. These issues will challenge current systems of funding and delivery.

One possible model for helping to guarantee sufficient vaccine supply is the Revolving Fund of the Pan American Health Organization (PAHO), a mechanism of vaccine purchase which helps assures more affordable prices (De Roeck, 2006). The Fund is discussed further below.

## Infrastructure needed to deliver an AIDS vaccine among adolescents and adults

Once an HIV vaccine becomes available it will probably be delivered initially through mass immunization programs that target adolescent and adult populations, as well as supplemental campaigns aimed at specific risk groups. Since mass vaccination is usually geared to infants or children, the limited past experience with adult vaccination, for example against rubella, provides insights that can be usefully extrapolated to future HIV immunization campaigns (Castillo-Solorzano, 2004).

In 1986, 16 years after the rubella vaccine was licensed in the U.S., only six countries in the Western Hemisphere (Canada, Costa Rica, Cuba, Panama, US and Uruguay) had introduced measles, mumps, and rubella vaccine (MMR) into their national immunization programs. In 1994, the year that the Region of the Americas was declared free of indigenous polio transmission, the PAHO Directing Council launched an initiative to eradicate indigenous transmission of measles from the Americas by the year 2000. This initiative has been very successful, and the last case of indigenous measles was detected in Venezuela in November, 2002 (Centers for Disease Control, 2003).

But intensified surveillance for fever and rash illnesses found that rubella was circulating widely in Latin America and the Caribbean, carrying the potential for major epidemics. In response, PAHO adopted strategies for accelerated rubella control and congenital rubella syndrome prevention (Castillo-Solorzando et al., 2003). The vaccination strategies being promoted include targeting women of childbearing age and adult males for vaccination.

In 1999, as a result of an outbreak that began a year earlier, reported rubella cases peaked at 1,610 cases. Of these cases, 75% were among people between 15–45 years of age. Consequently, Costa Rica decided to accelerate its rubella control strategies and in 2001 conducted an Adult National Measles-Rubella Campaign using measles-rubella-containing vaccine (Morice et al., 2003). To evaluate the implementation and impact of this campaign, the first ever to target adult males, a National Commission of Immunization was established, chaired by the highest health official in the country, the Minister of Health. Social mobilization activities engaged local political, union, and religious leaders, as well as national personalities, community associations, presidents of professional societies, educators, artists, entrepreneurs, the media, and local nongovernmental organizations. It was a mammoth undertaking, but it was also well-organized and well-coordinated with all sectors of society.

Several tactics were used to ensure that everyone was reached, including mobile posts, use of brigades, house-to-house vaccination, fixed posts and highly flexible hours over a 1-month period. Local teams evaluated progress daily and implemented corrective action immediately when they encountered problems. Continuous monitoring and supervisory support at all levels helped ensure that geographic and other barriers did not impede implementation. Coverage among all age groups reached more than 90% (except in the 30–34 year age group, where it reached 87%).

This was the first adult vaccination campaign conducted in Latin America. Compared with childhood vaccination campaigns, adult vaccination campaigns can be quite challenging. Flexible tactics are essential, as are proper planning, clear identification of the target population, social mobilization and good communication strategies, galvanizing political commitment at all levels and monitoring progress on a daily basis.

## The need for appropriate management and coordination

Another lesson learned from experience with disease control initiatives is the critical importance of a supportive infrastructure for technical and logistical collaboration, particularly across national borders. This should include technical advisory groups, interagency coordinating committees, and national plans of action that outline activities, outputs, expected results and budgetary requirements covering a multi-year period (usually 5 years). The infrastructure should also encompass private sector, medical associations and community interest groups, since the stigma attached to HIV/AIDS means that patients who can afford it often seek care from non-governmental sources.

In most countries the National AIDS Committee is headed by the office of the Prime Minister or President, with the Ministry of Health and other line agencies as members. Once an HIV vaccine is licensed this committee will confer political authority on initiatives to introduce HIV vaccines, and in many settings it determines access to government funds. So far, a major challenge for these committees has been the coordination of supporting partner agencies and non-governmental organizations, often due to the lack of clearly defined roles and responsibilities. Using models from WHO's Regional Offices, the national committees should also be supported by technical and financial coordinating bodies at the regional level.

Information on disease burden, risk groups, and cost-effectiveness are also fundamental to the introduction of new vaccines. Regional and country-specific information will be required to launch initial efforts, while country-level policy will need to address whether surveillance systems should be hospital- or provider-based. In either case, surveillance requires sufficient laboratory support, coordinated through networks of global, regional, and national accredited virologic laboratories with the capacity to monitor the genetic epidemiology of transmission and the impact of vaccine interventions.

Lastly, national regulatory authorities and control laboratories must develop and implement policies to ensure that safe, effective vaccines are deployed in-country, tasks that will require strengthening the existing infrastructure in most countries. These authorities should use the results from WHO assessments of manufacturers that are pre-qualified to supply vaccines to UN agencies, a step which would greatly facilitate the licensing process in many countries.

However, fundamental to any infrastructure for the successful introduction of HIV vaccines will be establishing high-quality supervision and management of immunization activities within national programs. Supervision and management must seek to improve services that cover the basic functions of vaccination practices and vaccine safety, accurate reporting of vaccination coverage, weekly reporting and surveillance of vaccine-preventable diseases, and programming and implementation of vaccination activities such as supplemental immunization campaigns and maintaining the vaccine cold chain.

## Who pays?

If the introduction of a new HIV vaccine is to avoid replicating past inequities in access to immunization, then developed countries will need to assist and partly finance vaccine introduction in poorer countries which lack the resources to absorb start-up and early maintenance costs. Several mechanisms can be institutionalized at the outset to help ensure sustainability of these efforts.

One is that procurement mechanisms should function not only to purchase vaccine, but also as a tool for a broad program of technical assistance that covers epidemiology as well as financial and logistical sustainability. Ultimately, this would ensure that everyone pays, particularly the governments purchasing the vaccines.

This is exactly what PAHO's Revolving Fund strives to do (Carrasco et al., 1983). The Fund, which began operations in 1979, provides countries with a reimbursement mechanism for the purchase of vaccines, syringes, needles and cold chain equipment. Its purpose was to ensure better and more efficient national planning; to avoid disruptions in vaccine supply and funding for their purchase; to allow purchase of vaccines in local currencies, which avoids delays and currency loss exchanges; to consolidate vaccine orders for economies of scale, translating into lower prices for countries; to assure vaccine quality; and to develop contracts with suppliers so that urgent orders can be delivered on short notice, while assuring suppliers of firm orders so they can plan production in advance.

Since 1979, PAHO has requested annual bids from vaccine manufacturers. Selection criteria for suppliers cover price, track record for quality and capacity to deliver on time, and an estimate of whether the purchase will encourage competition and avoid interference with country programs. The Fund began with a capitalization of US$1 million, which was increased to approximately US$4 million by 1982 through donations from collaborating agencies and countries such as UNICEF, the US and the Netherlands. It is important to note that PAHO does not sell the vaccines; rather it buys them on behalf of member countries, charging a fee of 3% of the cost, which goes towards the capitalization of the Fund. In this manner, the Fund's capitalization grew to over US$20 million in 2003. The number of countries participating has also grown from 19 in 1979 to 34 in 2003.

The concept of the Revolving Fund is appealing for several reasons, primarily because it provides a ready and continuous source of funds which, once committed for a purchase, become available for commitment again as soon as they are repaid. Prior to the establishment of the Fund, PAHO encountered enormous difficulties in trying to coordinate vaccine purchases. When orders were needed urgently they were placed without regard to price, solely on the basis of the supplier's ability to meet the request. At the same time, manufacturers found it difficult to plan their production in advance.

When placing orders, PAHO charges an average price, which lowers costs for individual countries and thereby maintains equity. If countries are delinquent in reimbursing the Fund, no further orders are placed on their behalf. PAHO has maintained this discipline over the last 24 years, guaranteeing lower prices for all countries while ensuring the manufacturer an affordable selling price.

But for such mechanisms to succeed, countries must demonstrate commitment to their national immunization programs. To that end, PAHO only allows countries to participate in the benefits of the Revolving Fund if they have a national budget containing a specific line item for the cost of vaccines and syringes, a comprehensive and realistic national plan of action covering multiple years and consistent with PAHO policies, and a national program manager with authority to develop and implement the national plan.

These criteria help ensure that vaccines are not only purchased, but actually delivered to the communities which need them most (Andrus, 2005). The advantages to participating countries are many, such as reduced vaccine prices, earlier introduction of vaccines, price stability, improved ability to estimate demand, a more orderly planning process, improved quality vaccines, established mechanisms to cover emergencies when outbreaks occur, and sustainability of vaccine purchase because of line item allocation in national budgets.

Could a revolving fund work in regions outside the Americas? If so, this could help catalyze efforts to ensure the sustainability of HIV vaccine introductions. One factor in the Fund's success was that many countries were already purchasing their own vaccines, and therefore had a line item for vaccine purchase in their budgets. This is not the case for countries in Africa or many countries in South Asia. However, the Global Alliance for Vaccines and Immunization (GAVI) and the Global Fund for HIV/Malaria and Tuberculosis could play an important role in mobilizing resources and promoting budgetary line items with Parliaments and Finance Ministers in countries which are most in need. This would require a concerted effort, and should ultimately include a vision for creating a Global Revolving Fund for Vaccine Purchase.

## Acceptance and uptake of HIV vaccines

Another issue raised by HIV vaccines (but not by childhood antigens) is that of achieving high coverage in adult populations with existing AIDS prevention strategies. A brief look at Thailand's success in raising public awareness early in its epidemic, leading to a rapid drop in unsafe sex (and new HIV infections), offers some interesting lessons on what is most important.

Thailand was able to reduce HIV incidence by 80% over the last 10 years because it had strong and consistent government leadership which committed national resources to control efforts (Curran, 2003). These efforts were highly successful in implementing strategies targeting sex workers and achieving behavior change with safer sex practices through expanded condom use. Some would characterize the turnaround in Thailand's epidemic as one of the most remarkable success stories in public health in the last 30 years. Clearly, condoms are not vaccines, but much could be learned about the marketing and operations that led to their widespread acceptance and rapid uptake, particularly in a society where the level of sexual openness was historically very high.

A key element of Thailand's strategy was its approach to communication and its successful mobilization of sex workers and of people who had unprotected sex with partners of unknown HIV status. Such social mobilization efforts will be essential when an HIV vaccine becomes available, particularly in countries with a growing anti-vaccine sentiment among some lay people.

To help increase acceptance of an HIV vaccine, health messages should be initiated now and targeted to community leaders who can begin to promote acceptance of already-available interventions and technologies. These leaders must openly acknowledge the epidemic and work towards reducing the stigma of HIV/AIDS, which requires that they are perceived as supportive of those with HIV disease.

## References

Andrus, J.K., and Fitzsimmons, J.W. (2005). Introduction of new and under-utilized vaccines: Sustaining access, disease control, and infrastructure development. PLoS Med. *2(10)*, e286.

Andrus, J.K., Fitzsimmons, J., Carrasco, P., di Fabio, J.L., Tambini, G., and Roses Periago, M. (2005). The Revolving Fund of PAHO: Sustaining immunization programs of the Latin America and the Caribbean. Chapter in Vaccines, Sera, and Immunizations in Brazil (Portuguese: Fundo Rotatorio de Imunizacao de Opas: Sustentabilidade de programas de imunizacao na America Latina e Caribe, en Vacinas, Soros, Imunizacas no Brazil), Eds. Buse PM, Temorao JG, da Rocha Carvalheiro J. Editora FIOCRUZ. pp. 405–411.

Andrus, J.K., Tambini, G., di Fabio, J.L., and Roses Periago, M. (2004). Anticipating new vaccines in the Americas. Pan. Am. J. Public Health (editorial) *16*, 369–370.

Castillo-Solorzano, C., and Andrus, J.K. (2004). Rubella elimination and improving health care for women. Emerging Infect. Dis. 10(11): 2017–21.

Carrasco, P., de Quadros, C., and Umstead, W. (1983). EPI in the Americas benefits from Revolving Fund. WHO Chronicle 37, 81–85.

Castillo-Solorzando, C., Carrasco, P., Tambini, G., Reef, S., Brana, M., and de Quadros, C.A. (2003). New horizons in the control of rubella and prevention of congenital rubella syndrome in the Americas. J. Infect. Dis. *187* (Suppl. 1): S146–S152.

Centers for Disease Control (2003). Public Health Dispatch: Absence of Transmission of the d9 Measles Virus—Region of the Americas, November 2002–March 2003. MMWR 52, 228–229.

Curran, J.W. (2003). Reflections on AIDS, 1981–2031. Am. J. Prev. Med. *24*, 281–284.

DeRoeck D.A., Bawazir S.A., Carrasco P., Kaddar M., Brooks A, Fitzsimmons J.F., and Andrus J.K. (2006). Regional group purchasing of vaccines: Review of the Pan American Health Organization Revolving Fund and the Gulf Cooperation Council Group Purchasing Program. Inter. J. Health. Plann. Mgmt. 21:23–43.

Homma, A., di Fabio, J.L., and de Quadros, C.A. (1998). Los laboratorios públicos productores de vacunas: el nuevo paradigma. Rev. Panam. Salud Publica 4, 223–32.

Morice, A., Caravajal, X., Leon, M., Machado, V., Badilla, X., Reef, S., Lievano, F., Depetris, A., and Castillo-Solorzano, C. (2003). Accelerated rubella control and congenital rubella syndrome prevention strengthen measles eradication: the Costa Rican experience. J. Infect. Dis. 187 (Suppl 1): S158–63.

Pan American Health Organization: Technical Advisory Group on Vaccine-Preventable Diseases; XV Meeting. Washington, D.C.; 22–23 November (2002). Available at http://www.paho.org/English/HVP/HVI/tag15_conclusions.pdf.

# The Potential Public Health Impact of Imperfect HIV-1 Vaccines

# 19

Roy Anderson and Stanley A. Plotkin

## Abstract

The many biological uncertainties regarding vaccination against HIV make it likely that the first available vaccines will be only partly effective. The most likely scenario is that these vaccines may not prevent the establishment of infection, but instead might work by reducing viral load and transmission to sexual partners. Mathematical models indicate that such partially effective vaccines will be valuable only if protection is long-lasting and risk behaviour amongst vaccinees does not increase greatly. Therefore, once efficacy is demonstrated in a controlled trial, long-term follow-up will be necessary to determine vaccine effectiveness. Another issue is the effect of vaccination on viral load if vaccinees become infected, with current data suggesting that decreasing viral load would delay the onset of disease and greatly reduce transmission. Despite some caveats, suboptimal vaccines that give persistent sterile immunity or that slow disease progression and diminish transmission could have major public health benefits if properly used, particularly in mass vaccination campaigns.

## Introduction

Expectations for current candidate HIV-1 vaccines are modest, in terms of both efficacy and duration of protection. However, experimental work in primate models; together with data from HIV-infected people, suggest that vaccines that induce cellular immunity may reduce viral load and slow progression to AIDS (Chapter 4).

The expectation of low efficacy and/or an infection-modifying effect raises three crucial questions. First, would a low-efficacy vaccine have significant public health impact in areas of high HIV prevalence? Second, will prior immunization modify breakthrough infection enough to have an impact at the population level? Third, will such vaccines lengthen the incubation period of AIDS and/or reduce infectiousness? These effects could be very important in terms of both net mortality induced by HIV/AIDS and HIV incidence.

The first question has been addressed previously using various mathematical models (Anderson *et al.*, 1991; McLean *et al.*, 1993; Blower *et al.*, 1994; Anderson *et al.*, 1995; Anderson

*et al.*, 1996; Owens *et al.*, 1998). The main conclusion from these analyses is that a low-efficacy vaccine could have significant public health benefits, provided those vaccinated do not greatly increase risk behaviors (Anderson *et al.*, 1996). The second and third questions have received less attention to date. However, preliminary analyses of vaccines that slow disease progression suggest that a measurable benefit could be achieved under some circumstances (Anderson *et al.*, 1991; McLean *et al.*, 1993; Blower *et al.*, 1994).

In this chapter we briefly review the mechanisms of vaccine effectiveness in general and the potential impact of a low-efficacy HIV vaccine that induces short-lived protection. We then turn to the question of how an imperfect vaccine with a measurable impact on viral load in vaccinees who become infected would influence HIV incidence and HIV/AIDS mortality in a given community with varying levels of vaccine uptake.

## Vaccines in general

### Mechanisms of effectiveness

Table 19.1 summarizes the various means by which existing vaccines protect against disease. These means are not mutually exclusive, and vaccines may act through any or all of them. it should also be borne in mind that we have little experience with vaccines against sexually transmitted diseases, with the exception of hepatitis B, in which sexual transmission is only one of several transmission routes.

**Table 19.1** Mechanism by which vaccines protect against disease

| |
|---|
| Increase immunity of vaccinees |
| Increase protection of unvaccinated by transmission blocking effect of vaccinated or by spread of vaccine virus from vaccinated |
| Decrease carriage of pathogen and therefore transmission |
| Decrease excretion of pathogen and therefore transmission |
| Decrease severity of disease in vaccinated |

All current vaccines provide substantial protection for the recipient, and many also provide some degree of protection to the unvaccinated. For example, rubella vaccination of infants decreases circulation of the virus in the community, and thus indirectly protects unvaccinated women of child-bearing age (although in good public health practice, they too are vaccinated) (Plotkin, 2004, Chapter 26). Another example is pertussis vaccine given in infancy, which induces protection that lasts throughout childhood and thereby reduces the risk of infection in newborn siblings (Plotkin, 2004, Chapter 21).

The classic example of such "herd immunity" is smallpox, which was successfully eradicated despite vaccine coverage rates well below 100% because vaccinees provided an effective barrier against viral spread to susceptible contacts (Plotkin, 2004, Chapter 9). another case of effectiveness exceeding efficacy is the live oral polio vaccine, which spreads from vaccinees to contacts and thereby induces active immunity in a portion of the unvaccinated population (Plotkin, 2004, Chapter 44).

For some vaccines, particularly those targeting bacterial diseases, herd immunity is mediated by reduction in carriage of the organism (i.e. bacterial load) rather than by resistance to disease. For example, the vaccine against *Haemophilus influenzae* type b lowers disease incidence well beyond the protection it affords the vaccinee by decreasing the rate of pharyngeal carriage of the organism (Plotkin, 2004, Chapter 14). This in turn reduces transmission from vaccinated to unvaccinated contacts, a situation analogous to that postulated for HIV vaccines that induce cellular immunity.

Another interesting example of how decreasing viral load affects transmission (and disease incidence) comes from the inactivated polio vaccine. The early years of its use in the US brought a precipitous drop in the number of polio cases despite a low vaccination coverage rate (Plotkin, 2004, Chapter 24). This occurred because the vaccine abolished pharyngeal excretion of the virus, the major transmission route in countries with good hygiene.

The essence of these indirect protective effects is that transmission is decreased to the point where on average each infected person transmits to less than one susceptible contact.

A last mechanism is that vaccine would not affect disease incidence at all, but only severity. Whereas all vaccines probably moderate disease severity when breakthrough infections occur, breakthrough is relatively uncommon except with varicella vaccination. Vaccinees who suffer mild varicella when exposed to wild viruses have fewer, less vesicular skin lesions, making them less infectious for unvaccinated contacts (Plotkin, 2004, Chapter 28). Rotavirus vaccines do not prevent infection but render them asymptomatic (Plotkin, 2004, Chapter 51).

## Duration of protection

Aside from efficacy, the most important characteristic of a vaccine is the duration of protection it affords. For example, while both hepatitis B and diphtheria toxoid vaccines are efficacious, the former gives long-lasting immunity, whereas the latter requires boosters (Plotkin, 2004, Chapter 16). The recent diphtheria epidemic in the former Soviet states occurred primarily in adults who had not received boosters and therefore had lost their immunity (Plotkin, 2004, Chapter 13).

The age of maximum risk for a disease plays a key role in the interplay of vaccine efficacy and duration of protection. While a hepatitis B vaccine that only protected newborns against maternal infection would be valuable, the fact that immunity is very long-lived means that vaccinees are also protected against later sexual exposure. Similarly, rubella vaccination of infants is predicated on protection later in life when the girls are pregnant and the boys are their consorts. The promising human papillomavirus vaccine intended to prevent cervical cancer (Plotkin, 2004, Chapter 45) will be optimally effective if its protection lasts throughout the entire period of peak sexual activity. Nevertheless, boosters remain an effective way to prolong vaccine immunity, although their uptake is often less than that of primary immunization.

### Partially effective vaccines

While vaccines used in childhood immunizations programs protect at levels of at least 80%, several important vaccines in public health use, such as inactivated influenza vaccine and pneumococcal polysaccharide vaccine (PPS), do not reach that level (Plotkin, 2004, Chapters 17 and 22). Nevertheless, both vaccines are highly recommended for general use, particularly in high-risk populations, for reasons of cost-effectiveness and reduction in disease incidence.

Although the PPS vaccine has frequently given disappointing efficacy against non-bacteremic pneumonia, its efficacy against bacteremic disease is about 75%. (Plotkin, 2004, Chapter 22). Despite variation in the ratio of bacteremic to non-bacteremic pneumonia, cost-benefit analyses in the US show that the proportion of pneumonia averted, and the resultant savings in medical costs, pay for the purchase and administration of the vaccine to all the elderly.

The efficacy of influenza vaccine in protecting high-risk individuals varies from year to year, up to about 60% protection (Plotkin, 2004, Chapter 17) Here again, cost-benefit analyses consistently demonstrate the economic benefit of preventing disease (Plotkin, 2004, Chapter 56). More controversial is whether decreased incidence in vaccinees results in decreased exposure of the unvaccinated, but at least in institutionalized populations the evidence is clear that vaccination can provide a cordon sanitaire for debilitated and therefore highly susceptible people.

## HIV vaccines

### Protective vaccines with low efficacy

The simplest deterministic models of HIV-1 transmission and the impact of vaccination typically include three groups of people: those who are susceptible (i.e., uninfected), infected/asymptomatic, immune (vaccinated) and those with AIDS. They typically ignore variables such as gender, age, and degree of mixing between people with different levels of sexual activity (Anderson et al., 1991). The most important result derived from this type of model is a simple mathematical expression relating the minimal level of vaccine coverage required for blocking HIV transmission to vaccine efficacy, duration of protection, and intensity of transmission in the community (Fig. 19.1).

The key insight revealed in Fig. 19.1 is that average duration of protection is as important as vaccine efficacy in determining the potential impact of a vaccine on a population: The shorter the duration, the higher the proportion of people who must be vaccinated, even in communities with a low intensity of transmission (i.e., the basic reproductive number, $R_0$—the average number of people infected by a single infected individual—is just above unity) (Fig. 19.2). Stated another way, mass immunization will have limited impact in communities with high transmission intensities (e.g., $R_0 = 10$) if the vaccine has only moderate efficacy (50%) and a short duration of protection (a few years), even at high levels of coverage. This point is not widely appreciated by those currently involved in HIV vaccine development and trial design. VaxGen's two completed

phase III trials were designed to detect a defined level of vaccine efficacy (30% efficacy as the lower confidence bound) as quickly as possible (within 3 years). However, measuring the duration of protection will require long-term follow-up of those immunized, with the time horizon defined not in years but in decades.

## Imperfect vaccines with an infection-modifying effect

We now turn to the more complex problem of assessing the potential public health value of vaccines that act by slowing progression to disease, rather than by blocking infection. We also examine the impact of reduced infectiousness in vaccinees who subsequently become infected (McLean et al., 1993; Blower et al., 1994).

First, a series of parameters must be defined (Fig. 19.3a) to capture the assumptions built into this model and outlined in the flow chart shown in Fig. 19.4. Expanding on the four

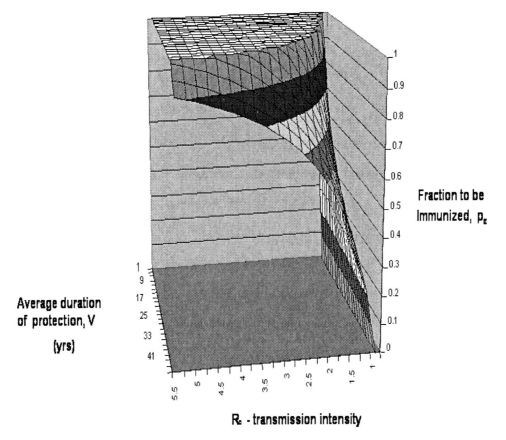

**Figure 19.1** Relationship between vaccination coverage, vaccine properties, and reducing transmission: simple model.

$$p_c > \frac{[1 - 1/R_0][1 + L/V]}{\varepsilon}$$

$p_c$ = **minimal proportion** of the population that must be immunized to block HIV transmission;

$R_0$ **(basic** reproductive number) = transmission intensity, expressed as the average number of people infected by a single (primary) infected person in a susceptible population;

$L$ = **average life** expectancy in the absence of AIDS;

$V$ = **average duration** of vaccine protection, in years;

$\varepsilon$ = **vaccine efficacy,** expressed as the fraction of immunized people who are fully protected upon exposure.

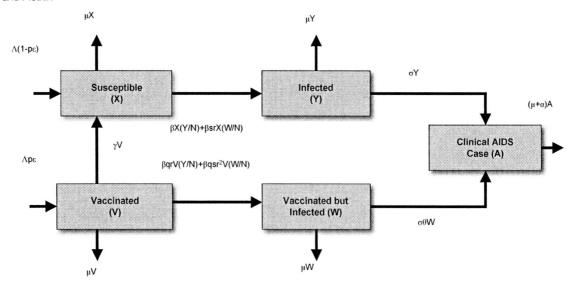

**Figure 19.2** Flow chart of the action of an imperfect vaccine with variable duration of effect and where vaccinated individuals can acquire infection.

different population subgroups (susceptibles, vaccinees, infecteds, AIDS cases), vaccinees are further divided into those who have not acquired infection ($V$) and who lose vaccine protection at a rate expressed as $\gamma$, and those vaccinees who have acquired infection ($W$). The formal structure of the model is presented elsewhere (Anderson et al., 1991; Blower et al., 1994; Hanson et al., 2004).

The key new assumptions relate to the vaccinees and how they acquire and transmit infection. First, it is assumed that they have a slower rate of progression to AIDS, with a crucial attribute of the vaccine (designated $\theta$) being the degree to which it delays disease progression. The second assumption is that vaccinees who seroconvert are less infectious (by a factor termed $s$) than unvaccinated, HIV-positive people, due to their lower viral loads. (However, this group may show increased rates of risk behavior, designated $r$, stemming from a sense of "vaccine optimism"). Third, even vaccines that fail to block infection may reduce the susceptibility of vaccinees (by a factor called $q$). Using these parameters, it is possible to calculate the HIV prevalence for immunized and unimmunized groups in a population with a particular vaccine in use, as well as the critical proportion of the population that must be immunized to block transmission (Fig. 19.3b).

The model has complex behaviour and predicts six possible equilibrium states in terms of HIV prevalence and population size, depending on vaccine properties. These are: (1) the trivial state of extinction of infection, due to a drop in transmission rate below that which sustains the epidemic (i.e., $R_0 < 1$); (2) $R_0 > 1$ with $P = 0$ (no vaccination), and infection prevalence at the vaccine-free equilibrium state (designated as $y^*$); (3) eradication of infection by vaccination where the equilibrium prevalence of infection (called $y_v^*$) = 0; (4) the first of three

states of persisting infection under vaccination, with $y_v^* < y^*$, and population size in the presence of vaccination ($N_v^*$) greater than that without vaccination ($N^*$); that is, $N_v^* > N^*$; (5) prevalence under vaccination greater than prevalence without (i.e., $y_v^* > y^*$), but with increased population size ($N_v^* > N^*$); and (6) the perverse outcome of increased prevalence and decreased population size in the presence of cohort-based vaccination ($y_v^* > y^*$ and $N_v^* < N^*$).

What does this tell us about the utility of vaccines that delay disease? One conclusion is that eradication of new infections by mass cohort vaccination will always be difficult to achieve using imperfect vaccines, even if vaccination significantly reduces infectiousness in immunized individuals who seroconvert. This is especially true for vaccines with only short-lived protection; as with the simpler model described above. Moderate transmission intensity and short-to-medium duration of vaccine protection give a value of $p_c$ that exceeds unity, meaning that each cohort must be repeatedly immunized to block transmission.

However, while complete eradication will be difficult to achieve with these vaccines, mass cohort-based vaccination can still have a significant public health impact. Cohort vaccination will always result in reduced prevalence of infection and net mortality from AIDS, as long as infected vaccinees transmit virus less frequently than unimmunized, infected people. This relationship is expressed mathematically as shown in Fig. 19.3c, and reflects the complex interplay between outcome (HIV prevalence), the vaccine's ability to reduce infectiousness and susceptibility and to slow disease progression, and changes in the risk behavior of vaccinees. An effective, imperfect vaccine should decrease infectiousness and susceptibility by at least a factor of 2, and must reduce the reproductive number of the

**Figure 19.3** Assessing public health impact of HIV vaccines that slow disease progression: complex models

*(a) The parameters*

$\sigma$ = rate of disease progression in infected, unvaccinated people

$\theta$ = factor by which prior vaccination slows rate of disease progression in infected people (value is between 0 and 1)

$\sigma\theta$ = rate of progression in infected, vaccinated people

$I_u$ = average incubation period of disease in infected, unvaccinated people, calculated as $1/(\mu+\sigma)$, $I_v$ = average incubation period of disease in infected, vaccinated people, calculated as $1/(\mu + \sigma\theta)$

$\beta$ = rate at which susceptibles acquire infection from infected, unvaccinated people (calculated as per partner transmission probability times the average rate of new sexual partner acquisition)

$s$ = degree of reduction in infectiousness in infected vaccinees relative to unvaccinated infected (value between 0 and 1)

$r$ = degree of increase in risk behavior in infected vaccinees relative to unvaccinated infecteds (value > 1)

$q$ = degree of reduction in susceptibility to infection in uninfected vaccinees, relative to unvaccinated people (value between 0 and 1)

$\gamma$ = rate at which protection in vaccinees is lost over time.

*(b) The critical fraction that must be immunized to block transmission ($p_c$):*

$L$ = life expectancy in the absence of AIDS

$\varepsilon$ = vaccine efficacy

$V$ = average duration of vaccine protection $(1/\gamma)$

$R_0$ = the basic reproductive number in unvaccinated people

$R_{0v}$ = the basic reproductive number in vaccinated people (McLean and Blower, 1993, 1994).

*(c)*

If $R_{0v} < R_0$ (infected vaccinees transmit less than unvaccinated infected people), then HIV prevalence will decrease and AIDS-induced mortality will decline relative to mortality in an unvaccinated population. This requires eq3 to be satisfied, where $I_u$ is the incubation period of AIDS in unvaccinated individuals and $I_v$, in vaccinated individuals).

$$1 > sqr^2 I_v / I_u$$

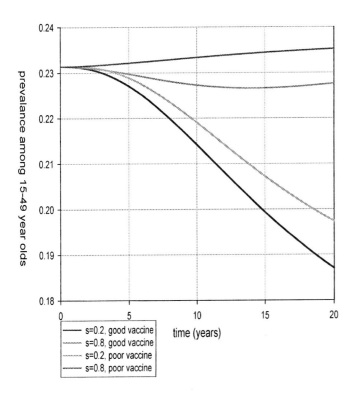 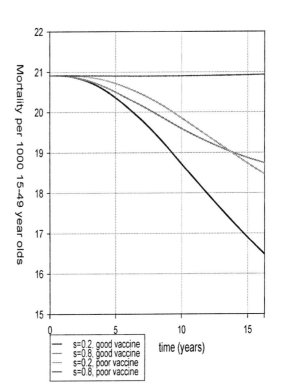

**Figure 19.4** Changes over time in the prevalence of HIV-1 in the 15–49 year old age group of both sexes (a) and the number of deaths per annum, per 1000 head of 15–49 year olds (b). In all cases in which the value of s is varied (relative infectiousness), the level of vaccine coverage is set at p=0.4. For values of s of 0.2, and 0.8, a good ($\gamma = 0.1$, 10-year duration of protection) and a poor ($\gamma = 0.2$, 5-year duration of protection) vaccine are compared (Hanson and Anderson, in preparation).

virus in vaccinated individuals ($R_{ov}$) as much as possible below that in unvaccinated people ($R_0$). On the other hand, delayed disease progression (which lengthens the time period when infected people can infect others), combined with increases in risk behavior, could act to offset any benefit.

Some insight into the relationship between decreased viral burden and disease progression can be derived from longitudinal studies of individuals from the time of seroconversion. They generally show that low viral loads are associated with longer incubation periods (Ogg et al., 1998; Dalod et al., 1998; Kalams et al., 1999; Fraser et al., 2001; and Chapter 4). In the absence of such data for any specific candidate vaccine, the relationship plotted in Fig. 19.5a suggests that a vaccine which lowers average viral load by two logs could greatly lengthen the incubation period to AIDS.

A related question is the degree to which lower viral load corresponds to reduced infectiousness. Data on this point are limited and derive largely from two studies, one by Quinn et al. (2000) and the other by Gray et al. (2001). The latter work suggests that a 1.4 log decrease in viral load (from 4.58 to 3.23,) lowers the probability of transmission (defined per act) by a factor 23, arguing that vaccines which substantially reduce viral load could be of great benefit. However, these data also hint at a non-linear relationship between viral load and transmission probability; hence the decrease in infectiousness

resulting from lower viral load will depend on the range of viral burden over which this decrease is induced.

Further insight into vaccine impact comes from assigning specific values to the degree of reduction in infectiousness and susceptibility of vaccinees (parameters $q$ and $s$) and to the fraction of each birth cohort immunized upon joining the sexually active age classes ($p$). These results are summarized in Fig. 19.5b and c, which show the ratio of HIV prevalence in a population with and without vaccination, at different levels of vaccine coverage and over a range of values for susceptibility and infectiousness ($q$ and $s$) that reflect a fairly modest vaccine impact on these properties. Assuming no change in risk behavior, these conservative assumptions show that imperfect vaccines can have a substantial public health impact, as measured by the equilibrium HIV prevalence. Similar conclusions emerge if we use population size or net AIDS-induced mortality as the outcome measure. For larger changes in the ratio $qs$, the data from Gray et al. (2001) suggest that the benefits would be much greater.

Even when the condition defined in Fig. 19.3c is not satisfied and HIV prevalence rises over that in the unvaccinated population (because infected vaccinees live longer), mass vaccination can still decrease net AIDS mortality. For example, in the conservative case where transmission in a vaccinated population is little changed ($R_0$ just greater than $R_{0v}$) but reductions

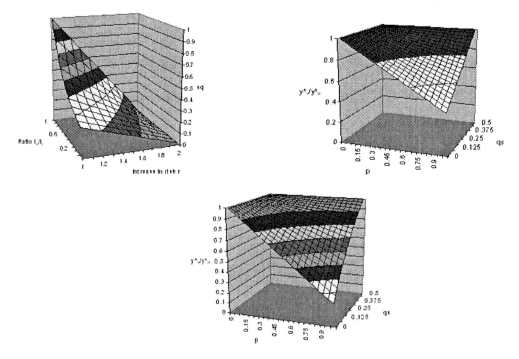

**Figure 19.5** (a) Boundary relationship as defined in Eqn 19.3 between the product of the degree of reduction in infectiousness ($s$) and the degree of reduction in susceptibility ($q$) of vaccinated individuals, qs, as a function of the ratio of the length, the incubation period of AIDS in vaccinateds divided by that in unvaccinateds, $L_v/l_u$, and the factor by which risk behavior increases in vaccinated individuals, $r$ ($r = 1$ denotes no change). Imperfect vaccines with properties defined by parameter value combinations that lie below lead to a decrease in prevalence and mortality from the values pertaining prior to immunization. Above the surface two regions exist—one with increased prevalence and decreased mortality and one with increased prevalence and mortality (see text). (b) and (c) Surfaces showing the equilibrium relationship (the exact relationship derived from numerical evaluation of the model equations) between the ratio of HIV-1 prevalence after cohort vaccination divided by that before ($y^*_v/y_u$), with the fraction $p$ of each cohort vaccinated and the ratio qs, which denotes the product ofthe proportional reduction in infectiousness times the reduction in susceptibility. In (b) $q$ is held fixed at a value of 0.5 while in (c) $s$ is held fixed at a value of 0.5. Other parameter assignments: $R_0 = 2.0$, $R_{0v} = 1.0$, $r = 1.0$ (no increased risk behavior), $\varepsilon = 1.0$, $V = 10.0$ years.

in susceptibility and infectiousness are substantial ($qs < 1$), net mortality due to AIDS (as reflected inversely by population size at equilibrium) will still decrease. This relationship is expressed mathematically in Eqn 19.1.

$$qsr^2 < \frac{I_u}{I_v} + qr(R_0 - 1)(1 - \theta) \qquad 19.1$$

More complex models that incorporate various refinements (such as age and gender structure, heterogeneity in sexual activity and different patterns of mixing between low- and high-risk groups) to better match reality can also be used to analyze the population-level impact of imperfect vaccines. Similar conclusions emerge to those derived from simple frameworks, but the quantitative detail varies according to the values assigned for the different parameters. One such analysis is presented in Fig. 19.6, which shows the temporal impact of an immunization program employing imperfect vaccines with different properties. Based on a cohort immunization program (initiated before the onset of sexual activity), the impact on net mortality and HIV prevalence emerges slowly over many decades.

## Discussion

High vaccine efficacy in a traditional prophylactic sense is the key long-term goal of HIV-1 vaccine development. However, given the relentless toll of the AIDS epidemic globally, less-than-perfect vaccines may be considered for use in the coming decade. Yet the question of what constitutes a "useful" vaccine is not easy to answer, as illustrated by the analyses presented here.

According to Johnston and Flores (Johnston *et al.*, 2001) the possible outcomes of immunization against HIV are sterile immunity, transient infection, controlled infection, or lack of transmission. The first two outcomes imply effective immunity akin to that seen with conventional vaccines, while control of infection is based on the idea that cellular immunity would suppress viremia to low or undetectable levels and preserve CD4$^+$ cell counts and other immune parameters. The last outcome should prolong the incubation period from HIV infection to AIDS, and should also diminish the viral excretion by the vaccinee, and thus the capacity to infect others. Mathematical models suggest that a vaccine with no protective efficacy in the traditional sense, but with a measurable impact on the course of infection in infected vaccinees, can be very beneficial in lowering net AIDS-induced mortality and, in some cases, HIV-1 prevalence. However, a beneficial outcome will require vaccines that delay progression to AIDS while reducing infectiousness over this lengthened period (Anderson *et al.*, 1991).

Taking into account the possibility of increased risk behavior in vaccinees, the condition for a beneficial outcome is simply that the vaccinated group shows reduced transmission. The degree of benefit, in terms of reduced mortality from AIDS, depends on both the degree to which transmission is reduced in vaccinees and on the relationship between reduced susceptibility plus infectiousness and increased incubation periods. If these vaccine attributes (for each candidate entering phase II trials), along with epidemiological parameters (in defined communities) can be measured as precisely as possible, the model can be used to assess which of the six possible equilibrium states for HIV-1 prevalence and population size correspond to the actual vaccine parameters.

However, moving from models to predictions based on real vaccine candidates will not be easy, partly because measuring these properties within phase III trial settings will be problematic. People and populations vary widely in their viral load

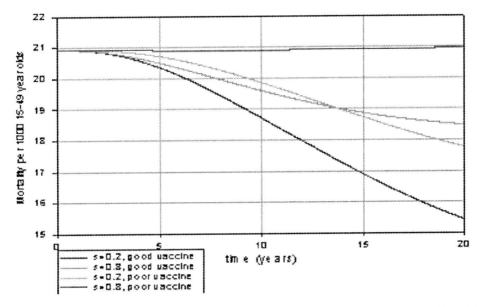

**Figure 19.6** Changes over time in the prevalence of HIV-1 in the 15–49 year old age group of both sexes (a) and the number of deaths per annum, per 1,000 15- to 49-year-olds (b). In all cases in which the value of s is varied (relative infectiousness), the level of vaccine coverage is set at $P = 0.4$. For values of s of 0.2, and 0.8, a good ($y = 0.1$, 10 year duration of protection) and a poor ($y = 0.2$, 5-year duration of protection) vaccine are compared (Hanson and Anderson, in preparation).

levels and rate of progression to disease—a "noisy" background against which vaccine-induced changes must be detected and assessed. Other heterogeneities, such as the diversity of HIV strains and individual genetic differences in susceptibility to infection, also complicate this analysis.

Although examples of vaccines other than HIV are partly useful, AIDS vaccines break new ground, and surprises can be expected. Nevertheless, the importance of high immunization coverage appears fundamental: only if there is wide acceptance of an AIDS vaccine among sexually active young adults can a partially effective vaccine have much impact.

High coverage, in turn, will be achieved in poor countries only if vaccine is distributed at a low price by governments or some multilateral organization and used in well-organized vaccination campaigns. The latter will be necessary because of the notoriously poor uptake of vaccines when given casually or sporadically to adults by individual physicians, even in developed countries. Moreover, health authorities will also have to educate vaccinees about the need to use additional risk-reduction measures, such as condoms. Overoptimism among vaccinees that leads them to take increased risks because they believe themselves protected can counteract the effect of the vaccine, as the models discussed here demonstrate

The models also underscore the importance of duration of protection. An effective vaccine should ideally protect during the entire period of high sexual activity. However, while this is the ideal, it is not inconceivable that AIDS vaccine booster shots could be given. A vaccine that protects for 5 years might still have value if the population were to accept a booster that would extend protection for another 5 to 10 years. However, the more vaccine doses required, the less cost-effective vaccination will be (Bos, 2001).

Returning to Table 19.1, we can now appreciate that even partially efficacious AIDS vaccines could limit the epidemic by directly protecting vaccinees or by reducing viremia (and concomitantly transmission) to levels that indirectly protect contacts of vaccinees. Results with experimental vaccines in monkeys suggest that the reduced viremia at least is possible. As the risk of infection through heterosexual coitus has been estimated as 1:500–1:1,000 (Royce, 1997; Gray et al., 2001), a 10-fold reduction in this risk would be extremely important in a public health context.

It is well known, as other chapters in this book portray, that a completely effective AIDS vaccine is not just around the corner. Yet even a partly effective vaccine would have great public health consequences if properly applied. This is both an optimistic and realistic conclusion, which should lend heart to the AIDS vaccine enterprise.

## Acknowledgment

R.A. gratefully acknowledges financial support from the Wellcome Trust.

## References

Anderson R.M., Gupta, S. and May, R.M. (1991). The potential of community-wide chemotherapy or immunotherapy to control the spread of HIV-1. Nature 350, 356–359.

Anderson, R.M. and Garnett, G.P. (1996). Low efficacy HIV vaccines, potential for community-based intervention programmes. Lancet 348, 1010–1013.

Anderson, R.M. and May, R.M. (1991). Infectious Diseases of Humans, Dynamics and Control. Oxford University Press, Oxford.

Anderson, R.M., Swinton, J., and Garnett, G.P. (1995). Potential impact of low efficacy HIV vaccines in populations with high rates of infection. Proc. Roy. Soc. Ser. B 261, 147–151.

Blower, S.M. and McLean, A.R. (1994). Prophylactic vaccines, risk behaviour change and the probability of eradicating HIV in San Francisco. Science 265, 1371–1373.

Blower, S. (2005). Modeling the potential public health impact of imperfect HIV vaccines. J. Infect. Dis. 192, 1494–1495; author reply (1495)–146.

Blower, S.M., Bodine, E.N. and Grovit-Ferbas, K. (2005). Predicting the potential public health impact of disease-modifying HIV vaccines in South Africa, the problem of subtypes. Curr. Drug Targets Infect. Disord. 5, 179–192.

Bos, J.M. and Postma, M.J. (2001). The economics of HIV vaccines, projecting the impact of HIV vaccination of infants in sub-Saharan Africa. Pharmacoeconomics 19, 937–946.

Dalod, M., Harzic, M., Pellegrin, I., Dumon, B., Hoen, B., Sereni, D., Deschim, J.C., Levy, J.P., Venet, A., and Gomard, E. (1998). Evolution of cytotoxic T lymphocyte responses to human immunodeficient virus type 1 in patients with symptomatic primary infection receiving antiretroviral triple therapy. J. Infect. Dis. 178, 61–69.

Gray, R.H., Wawer, M.J., Brokmeyer, R., Sewankambo, N.K., Serwadda, D., Wabire-Mangen, F., Lutalo, T., Li, X., vanCott, T., Quinn, T. and the Raki Project Team. (2001). Probability of HIV-1 transmission per coital act in monogamous, heterosexual, HIV-1-discordant couples in Rakai, Uganda. Lancet 357, 1149–1153.

Anderson, R.M. and Hanson, M. (2005). Assessment of the potential public health impact of an "imperfect" HIV-1 vaccine in a high prevalence country in sub-Saharan Africa. J. Infect. Dis. 191, S86–S95.

Johnston, M.I. and Flores, J. (2001). Progress in HIV vaccine development. Curr. Opin. Pharmacol. 1, 504–510.

Kalams, S.A., Goulder, P.J., Shea, A.K., Jones, N.G., Trocha, A.K., Ogg, G.S., and Walker, B.D. (1999). Levels of human imunodeficiency type 1-specific cytotoxic T-lymphocyte effector and memory response decline after suppression of viraemia with highly active antiretroviral therapy. J. Virol. 73, 6721–6728.

McLean, A.R. and Blower, S.M. (1993). Imperfect vaccines and herd immunity to HIV. Proc. R. Soc. Lond. B Biol. Sci. 253, 9–13.

Ogg, G.S., Jin, X., Bonhoeffer, S., Dunbar, P.R., Nowak, M.A., Monard, S., Segal, J.P., Cao, Y., Rowland-Jones, S.L., Cerundolo, V., Hurley, A., Markowitz, M., Ho, D.D., Nixon, D.F. and McMichael, A.J. (1998). Quantitation of HIV-1- specific cytotoxic T lymphocytes and plasma viral load. Science 279, 2103–2106.

Owens, D.K., Edwards, D.M. and Shachter, R.D. (1998). Population effects of preventive and therapeutic HIV vaccines in early- and late-stage epidemics. AIDS 12, 1057–1066.

Plotkin, S.A. and Orenstein, W.A. (eds.) (2004). Vaccines. Philadelphia, Elsevier.

Quinn, T.C., Wawer, M.J., Sewankambo, N., Serwadda, D., Li, C., Wabwire-Mangen, F., Meehan, M. O., Lutalo, T., and Gray, R.H. for the Rakai Study Group. (2000). Viral load and heterosexual transmission of human immunodeficient virus type 1. N. Engl. J. Med. 342, 921–929.

Royce, R.A., Sena, A., Cates, W., Jr., and Cohen, M.S. (1997). Sexual transmission of HIV. N. Engl. J. Med. 336, 1072–1078.

Smith, R.J., and Blower, S. (2004). "Could disease-modifying HIV vaccines cause population-level perversity?" Lancet Infect. Dis. 4, 636–639.

# Index

7473641

3 1378 00747 3641

Printed in the United States
67688LVS00003B/1-178

9 781904 455110